KNOWLEDGE TRANSFORMATION IN HEALTH AND SOCIAL CARE

The term 'mindlines' has become common currency in the world of research implementation and evidence-based practice. This book updates, develops, and applies the mindlines model more widely. It sheds light on how we can realistically mobilise and transform research-based evidence into practice in context.

This illuminating book shows how the mindlines model can be put to work. It highlights how practitioners collectively share and internalise implicit, flexible ways of rapidly handling complex clinical situations. Drawing on research and reflective studies from practice, education and guidelines development across a wide range of international health and care settings, the authors unpack the general components of mindlines. They find practical ways to uncover, bring together, and apply specific mindlines to improve practice, and to develop evidence-based healthcare policy, practice and education in ways that capitalise on the crucial role of mindlines. Closely edited by the originators of the mindlines model, this book brings together the work of a cohesive group of researchers and practitioners to showcase and develop its theory and consequences.

It is an essential read for all those interested in knowledge mobilisation, evidence-based practice, and research implementation both within healthcare and beyond.

John Gabbay is Professor Emeritus of Public Health and former Director of the Wessex Institute at the University of Southampton. He is also Honorary Senior Visiting Fellow at Cambridge Public Health, University of Cambridge and a Senior Member of Darwin College, Cambridge. Until recently, he was Implementation Co-lead at the National Institute of Health and Care Research (NIHR) East of England Applied Research Collaboration, UK.

Andrée le May is Professor Emerita of Nursing at the University of Southampton. She is Editor-in-Chief for the NIHR's Journals Library for the Health and Social Care Delivery Research, Public Health, Global Health and Programme Grants for Applied Research journals. She is also Co-editor of the *Journal of Research in Nursing* and Honorary Visiting Senior Fellow at Cambridge Public Health, University of Cambridge. Until recently, she was Implementation Co-lead for the NIHR East of England Applied Research Collaboration.

KNOWLEDGE TRANSFORMATION IN HEALTH AND SOCIAL CARE

Putting Mindlines to Work

Edited by John Gabbay and Andrée le May

Routledge
Taylor & Francis Group
LONDON AND NEW YORK

First published 2023
by Routledge
4 Park Square, Milton Park, Abingdon, Oxon OX14 4RN

and by Routledge
605 Third Avenue, New York, NY 10158

Routledge is an imprint of the Taylor & Francis Group, an informa business

British Library Cataloguing-in-Publication Data
A catalogue record for this book is available from the British Library

ISBN: 978-0-367-74618-6 (hbk)
ISBN: 978-0-367-74616-2 (pbk)
ISBN: 978-1-003-15872-1 (ebk)

DOI: 10.4324/9781003158721

Typeset in Bembo
by SPi Technologies India Pvt Ltd (Straive)

CONTENTS

FIGURES

TABLES

BOXES

CONTRIBUTORS

Maria Nordheim Alme is Associate Professor and Head of Section in Global Health and Rehabilitation at Western Norway University of Applied Sciences, Bergen, Norway. She has a background in neuroscience research, and currently, her work is focused on building competence for healthcare professionals in topics related to global health.

Kate Beckett is a Senior Research Associate at the University of Bristol. Her mindlines work stems from her recent National Institute for Health Research Knowledge Mobilisation Research Fellowship (sponsored by the University of the West of England). A qualitative researcher, with experience in National Health Service (NHS) nursing, she uses coproduction and creativity to improve NHS care.

Marianne Brattgjerd was enrolled as a PhD student at Nord University's programme for PhD in Professional Praxis when she conducted the fieldwork on mindlines. She is currently working as an Associate Professor at Nord University. Her areas of research interest are sociology of professions, practical cognition, standardisation, death, and dying.

Jane Bye is Associate Dean of Learning and Teaching in the School of Business, Western Sydney University. She is an experienced learning facilitator with teaching and supervision interests in workplace learning in a variety of professional contexts. Her current research focuses on graduate employability, human resource development, and lifelong learning.

Fiona Cowdell is Professor of Nursing and Health Research, Birmingham City University, UK, and was a National Institute for Health Research Knowledge

Mobilisation Research Fellow when she conducted the eczema mindlines study. She is a qualitative researcher who generates impact in clinical practice using knowledge mobilisation and implementation methods.

Ann Dadich is Associate Professor of Human Resources and Management with the Western Sydney University School of Business. She studies health-service management, notably knowledge translation and brilliant healthcare, clarifying how different kinds of knowledge can coalesce to enable and sustain healthcare experiences that exceed expectations, bringing joy and delight.

John Gabbay has focussed on mindlines since becoming Emeritus Professor of Public Health at the University of Southampton, UK. He was until recently the Implementation Co-lead at the East of England Applied Research Collaboration. He is a qualitative healthcare researcher with a particular interest in knowledge utilisation for healthcare development.

Michael Hodgins carried out this work as part of his PhD at Western Sydney University entitled "Emotion and Mindlines: A Community-Based Palliative Care perspective". He is currently a Senior Research Associate at the School of Clinical Medicine at the University of New South Wales studying the implementation of complex interventions.

Judith Hughes was a PhD candidate at the University of St Andrews when she conducted her mindlines work as part of her PhD research. Until recently, she was a Research Fellow there in the School of Management. Currently, she is an independent researcher with an interest in qualitative health research.

Dominic Hurst was a DPhil student at the University of Oxford and Senior Lecturer in Adult Oral Health at Queen Mary, University of London when he carried out his fieldwork into how knowing is generated in practice. He is an academic dentist conducting qualitative research into various aspects of practice.

Andrée le May is Emerita Professor of Nursing, University of Southampton, UK. She conducted the original mindlines research with John Gabbay. Until retiring, she was the Implementation Co-lead at the East of England Applied Research Collaboration. As a qualitative researcher, she is interested in knowledge utilisation and communities of practice.

Elizabeth Matovinovic is a CauseHealth member in NMBU Norway (Norwegian University of Life Sciences) and consultant epidemiologist in the Faculties of Medicine/Dentistry at Chiang Mai University (Thailand). She is a freelance epidemiologist with clients in academia, pharmaceuticals, and public health, and has been active in the Guidelines International Network (GIN).

Tony McBride is a theatre director, facilitator and trainer, exploring theatre as a catalyst for learning with communities and organisations. Expert in participatory theatre techniques, including Forum Theatre, Tony has developed community consultation and training models for Education, Health, and Housing, engaging everyone from marginalised groups and individuals to CEOs.

Edward Suh is Associate Professor of Emergency Medicine at Columbia University Irving Medical Center and the Director of Evidence Based Practice for the Department of Emergency Medicine. He was interim Medical Director of the Emergency Department at New York-Presbyterian Allen Hospital in northern Manhattan during the COVID-19 crisis in 2020.

Tricia R Tooman was a doctoral student, research fellow and managing editor of a health education journal when she conducted her study. She is presently a postdoctoral research fellow and tutor at the University of Dundee. She is a qualitative health services researcher, interested in knowledge mobilisation, networks, and health-provider well-being.

Sietse Wieringa is a general practitioner and hospitalist working in the Netherlands and the UK. He conducted his ethnographic study as part of his DPhil in Evidence-Based Medicine at the University of Oxford. As a clinical research fellow, he is interested in guidelines, the philosophy of evidence-based medicine, and sustainable healthcare.

Joost van Wijchen leads the Bachelor Physiotherapy Programme, Western Norway University of Applied Sciences, alongside continuing as a Senior Lecturer in Physiotherapy, HAN University of Applied Sciences, the Netherlands. The latter is where his mindlines journey started. He is an educational designer and action researcher connecting learning health and the future.

Peter C Wyer is Associate Professor of Emergency Medicine at Columbia University Irving Medical Center and the Co-chair of the Section on Evidence Based Health Care of the New York Academy of Medicine. He publishes extensively on matters related to maximising the value of clinical research in medical practice.

1

INTRODUCING MINDLINES AND THIS BOOK

John Gabbay and Andrée le May

It's now well over a decade since our book *Practice-Based Evidence for Healthcare: Clinical Mindlines* was published (2011) and 20 years since our first publication introducing the concept of mindlines appeared in the *British Medical Journal* (Gabbay & le May 2004). We always hoped that the ideas we put forward would have a life beyond the page and so have been meeting, for the last few years, with a group of people interested in and working with the mindlines model. We like to call this group the Darwin Mindlines Group largely because we met regularly in Darwin College, Cambridge, but also because this group has helped the mindlines model evolve through their lively discussions and actions, and through their work. It is these deliberations that have nurtured this book into being and their work that largely fills its pages.

When we first mooted mindlines in 2004, we had no clue whether the concept would catch on. It was one of those ideas that in retrospect seems obvious, almost banal, and yet also too enigmatic to explain. The *BMJ* editors may well have had similar concerns, but, luckily, they decided to publish it. We took heart from that, and from the fact that the history of science is littered with concepts that explain phenomena while themselves being intrinsically inexplicable. And it turned out that the mindlines model took hold – partly because it helped explain why, despite all best efforts, it is often so hard to implement research-based evidence, but partly also because it apparently resonated with people's lived experience as practitioners/clinicians (we use these descriptors interchangeably in the book). And so, now nearly 20 years later, we hear people using the term widely, and we see hundreds of academic articles that quote our mindlines work (and sometimes misquote it …), but more of that later.

First though, let's explain how the mindlines model emerged.

DOI: 10.4324/9781003158721-1

How and why mindlines research began

For decades, we both independently struggled with the same cluster of problems. How does one get practitioners to make use of important research evidence? Why don't they seem to use it? How does one justify the time and effort spent on research, including our own, if it's not used? And what makes research evidence so special anyway? Working to help nurses and other clinicians make better use of research, AlM had consistently found that they used a very wide range of other evidence and that this was not always the 'Bad Thing' that the purist Evidence-Based Medicine movement of the time declared it to be. Sometimes some of the other sources that they called upon could be misleading, but often they could be useful in helping manage a particular patient or circumstance, not least because there was often no alternative – often there *was* no relevant research evidence available. Meanwhile, JG, having spent a few years grappling with the history and philosophy of medical knowledge, had come to the conclusion that the knowledge used by clinicians is always a contextually-situated social construction. Then, having returned to the world of practice and policymaking, he had seen how hard it was to help research make the impact it so often deserved. And yet research-based knowledge is what drives medical progress forward.

Such concerns were also beginning to dawn on the healthcare research establishment; in the UK in the 1990s, the NHS R&D Programme began offering grants aimed at helping at understanding how research could be applied more often than it was. In 2000, we secured such a grant to work with policymaking groups – including clinicians, public servants, and the public – to help them decide in an 'evidence-based' manner what most needed doing to improve their local services for older people. We offered them a dedicated librarian to help them track down and use any research that might inform their policies, and we observed what happened as they used that evidence in their deliberations. We had expected that the participants would immediately recognise its relevance and simply build it into the policies they were developing. To the dismay of our funders, what we found was far from any kind of linear pathway or logical deliberation (Gabbay, le May, Jefferson et al. 2003) (Figure 1.1).

When we analysed their discussions, it was clear that – far from taking research and carefully appraising, adapting, and incorporating it into their thinking – they were bouncing it around and distorting it in all sorts of ways that relied on the happenstance of who was attending the meetings, how influential they were, what jargon they understood and used, and what prior beliefs, experiences, and interests – even prejudices – they were bringing to the table. Even when the group was being encouraged to make the most of the available evidence, its eventual link to the policy decisions they made was usually tenuous. A moment's reflection, however, would tell anyone who has sat in a committee meeting that we really should not have been too surprised, especially when people from such different backgrounds, and with differing views of what counts as good evidence, are brought together to agree on policy in a contentious area. However, this finding had serious implications for the whole business of using research evidence to inform health and social care policy.

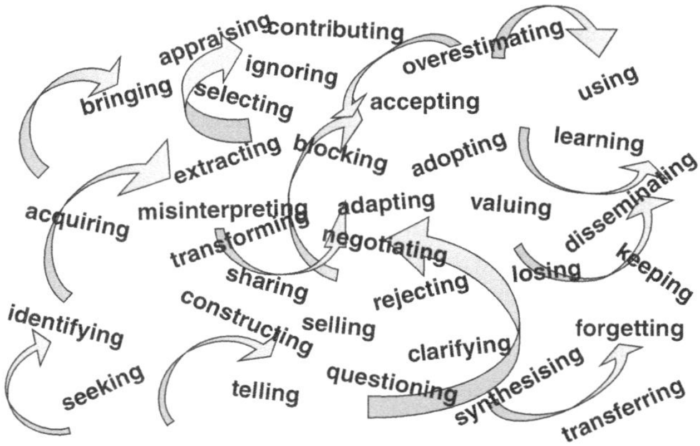

FIGURE 1.1 What a multisectoral group did with the research evidence presented to them (adapted from Gabbay, le May, Jefferson et al. 2003).

The next question, then, was to see if anything similar happened when a group of practitioners was deciding how to practise. Even more interestingly, we wanted to answer the obvious key question that no-one had really looked at before: How *do* clinicians, when making decisions about patients, put their knowledge into practice? Rather than trying to derive idealised analyses of clinical decision-making – which is where much of the existing research had been – our approach required just watching, listening, and probing to try and see what actually goes on, day to day. We wanted to do what anthropologists do – try to get beneath the surface of a culture and understand how and why it works as it does.

A further small grant from NHS R&D allowed us to begin just such an ethnography, initially working over the course of one year to observe how a very highly regarded primary care team, "Lawndale", developed their treatment policies and routines and how they put them into practice. It was this ethnography that led to the publication of the 2004 *BMJ* paper in which we first proposed the notion of mindlines. The research thereafter turned into what must be one of the most cost-effective grants ever; JG retired from his day job, and the Lawndale partners invited us to stay on – a situation that gave us the freedom and the time to voluntarily continue the ethnography. So, for a further five years, we regularly joined practice meetings and other key events, sat for hours in the coffee rooms, chatted to the staff, and generally became part of the furniture. In addition, JG was now free to carry out short informal periods of non-participant observation of another very different practice in the UK, followed up with shadowing US hospital doctors and observing UK medical students' teaching sessions to check out our emerging findings. It was this prolonged ethnographic work that led to *Practice-Based Evidence* (2011), in which we presented a much more thought-through analysis of mindlines than had been possible in the brief, and by then merely preliminary, *BMJ* paper.

In the abstract of our early paper in 2004, we defined mindlines as

> collectively reinforced, internalised, tacit guidelines. These were informed by brief reading but mainly by their own and their colleagues' experience, their interactions with each other and with opinion leaders, patients, and pharmaceutical representatives, and other sources of largely tacit knowledge. Mediated by organisational demands and constraints, mindlines were iteratively negotiated with a variety of key actors, often through a range of informal interactions in fluid 'communities of practice', resulting in socially constructed 'knowledge in practice'.
>
> *(p. 1)*

We derived the term *mind*lines from "guidelines" because healthcare was, and still is, tussling with the content and use of guidelines in the real world of practice, and we wanted to show how practitioners melded different types of knowledge (including guidelines) in their minds to create knowledge they could use in practice in varying contexts. Later, we referred to this as knowledge-in-practice-in-context (2011). In 2011, we refined our definition of mindlines to

> internalised, collectively reinforced and often tacit guidelines that are informed by clinicians' training, by their own and each other's experience, by their interactions with their role sets, by their reading, by the way they have learnt to handle the conflicting demands, by their understanding of local circumstances and systems, and by a host of other sources.
>
> *(p. 44)*

By now we'd analysed all our ethnographic data and could confidently say that the mindlines model helped to explain how practice occurs and why the implementation of research and guidelines is not straightforward. We were also able to describe individual mindlines *and* collective mindlines in more detail in a series of practice-derived vignettes.

In Chapter 2, we summarise that work to help give the context for the rest of the book, and then in Chapter 14, we detail how others have used the model. But first, we should introduce the authors of the bulk of the chapters and outline how each of them has helped to put mindlines to work in practice, education and research.

Working with mindlines: a foretaste of the chapters

The first five of their chapters focus largely on different aspects of practice and care. In Chapter 3, Kate Beckett and Tony McBride explain the use of Forum Theatre (FT) – a form of participatory drama – to mobilise diverse knowledge and catalyse change in post-injury psychological care, an aspect of care that has been neglected despite the evidence about its importance. They show how FT can replicate and enhance the ways in which mindlines are effectively learned, modified, and transmitted to enable multi-level improvements in practice, behaviour, and research.

Dominic Hurst, in Chapter 4, explores concepts of practice in dentistry and suggests that performed practices are those, guided by our mindlines, in which we interact, moment to moment, with people *and* things. Using a variety of techniques to meet the challenges of analysing videos taken in the dental surgery, his work has developed into an innovative approach to exploring practice. The method might enable us to find new ways to understand in precise detail how social and material interactions develop in an encounter with a patient, pointing to insights that will help health professionals learn how to practise better.

In Chapter 5, Fiona Cowdell focuses on childhood eczema, emphasising the need to develop a greater understanding and a shared language between child, parent, and healthcare practitioner. For too long there has been undertreatment of eczema because all three parties have had, in effect, misleading mindlines about its management. She describes several novel and relatively low-cost approaches to eliciting and amending eczema mindlines within and across lay-practitioner-wider-society boundaries, and reports on work that is beginning to show a real impact on the lives of children with eczema and their families.

Michael Hodgins, Ann Dadich, and Jayne Bye in Chapter 6 present findings from a study in community-based palliative care that reminds us of the important role of emotion in mindlines – a role too often ignored. Their observations of the ways practitioners talk about their patients demonstrate how emotions are assembled within mindlines to help them to cope with dilemmas, to persuade their peers towards different approaches to the care of dying patients, and to establish, and come to terms with, the limits of care. The chapter ends, therefore, by advocating more room for clinicians to engage with their emotions during clinical discussions, which could well benefit the patient and the practitioner.

Chapter 7 presents Marianne Brattgjerd's exploration of the thinking behind nurses' practice when they are using a standardised instrument, the Liverpool Care Pathway. The pathway has been controversial but is still widely used in many countries. Drawing on well-established ancient and modern philosophical approaches, she shows how important it is to ensure that nurses do not simply stick rigidly to the pathway as a standardised instrument. They can and do, however, work successfully with it in ways that ensure that their practices remain flexible, individualised, and are instilled with due thought and kindness.

The next two chapters specifically focus on education. In Chapter 8, Tricia Tooman uses a longitudinal case study of sepsis-focused knowledge to understand more about the connections between continuous professional development, clinical practice, and mindlines. She studied three interconnected research, policy, and practice communities to uncover structures important to mindlines development and enhancement. Her work traces the way in which new, life-saving developments in the care of sepsis were 'shepherded' into practice over decades of innovation as collective mindlines shifted and grew.

At the other end of the educational spectrum, Joost van Wijchen and Maria Nordheim Alme in Chapter 9 describe a revolutionary approach to the education of physiotherapy undergraduates, based on the assumption that they begin developing their mindlines from the very start. The course has been designed with an innovative shift in learning philosophies, environments, and experiences; it does away with a formal curriculum – learning occurs through varied collaborative, reflective experiences to encourage collective mindlines. The students who qualify through that course feel more confident and energised in their practice and their learning than previous cohorts did.

Next is a clutch of chapters focusing on guideline development. In the first of these (Chapter 10) Sietse Wieringa presents his findings from an ethnographic study of guideline panels across three countries, showing how they used (or did not use) mindlines in their deliberations and how this – and therefore the resulting guidance – varied. The panels all struggled with a fundamental problem, namely that the rules expected them to eliminate mindlines from knowledge translation and use only explicit, formally appraised knowledge, but due to limited available research evidence, the clinicians had little choice but to call upon their own mindlines. He suggests some ways of dealing with the implications of this finding, both philosophically and practically.

Judith Hughes in Chapter 11 uses a mindlines lens to reveal the social processes that led a guidelines committee to their consensus decisions about the guidance and recommendations. She too found that group members were using and changing their clinical mindlines as the discussions proceeded over a series of meetings. However, her observations particularly focused on how the members of the committee developed and used 'process mindlines', including 'chairing mindlines", in their deliberations. This emergent collective way of "doing" the guideline development process impacted on the resulting guidance.

In Chapter 12, Elizabeth Matovinovic, an epidemiologist whose work entails reviewing and appraising the evidence used to formulate guidelines, reflects on the philosophical limitations of the scientific rationale underpinning that work. She concludes that if guidelines are to serve practitioners and patients well, they need to develop methods to understand, legitimise and build on the sorts of evidence found in collective mindlines. These methods need to include collective ways to render such evidence reliable and usable. She discusses how guidelines developers may need to recognise and build on philosophical principles such as 'common sense' and 'evidentness'.

By contrast, Chapter 13 presents an illuminating example of the role of mindlines in ensuring the best care for patients in a rapidly evolving, non-guideline-dominated situation – the devastating early months of the unfolding COVID-19 pandemic in New York. Edward Suh and Peter Wyer's chapter shows vividly how healthcare systems and clinicians developed and relied upon new, silo-breaking networks of communication to undertake their drastically changing everyday practice. Clinical teams transformed published recommendations and the interpretation of research findings in ways that addressed the immediate patient-care needs they faced during the pandemic surge. It was a context-bound process that epitomised the mindlines model in clinical practice and which suggested some ways to improve guideline production in future.

Chapter 14 is our update on how the mindlines model has been used since it was introduced. We base this on a review of some 1,000 publications and on a series of interviews. We ask how the advent of easily accessed online information has impacted on the model, before exploring how its different facets have been used in other people's research and thinking, and how the model has been used to explain and improve suboptimal care. We end by warning that mindlines are not just a simple 'fast and frugal' form of thinking, as some have assumed; they are fast thinking that is slow and arduous to learn and update. Mindlines, therefore, are not subject to the same errors as heuristics.

Finally, Chapter 15 is a foray into the unknown, where we explore mindlines beyond the world of health and social care. Based on conversations with people from occupations ranging from designing buildings to driving tanks, we conclude that the features of mindlines are visible in all of them. There is nothing special about clinical mindlines. The question is why something so obvious and universal had been so ignored by so many proponents of evidence-based practice.

Where next?

Readers will notice some common themes emerging across the chapters. For example, in their different ways, several of the contributors have had to struggle with the problems of uncovering the detailed processes by which mindlines are formed, enacted, shared, and elicited – be it in the context of practice, policy, or education. Several chapters also explore ways of using the mindlines model to understand how care can be improved at different levels of the system and to evaluate the impact of doing so. What they would all agree is that there are plenty of questions still to be answered about the how, why, and what of mindlines. Much more still needs to be done to put the model to work in the guidelines-development, education, training, and quality-improvement worlds, among others. For researchers and funders too, the mindlines model may play a part in improving the implementation of their findings. It may help to resolve the tensions between methodological paradigms and the everyday need for practical knowledge. The co-productive and collaborative methods, now widely encouraged, may allow the knowledge held in mindlines to nurture research and vice versa. That in itself can be a key way to improve research implementation, as contributors to this book have demonstrated. However, as we once stated,

> [H]ow ironically inconsistent we would be if we now tried to dictate how [the mindlines model] should be put into practice! If our conclusions are to change anything, it will not be because we the writers but you the reader

> who is engaged in the practical realities will have worked through the implications of our analysis.
>
> *(Gabbay & le May 2011, p. 199)*

The findings of mindlines researchers will, like all research, be collectively interpreted, transformed, and implemented according to context. We will therefore not end with a list of things that now need to happen. That is for others to decide.

Nonetheless, we will make one key point here. From our own practice in implementing research, and from our readings, thinking, and discussions with others, it has become clear that some fundamental essentials need to be nurtured for the development and sustenance of mindlines. These essentials are largely *relational.* They revolve around creating the space, time, and ethos for focused and action-oriented social interaction – we have found, even in the busiest of overworked healthcare organisations, that this can pay dividends. Figure 14.1 in Chapter 14 illustrates that social interactions take many forms (e.g., networks, communities of practice, chance encounters with influencers), but we suggest that regardless of form, they need to foster certain characteristics that enable mindlines to be exposed, appraised, and replenished with new insights, or discarded when they become dated or dangerous. These characteristics include an ethos of collectivity, collaboration, and flexibility; a shared 'language' that is inclusive and respectful of different types of knowledge; and the ability to have the respectful critical conversations that are needed to nurture people's mindlines. We hope that the work of the Darwin Mindlines Group will illustrate what this can mean.

Acknowledgements

We thank Darwin College, Cambridge for kindly hosting the Darwin Mindlines Group meetings.

References

Gabbay J, le May A. 2004. 'Evidence based guidelines or collectively constructed "mindlines?" Ethnographic study of knowledge management in primary care'. *BMJ*, 329(7473):1013.

Gabbay J, le May A. 2011. *Practice-based evidence for healthcare: clinical mindlines'* Abingdon: Routledge.

2

WHAT (AND WHY) ARE MINDLINES?

John Gabbay and Andrée le May

Acquiring many types of evidence

When people find themselves having to deal efficiently with complicated situations, they bring to bear a wide (and often deeply embedded) range of knowledge that enables them to do what is needed then and there. It is not always appropriate to go back to the textbook, to carefully follow the instruction manual, or to stick meticulously to the rules. People also draw upon their experience, the routines and shortcuts that they have learnt to rely on, and the stories they have heard from others about how they dealt with similar situations. And so it is for clinicians.[1] Every time they see a patient, they must rapidly weigh up that individual case with its own special circumstances. They must apply what they know about the accepted, scientifically-grounded solution for that problem in general, even when this particular version of it may not fit the general mould.

This limits the immediate value of clinical guidelines, which are developed for typical, average patients when everyone (including, of course, the guideline writers) knows that patients and their circumstances are so often neither typical nor average. Moreover, it is rarely feasible to consult the plethora of available guidance. As two junior doctors pointed out in the *Lancet*, during one night on call, they dealt with "8 patients with a total of 44 diagnoses. The guidelines that the on-call physician should have read, remembered and applied correctly for those conditions came to 3,679 pages." They calculated that reading them would have taken them 122 hours (Allen & Harkins 2005). What they didn't add was that those guidelines would all be designed for patients who had a single diagnosis. Such guidelines would probably therefore not even apply straightforwardly to their patients, who would each have had several different diagnoses, any or all of which might require the guidance to be modified.

DOI: 10.4324/9781003158721-2

Moreover, it is not simply the *clinical* problem that the practitioner must solve. They also need to balance the demands and constraints of their jobs, the many roles they are required to play (clinical vs managerial, individual health vs population health, treatment vs prevention, etc.), and the resources they have to manage – and manage within. These include the limited time they have; the staff they employ; the colleagues they happen to work with; the views of patients, their families, and carers; the equipment that is available or not; the information technology they must grapple with; the economies they must make; the regulations and targets they must conform to; and the professional standards and personal standing that they feel impelled to enact and be seen to enact. No clinical guideline can help with that degree of conflicting complexity.

Knowledge-in-practice-in-context

To handle all that at once, practitioners need an efficient, elegant, and timely way of understanding what needs to be done across a whole range of predictably unpredictable situations. That guidance, which they use day to day, is not – and cannot be – mere theoretical knowledge (Polanyi 1983; Schön 1983; Hunter 1991). Rather, it is what we have called their 'knowledge-in-practice-in-context'. It exists in their heads; it is readily and rapidly accessible to them; it is flexible, malleable, and practical; it is what they know is likely to work for the context they are faced with. Such knowledge does not come just from science-based guidelines, still less from reading research papers or systematic reviews. If they are competent practitioners, the relevant research will surely still be at the heart of their knowledge-in-practice-in-context, but it is melded with many kinds of knowledge from many diverse sources.

Practitioners spend their whole careers absorbing and processing the many kinds of knowledge and evidence that they are exposed to:

1. the sciences and practices they learnt at school and university;
2. the principles and facts they read in their textbooks;
3. the lessons they learnt from their trainers;
4. the mentors and role models they emulate;
5. the updates given to them by educators and trainers;
6. the articles they have read in journals and professional magazines;
7. the guidelines – national or local – that they have read or heard about;
8. the views of the local experts whom they trust and respect;
9. the practical and technical skills they have assiduously acquired;
10. the procedures and protocols their employers/organisations require of them;
11. the information they have had from pharmaceutical, devices, and other reps; and
12 so on and on.

They add to that mix their own experience, the opinions and experiences they have heard from colleagues, and the views, experiences, and expectations of the patients (and their families) in front of them. As they are acquiring and melding all of that, they are also learning the accepted ways of behaving, the values, the emotional control, the ethics, the professional image or 'face' they are expected to display – even the speech patterns, writing styles, and dress codes – all of which will alter the way in which they can or cannot use that potent blend of accumulated knowledge.

Somehow, all that material needs to be amalgamated into a form that can help guide the practitioner's actions in any given situation. We often liken the blending process to a compost heap: the gardener deposits all manner of stuff into the compost bin and, provided it is continually watered, aerated, and turned over, something extraordinarily useful emerges at the end of a complex and mysterious process. The original contents are no longer identifiable, but that final product could not exist without that diverse mix of ingredients, nor could it have materialised without being given the right conditions for the metamorphosis to occur. Similarly, practitioners spend their whole careers absorbing all kinds of knowledge that merges and morphs into their instantly accessible internalised guidelines-in-the-head: their mindlines.

Individual mindlines and contextual adroitness

In 2011, we described mindlines as

> internalised, collectively reinforced and often tacit guidelines that are informed by clinicians' training, by their own and each other's experience, by their interactions with their role sets, by their reading, by the way they have learnt to handle the conflicting demands, by their understanding of local circumstances and systems, and by a host of other sources.
>
> *(Gabbay & le May 2011, p. 44)*

For all but the most unusual or novel clinical problems, practitioners are immediately able to call on the relevant set of mindlines to guide their actions. It is their mindlines that allow rapid decision making, not – as is often supposed – some kind of instinctive 'clinical intuition', but a long and hard-won possession. Nor is that ability down to simple pattern recognition. Educationists have long been aware that clinicians learn to rapidly recognise patterns, known variously as 'illness scripts' (in a man with tight, radiating chest pain, shortness of breath, sweating, nausea: think myocardial infarction), 'heuristics' or 'rules of thumb' (if there's a raised ST segment on the electrocardiogram, call coronary care). These play their part but are only a small portion of mindlines; they go nowhere near the level of nuanced and multifaceted thinking required. Mindlines deal not simply with clinical problems but also intricately complex challenges that may well include the psychosocial, organisational, and even the socio-political, ethical, or economic aspects of a clinical situation in a specific context. Very often in practice, one requires a rapid solution to much more nuanced problems that no guideline or formal training can provide

("Which of the three busy local coronary care units do I call for this homeless malnourished elderly man with dementia who has developed chest pain in a rural village?").

The doctors at Lawndale, where we did our main ethnography, would have immediately known the answer to such a question, but were it to be posed to a general practitioner (GP) from another part of the country, they would struggle with it. Both they and the Lawndale GP are expert generalists. They could have been at the same medical school, studied the same textbooks, passed similar exams, seen the same guidelines, and imbibed the same moral, behavioural, and social attitudes of their profession during their early training, but the mindlines that they must now use to solve this typically real-world problem will rely on the innumerable other, differing, sources they have accumulated throughout their subsequent careers, specific to their divergent contexts. Like anyone with professional expertise, each of them, when they began practising, would have stuck closely and carefully to what they had been taught – 'going by the book'. Gradually, as they learned the ropes, they would have moved from wary, slow 'novice' behaviour through the 'advanced beginner' stage to the 'competent' practitioner, by which time they would have been able to recognise patterns and get quickly to the core of a clinical problem, perhaps bending some rules but still acting logically and systematically within the formal guidance. Much of that newly acquired practical knowledge would have been steeped in the context where they were assimilating it. Then, learning shortcuts and ruses that get the job done effectively, they would have become 'proficient', making the leap from orderly, logical thinking to being able to tackle complex problems so slickly that it can be mistaken for being intuitive. Only when they had developed such a knack could they have achieved the status of being regarded as 'expert' – a person who can be relied upon to know all about both the theory and the practice. These stages, first described in nurses by Benner (1984) in a richly nuanced description of the progression, have often since been oversimplified. There has been a tendency to underplay not only how easily one can be simultaneously at different 'stages' for different aspects of one's job but also the crucial part played by the context where one's learning takes place; hence, a change in circumstances can leave a person floundering, however expert they are. That is why someone unused to the Lawndale context would struggle to answer questions as subtle as the one about the homeless man's chest pain on a busy night. In a new role or a new place, even the most expert practitioner will need to relearn some of the ropes like a novice again.

In our ethnographies – which also included observations of nurses, medical students, and trainee hospital doctors – we found ourselves watching that progression. We were able to see how each stage from novice to expert required the laying down of ever richer mindlines – and also watch, for example, how a highly skilled hospital doctor needed rapidly to adjust his mindlines when retraining in primary care. Some of the knowledge embodied in those mindlines was transferable, even universal. But a great deal of it was about knowledge-in-practice-in-context. Their mindlines took them beyond mere expertise to what we have labelled 'contextual adroitness'. This is what enables a hospital ward manager to shine in her world but be hesitant if suddenly placed in a district-nursing role, and vice versa. Learning within the locality is partly about knowing the local resources and routines, but partly also about knowing the place, the people, their culture, expectations, and norms. That is what confers 'contextual adroitness'.

Collective mindlines, communities of practice, sensemaking, and identity

The process of developing one's mindlines is anything but solitary. The information being gathered, whether written, oral, or experiential, inevitably results from interactions with others. A moment's refection will reveal that – for all of us – our knowledge and skill in handling complicated problems have mostly come from what we have learned from or with other people. Moreover, if we're stuck, who better to turn to than someone we know and trust to advise us or jog our memory? So it is for clinicians. For a GP, those 'other people' might, for instance, be remote (guideline committees), immediate (the patient's mother), continual (one's immediate colleagues, including, e.g., practice nurses), intermittent (the senior cardiologist), formative (the early role model), long past (that never-forgotten tragic case), or recent (yesterday's Continuing Professional Development lecturer), but they have all played their part. When, during our ethnographies, we observed the practice nurses, GPs, medical students, or trainee hospital doctors talking about their practice, we were witnessing practitioners continually disclosing to each other little snippets of their knowledge-in-practice-in-context, and in doing so shaping each other's mindlines.

Clinicians talk or write about their practice, telling each other stories ("anecdotes with a purpose"), comparing notes, listening to what is being said, and almost unconsciously checking out whether what they are hearing now obliges them to adjust their own practice. When they do so, whether formally or informally, they are exchanging thoughts, practices, and experiences that feed and fine-tune each other's mindlines. Sometimes they back up what they are saying, or check out what they are hearing, by referring to the written sources or to other knowledgeable colleagues they have learnt to rely on. Sometimes they just take what they hear on trust. Depending on how much they trust the source, their own individual mindlines are affected to a greater or lesser extent. But during this process of learning through social interaction, something more mysterious is going on beyond the individual. They are developing collective mindlines.

The collective mindline provides the shared framework of principles and practices, and the boundaries within which practitioners can discuss their individual discrepancies. Like the individual mindline, it is complex, multifaceted, fuzzy, flexible, contextualised, and contingent on the people involved. Collective mindlines might be very widely shared across a profession, and/or within a limited group of people. Locally, such mindlines develop when a group of colleagues spend time attending meetings together or just chatting, hearing others' experiences and opinions, directly or indirectly observing each other's practices, following each other's patients – learning from each other in many ways. In doing so, the colleagues adjust their individual mindlines but also influence their collective ones. Usually – because all the individuals share similar training within an accepted paradigm – the core of collective mindlines is relatively stable and has evolved to adapt to the local context. Some aspects of mindlines (we should not prescribe antibiotics unnecessarily) are so embedded that they never get discussed, but more uncertain aspects (exactly what is the threshold for prescribing an antibiotic for a child's sore throat?) are much more likely to be talked about and to change as a result. Local collective mindlines usually tend to change only in relatively minor ways until a major new finding comes along, when they can be rapidly revised.

If clinicians interact with the same colleagues all the time, a form of 'subspeciation' of mindlines can occur – for instance, two neighbouring hospitals can evolve such that they treat the same patients differently, perhaps through the necessity of their distinctive context or resources, or perhaps because key local individuals ('opinion leaders') have undue influence. Indeed, there can be an echo-chamber effect that results in a local collective mindlines veering away from more widely accepted collective mindlines, for good or ill. As we have pointed out, "Mindlines can spread collective folly" (Gabbay & le May 2011, p. 203). However, the practitioners that we observed all belonged to many different collections of colleagues, which helped to obviate that potential problem since they could modulate the collective and individual views of each group by bringing ideas from their other groups. That openness and permeability of clinicians' multiple groupings and networks helped to avoid the echo chamber.

There has been increasing interest over the past three decades in loose groupings of people, known as communities of practice, who share a passion or an interest, face similar problems, and can learn together by informally exchanging their experiences and views (Wenger 1998). They enhance not only their individual and collective ability to solve problems and improve what they do but also to own a shared sense of identity, meaning, and belonging. Such groups also, crucially, over time, help their members develop a feeling for whose opinion to trust on what subjects. Communities of practice, wherever they emerge, play a vital role in mindline development. We saw the key features of a community of practice – often referred to as "joint enterprise, mutual engagement, and shared repertoire" (le May 2009) – when we witnessed the Lawndale practitioners in the many places where they were swapping stories and sharing information, such as the coffee room, the nurses' treatment room, the corridor, the lunch table, the dining club, and the conference bars. (Nowadays this would also include online chatrooms and WhatsApp groups). A community of practice can rapidly foster new ideas, good or bad, but runs the risk of confining that spread within the group of participants. And as we have seen, it runs the risk of becoming an echo chamber, a risk that is mitigated not only by its members belonging to a range of other communities of practice (as most practitioners do) but also by fostering an atmosphere where it is easy to challenge ideas with good humour and openness. We have found that an essential quality of high-functioning communities of practice is to ensure an ethos of respectful critical conversation, by which we mean a form of dialogue that encourages neither competitive argument nor acquiescent agreement but instead fosters open enquiry and evaluative exploration (Littleton & Mercer 2013).

This collective process of formulating mindlines leads to two further consequences. First, when faced, for example, with an anomalous or unusual situation, the process of talking about it with like-minded colleagues helps practitioners make sense of it together. (Why is the patient not responding to the treatment as expected? Why does the latest guideline seem to fly in the face of how we seem to do things successfully here?) The ensuing dialogue, which is often an exchange of knowledge gleaned from many sources, including experience, helps to give meaning to such situations. As a result, a collective view emerges – be it at a profession-wide or a local level – on how to deal with this unfamiliar situation. This process of collective sensemaking (Weick 1995) is fundamental to the development of collective mindlines. The second consequence of such collective thinking is that through such dialogue the participants gradually grow a sense of collective identity. Without being conscious of it, the people involved in such exchanges will develop ways of thinking and behaving that not only shape their practice but who they are. This can happen across a whole profession (physiotherapists thinking, behaving, even dressing differently from occupational therapists), across specialities (the differing ethos of surgeons and physicians), or across localities (again, the example of 'subspeciation' between hospitals). Collective mindlines are closely bound up with collective identity.

Codifying mindlines?

We have suggested that, through their discussions, practitioners expose the relevant snippets of their mindlines at the relevant moments. They do this largely through telling each other stories about their experiences, revealing each time an aspect of their mindlines that will help in a specific situation. But what if we could get them to 'download' the whole set of mindlines? If we managed to do that, could we not use the mindlines of excellent practitioners to train others, or to systematically upgrade deficient ones, or to share them across disciplines or with patients? Sadly, it is simply not possible to expose an entire set of mindlines, only the bits of them that are relevant to the immediate problem. It is, of course, possible to reveal *portions* of a mindline, including the tacit knowledge, which is deeply embedded and difficult to articulate. But because a person's mindlines are so bound up in the unique knowledge, context, experiences, and behavioural characteristics that have made them the practitioner they are, it is too complex to reveal all its different facets, especially when every use of a mindline varies according to the exact circumstances. Any attempt to unpack a complete set of mindlines for a given condition would either end up selecting an unreliable subset of its contents or producing an unfeasibly huge tome that explores every possible contingency; neither would be much use to anyone. Worse the 'download' would make no sense to someone who did not share that practitioner's professional evolution and – Catch-22 – if they did share it, they wouldn't need to have the mindline explained to them. Besides, a mindline is not a static entity; it is a constantly evolving set of dynamic processes. One can therefore no more capture a whole mindline than one can depict how to climb a mountain (especially when the weather closes in) by documenting an expert mountaineer's view of every conceivable safe route and technique. The best one can do is to help people expose *some* of the key relevant facets of their mindlines – possibly through the kinds of dialogue previously described – and to use that to help others understand how and why to respond to a particular problem. (Perhaps that is why mindlines are a precious form of intellectual and professional capital only available to those who have gone through the process of becoming a member of the group that formulates them.)

Through such dialogue, collective mindlines can become incorporated into local policy and guidance. At Lawndale, for example, writing a practice policy for any given clinical condition always relied not just on a review of guidelines and other explicit sources but also on the many discussions that revealed the once-tacit knowledge, the collective mindline, and the acceptable individual variants within it. This is not unusual; it is now widely accepted in business circles that the 'tacit' knowledge that staff carry in their heads can be invaluable to an organisation and should be made explicit where possible. Based on what is known as the *SECI* Cycle (*Socialisation, Externalisation, Combination, Internalisation*) (Nonaka & Takeuchi 1995), management gurus advocate bringing people together and enabling them to exchange ideas freely, so they can express their tacit knowledge, usually through telling each other stories about their experiences. As the tacit knowledge is exposed, it can be blended with many other sources of information, perhaps into an explicit document which everyone can internalise. This model oversimplifies matters, but it usefully encapsulates how the Lawndale mindlines were not only collectively shared but incorporated into formal policy. The key to linking the explicit, formal knowledge of a guideline to the tacit, informal knowledge of a mindline is, again, the effective use of respectful critical conversation.

The social construction of disease and illness, the patient mindline, and the negotiating space

When people interact, they shape each other's understanding and knowledge; so much so that social scientists have long accepted that – to a greater or lesser extent – we are all continually, between us, constructing our view of the world around us. It can even be argued that, given that we have no access to the world other than how we perceive it and collectively think about it, everything is a culturally specific social construct (Berger and Luckmann 1966). By that view, all clinical knowledge must also be a social construct (Wright & Treacher, 1982). The mindlines model presupposes that there is a difference between what exists out there in the world (that which is actually happening to the patient), how each individual person (e.g., the clinician or the patient) perceives that problem (within their individual mindlines), and how that person's view relates to how other relevant parties (e.g., local networks or national guidelines writers) collectively perceive it.

One need not go that far, however, to accept that when, say, a group of physiotherapists or a multi-disciplinary team share their different perspectives about a clinical condition, the result may confirm or amend an individual's or a group's view of the problem concerned and its management. Moreover, each person may leave that discussion having adjusted their mindlines. If only in that sense, the collective and individual mindlines are socially constructed. We observed this happening during our Lawndale ethnography, for example when the GPs debated how to define and manage early chronic kidney disease. As a result of those discussions, they collectively re-defined the nationally endorsed view of the disease to better suit their local context, and then each GP adjusted how they managed individual patients who met the national but not the local criteria. Some would see that as the social construction of renal disease, but there is no need to enter such philosophical terrain (though some do!) to see that when people discuss a clinical or social problem, they can only do so in terms of their differing conceptions of the matter in hand and its possible remedies.

Nowhere is that phenomenon more important than in the crucial moment when the practitioner's mindlines come up against what some are now calling the 'patient mindlines'. Both parties come to the discussion with their own understanding, their own construct, of the problem. We have seen how the practitioner draws on the collective mindlines of their wider profession and their groups of colleagues. But the patient also draws on theirs; they may have come across ideas from their families, friends, communities, or social media, from articles they have read, podcasts they have heard, and their own and vicarious experiences. These sources and many more will have shaped their expectation of what is wrong with them and what could be done about it. As the consultation proceeds, much depends on the degree of overlap between the two sets of mindlines – the patient's and the practitioner's. In other words, their conversation can be described as two people using their mindlines to negotiate their joint best shot at how to proceed in dealing with the problem before them. There may be sufficient concordance for an easily agreed plan of action, but there may not. (Think of conversations about long-COVID or the value of COVID vaccination.) That degree of overlap determines how big a 'negotiating space' is available for the practitioner and patient to agree on the nature of the problem and a course of action. (We use the word 'negotiation' in its broadest sense (Strauss 1978) of the way in which we all, in the to-ing and fro-ing of our daily discourse, negotiate the way we understand the world.) Of course, depending on the consultation style and personalities, and the relative power that each has in the consultation, the degree of 'jointness' may vary greatly; but that is another story. Nevertheless, the outcome for both, which is rooted in their individual mindlines, is a bilateral construction of this instance of what is wrong and what to do next.

There is a myriad of interactions that impact upon a practitioner's mindlines – colleagues, teachers, pharmaceutical and devices reps, mentors (not to mention, journalists, health ministers, local authorities, health commissioners, scientists, service managers, journal editors, and the rest), and also patients and their families and carers. Every one of this multitude of actors (Latour, 1987), all with their own communities of practice, all with their own varied views, can, through their interactions, influence the matter in question. Each actor uses what they know or believe about it – or, as some have said, 'performs' it (Mol 2002) – in a different way. Each interaction between any of these actors, just like the one between patient and practitioner, consists of two or more people with differing mindlines negotiating a common – or compromise, or contradictory – view on how to handle it. Now imagine introducing research findings or a new guideline into this mêlée, and it becomes clear why research is so hard to move into practice.

Research transformed

When a research finding starts being moved into practice, at every turn, it will be melded with people's existing ideas, with other evidence that they think matters, with unexpected aspects of their contexts and interests – in short with the mindlines of a host of different actors. We often liken this scenario to a pinball machine in which the research finding is a pliable ball being flipped around this network of actors. Not only is there an element of chance as to whom it encounters and how it bounces around, but at each interaction between them, it changes its shape. The result – akin to what some have called the social life of information (Brown & Duguid 2000) – is that even if the new knowledge is taken on board, it gets altered, adapted, or transformed into something different that is absorbed into their mindlines in ways that suit the context where they 'perform' it. The result is that the influence or impact of the research may no longer be easily recognisable. This happened for example in our research with health service commissioners (Gabbay, le May, Pope et al. 2020).

This clearly has implications when one tries to develop and monitor evidence-based practice. If one is trying to promote the uptake of the research but also accepts that practitioners use mindlines that have transformed that research, then it makes no sense to look for close adherence to the original research findings. Research implementation and the monitoring or audit of research impact will need to be much more nuanced than it has been to date. It will need to take account of what happens in the everyday world of practice, and why.

Why do mindlines matter?

We interviewed 15 scholars (not including the original[2] contributors to this volume) who have written about our work and asked them what they have found useful or not about it. Almost all of them began by explaining that the main attraction was how the mindlines model resonated with people's perception of everyday practice in an empirically and theoretically well-supported way. A senior nurse-researcher spoke of how, on reading our study, she and her colleagues who were developing research implementation methods, could finally see "how the melding works" between research and the many types of evidence that they had found most people used in practice. An experienced social worker expressed relief at how the mindlines model had resonated with his experience of the realities of practice and policymaking – in contrast to previous attempts that had diminished his profession by "taking something that's really complex and contextualised, and trying to standardise it all". As another interviewee, a very senior academic GP, put it, the real nature of practice had hitherto been "hidden away"; – it was "liberating" to have clear evidence that good clinical practice was not achieved in the over-rationalised way that the guidelines movement demanded. In summary, the 15 'scholar interviews' implied that the notion of mindlines opens several doors. First, it allows honest, critical self-reflection about where one gets the evidence that informs one's own mindlines (e.g., a doctor-turned-researcher said that when he first read our work he realised how and why he had so easily fallen into the trap of uncritically using an unsupported erroneous local collective mindline and felt empowered to question it). Secondly, our findings "give permission" – as a senior medical educator said – to modify and adapt official guidelines without worrying about thereby falling inevitably into bad practice. It allowed practitioners to recognise that they are often trying to "fit square peg guidelines into round holes" and to acknowledge and develop the important role of knowledge-in-practice-in-context. Thirdly, and relatedly, many of the interviewees described to us how our model justifies the persistent doubts about the usefulness of guidelines; it explains why practitioners so often appear not to follow them 'properly'. Our interviewees found this helpful, one even called it "therapeutic"; it helped to restore the professional autonomy and clinical judgement that many felt has been increasingly undermined by the growing imposition of external guidance. In short, it had been a relief – in the face of always having been told unrealistically how things *ought* to be – that we had "told it like it really is". But had we? We explore the answer to that question in Chapter 14, where we review what subsequent researchers, scholars, and practitioners have written about mindlines.

Meanwhile, it is time to turn to the chapters that describe where the Darwin Mindlines Group has taken the mindlines model.

Summary

- The mindlines model, which we based on our ethnographies of practice and a wide variety of influential theoretical literature, has several key implications:
  - Practitioners rely on a wide variety of sources and types of evidence that they must meld together to help them deal with the situations they face.
  - Rather than relying simply on science-based guidelines or other formal, theoretical knowledge, practitioners deploy their knowledge-in-practice-in-context.

- They rely on their mindlines – flexible, malleable, rapidly accessible internalised, collectively reinforced, and often tacit guidelines-in-the-head – that they accumulate throughout their careers.
- Well-developed mindlines can eventually give the practitioner the contextual adroitness to cope efficiently with complex problems.
- Mindlines are not just individual but are the result of a collective process – often occurring in communities of practice – that involves collective sensemaking and is closely bound with professional identity and professional capital.
- The development of collective mindlines is a form of social construction of knowledge, highly dependent on the social relations that shape people's understanding of illness and disease.
- The mindlines model helps explain how formal knowledge becomes transformed when put into practice, and why the implementation of research and guidelines is not straightforward.

Acknowledgements

We thank our 'scholar interviewees' for their critical engagement with the mindlines model and their generous contribution of time for the interviews.

Notes

1 We use the term 'clinician' for anyone practising healthcare.
2 The one exception is Peter C. Wyer, who was not linked to the Darwin Mindlines Group that led to this book (Chapter 13). As a result of what he told us in our interview, we invited him to write a chapter about the COVID response, which he then co-authored with Edward Suh.

References

Allen D, Harkins KJ. 2005. Too much guidance?, *Lancet*, 365: 1768.

Benner PE. 1984. *From novice to expert: excellence and power in clinical nursing practice*. Menlo Park, CA: Addison-Wesley.

Berger PL, Luckmann T. 1966. *The social construction of reality: a treatise in the sociology of knowledge*. London: Allen Lane, the Penguin Press.

Brown JS, Duguid P. 2000. *The social life of information*. Boston: Harvard Business School Press.

Gabbay J, le May A. 2011. *Practice-based evidence for healthcare: clinical mindlines*. Abingdon: Routledge.

Gabbay J, le May A, Pope C, Brangan E, Cameron A, Klein JH, Wye L. 2020. 'Uncovering the processes of knowledge transformation: the example of local evidence-informed policy-making in United Kingdom healthcare'. *Health Research Policy and Systems*, 18: 110. https://doi.org/10.1186/s12961-020-00587-9

Hunter KM. 1991. *Doctors' stories: the narrative structure of medical knowledge*. Princeton: Princeton University Press.

Latour B. 1987. *Science in Action: how to follow scientists and engineers through society*. Milton Keynes: Open University Press.

le May A. 2009. 'Introducing communities of practice', in A le May (Ed.) *Communities of practice in health and social care* (pp. 3–16). Oxford: Wiley Blackwell.

Littleton K, Mercer N. 2013. *Interthinking: putting talk to work*. London: Routledge.

Mol A. 2002. *The body multiple: ontology in medical practice*. Durham and London: Duke University Press.

Nonaka I, Takeuchi H. 1995. *The knowledge-creating company*. New York and Oxford: Oxford University Press.

Polanyi M. 1983. *The tacit dimension*. Gloucester, MA: Peter Smith.

Schön DA. 1983. *The reflective practitioner: how professionals think in action* (2nd edition, 1991). Aldershot, Brookfield, Singapore, and Sydney: Ashgate Arena.

Strauss A. 1978. *Negotiations: varieties, processes, contexts and social order*. San Francisco and London: Josey-Bass Publishers.

Weick KE. 1995. *Sensemaking in organizations*. Thousand Oaks: Sage Publications.

Wenger E. 1998. *Communities of practice: learning, meaning and identity*. New York: Cambridge University Press.

Wright P, Treacher A (Ed.). 1982. *The problem of medical knowledge: examining the social construction of medicine*. Edinburgh: Edinburgh University Press.

3

MAKING EVIDENCE RICH, RELEVANT, AND REAL

Using theatre-based knowledge mobilisation strategies to enhance mindlines and hence practice

Kate Beckett with Tony McBride

Introduction

The potential for research to improve healthcare quality is rarely disputed, but neither are the difficulties of implementing scientific evidence into clinical practice (Greenhalgh & Papoutsi 2018; Nutley, Boaz, Davies et al. 2019; Oliver & Boaz 2019). This has given rise to diverse methods aimed at improving the uptake of research. They are mostly linked with the emergence of Knowledge Mobilisation (KM) as a field that explores how to tackle this persistent problem by combining diverse forms of knowledge to effect change. Debate has increasingly moved from how to implement evidence better to how to blend scientific evidence with contextual and experiential realities – and how to conduct complexity-informed research (Beckett, Farr, Kothari et al. 2018; Greenhalgh & Papoutsi 2018). Alongside this are calls to learn and share ideas with other disciplines, e.g. creative arts, design sciences, psychology (Langley, Wolstenholme & Cooke 2018; Nutley, Boaz, Davies et al. 2019; Oliver & Boaz 2019), to "generate rich pictures of complex phenomena" (Greenhalgh & Papoutsi 2018, p. 4) by capturing data from multiple sources, to create locally adapted solutions, and to generate new agile methods for healthcare research. In short, to fundamentally alter the dominant research paradigm and replace it with one(s) which emphasises collaboration, co-production, and puts complexity, human creativity, and experience at the heart of research (Rycroft-Malone, Burton, Bucknall et al. 2016; Beckett, Farr, Kothari et al. 2018; Langley, Wolstenholme & Cooke 2018; Beckett, Deave, McBride et al. 2022). But how?

The mindlines model reframes this problem (Gabbay & le May 2004, 2011); it provides rich material for improving the uptake of research and for understanding how to put it to work. In this chapter, we explore how theatre-based KM approaches (Boal 1979; Bleuer, Chin & Sakamoto 2018) can aid that process and demonstrate, using a case study, how improving research's fit with mindlines

DOI: 10.4324/9781003158721-3

content and transmission enhances impact, seeds creativity and innovation, and helps eliminate gaps between evidence, knowledge, and action. Our research entitled "The Enhancing Post-Injury Psychological Intervention and Care (EPPIC)" study used Forum Theatre to mobilise knowledge about post-injury psychopathology and improve National Health Service (NHS) trauma care. It illustrates how Forum Theatre can replicate (and enhance) the way in which mindlines are effectively learned, modified, and transmitted, leading to contextually situated impactful research.

The EPPIC case study

KB's mindlines journey started when, as an applied health researcher/nurse, she had recently completed a three-year research post with the Impact of Injury study (IOIS), a multi-site mixed-methods programme of research investigating the social, psychological, and economic impact of physical injuries on working-aged adults. This study confirmed and extended what is known (and by whom) about the impact of psychological disorders on recovery from injury (see Box 3.1).

BOX 3.1 THE PSYCHOLOGICAL IMPACT OF UNINTENDED INJURIES – WHAT IS KNOWN AND BY WHOM?

Unintentional injuries are a leading cause of disability worldwide (Kendrick, Kelllezi, Coupland et al. 2017). Annually, in the UK, they account for over 800,000 hospital admissions (Hospital Admitted Patient Care Activity 2019–2020) and cost English healthcare commissioning groups more than £1.53 billion per year (Kellezi, Baines, Coupland et al. 2016). Globally, evidence regarding the impact of psychological problems on recovery from injury is pervasive, compelling, and consistent (Bryant, O'Donnell, Creamer et al. 2010). Successive studies have shown that approximately 30% of adults admitted to hospital following a traumatic injury will develop a clinically significant psychological problem (e.g., post-traumatic stress disorder: PTSD) within 12 months and that these have a marked effect on the extent and duration of recovery and on individual, healthcare, and societal costs (Kendrick, Kellezi, Coupland et al. 2017; Bryant, O'Donnell, Creamer et al. 2010). Amongst clinicians working in trauma care, this knowledge is also tacitly, experientially, and sometimes more formally known. Those with lived experience (as patients or carers) of moderate to severe physical injury also relate how it impacts on body and mind, and how the slow route to recovery creates significant challenges for both. Yet despite being so widely 'known', this evidence has had little impact on practice, and injured patients' psychological needs are poorly met within trauma care. This contributes to under-recognition, delayed treatment, and increased costs.

At the end of the IOIS, an opportunity arose to apply for a National Institute for Health Research (NIHR) Knowledge Mobilisation Research Fellowship (KMRF) – a funding stream which explicitly invites creative research/ers to develop innovative means to transform knowledge into action. Simultaneously, several IOIS patient and practitioner participants got in touch, asking if, and how, the study would change anything (and what they could do to help). So, this initiated our collaboration and KBs immersion in the KM literature which – though inspiring – made it clear that any solutions are unlikely to be universally applicable and that more creative, inclusive, and innovative KM methods are urgently required (Nutley, Boaz, Davies et al. 2019; Oliver & Boaz 2019; Greenhalgh & Papoutsi 2018).

Then a chance encounter with Gabbay and le May's (2004) original mindlines paper shone a different light on the 'implementation problem' – by illustrating what KM mechanisms already work in the healthcare context. The challenge, we concluded, was to develop a new KM approach which replicated (or enhanced) those in which mindlines are already effectively modified and transmitted.

How mindlines informed EPPIC's methods

Informed by what mindlines tell us about the knowledge required for effective practice and how it is communicated, the NIHR KMRF funded EPPIC study (Beckett, Deave, McBride et al. 2022) developed and tested a new research method to mobilise the content of diverse stakeholders' mindlines, and scientific research, about the impact and costs of post-injury psychopathology. In devising EPPIC's methods, four elements derived from mindlines and KM principles were regarded as key:

a) generating a rich pool of diverse evidence (patient, practitioner, and research),
b) using social interactive means to transmit it,
c) storytelling (an essential means, in practice, of making sense of and communicating complex knowledge (Gabbay & le May 2011)), and
d) creating opportunities for practitioners to actively relate and shape this diverse knowledge to the NHS context. Since mindlines' flexibility, applicability, and utility also depend on constant interaction between different types of knowledge, stakeholders, and contexts, we also needed to incorporate these dynamic elements throughout EPPIC's processes and intervention.

Forum Theatre

Isolating these factors suggested a form of participatory theatre (Boal 1979) called 'Forum Theatre' (FT) as a KM approach that incorporates mechanisms used in mindlines transmission. So, the next step was to find an experienced FT director to collaborate with. Enter Tony McBride (TMcB) see Box 3.2.

FT has been used in multiple settings to convey diverse knowledge, stimulate debate, and catalyse change. In FT, a play (or FT model) depicting a story about a social issue with unsatisfactory outcomes is co-developed by key

BOX 3.2 REFLECTIONS ON FT AND ITS USE WITHIN EPPIC (TMcB)

I was delighted to be invited to collaborate on EPPIC. Having worked for many years in various community settings, it was a perfect opportunity to further explore FT within the health context and to use it in a novel way. Ordinarily, an FT model is developed from stories shared directly by people with lived experience of an issue. Within EPPIC, I discovered that a similarly authentic FT model can be created using well-researched case studies framed within the scientific literature. This permits creation of a dual-perspective model, representing patient and practitioner experience alongside the research evidence. The FT-making process brought these contrasting perspectives to life, provided a focal point, a story for stakeholder audiences to gather around: watch, consider, debate, and, importantly, change. It allowed for diverse stakeholder experiences, opinions, ideas, and strategies to be heard and explored in a non-judgemental and solution-focussed manner. This opened minds to the perspectives of others and the potential of progress towards a shared goal of – "providing care and services that we and our families would want to use".

stakeholders – those with experience of the issue and who have a vested interest in change (Boal 1979). Traditionally, the story is told from the perspective of a single protagonist whose story reflects (or represents) those of others. An audience for whom it resonates (from the same stakeholder groups) is invited to an FT workshop where the play is enacted straight through once, and then the audience members discuss what they have seen. The play is performed again; this time audience members are invited to stop it at any point, step into the role of the protagonist, and try out different ways of doing things. The remaining actors/characters skilfully improvise what changes as a result – so the audience can test and see the positive and/or negative consequences of their ideas/re-enactments. Multiple interactions with the whole audience and with the play follow, until a range of possible solutions has been explored, from a variety of perspectives. In this way, spectators become active transformers, develop new understanding, and rehearse solutions to complex issues in the real world. FT offered a means to mobilise knowledge which 'fits' with fundamental properties of mindlines' content and transmission. However, in contrast to usual FT methods, EPPIC aimed to create a dual perspective/protagonist model (foregrounding both patient and practitioner stories) for use as a transferable intervention which mobilised diverse knowledge garnered from systematic research – one that conveyed generalisable truths about the issue but could be used in different NHS contexts to inform locally implementable evidence-informed recommendations.

EPPIC was co-produced by a study team including patients, clinicians, applied health researchers, and theatre practitioners, including TMcB from Cardboard

Citizens – the UK's leading FT proponents (https://cardboardcitizens.org.uk/). The same key stakeholder groups provided evidence to inform the play and FT workshop audiences – so interaction between these disparate voices (and their individual/collective mindlines)[1] was continuous and created multiple opportunities for change to occur – and potential change agents.

Method

Based on this evidence and study team deliberations, EPPIC used the following three-stage KM approach: **Stage-1**: FT play (or intervention) development, **Stage-2**: FT workshop (or intervention) delivery, **Stage-3**: analysis of study outcome data to see what changed, how and why (see Figure 3.1):

Stage-1 FT play development

Stage-1 was to **capture** patient, practitioner, and research perspectives on post-injury psychological needs and care; we interviewed patients (53), practitioners (40),[2] experts in post-injury psychopathology (3), ran three practitioner focus groups (22 participants total), and completed a literature review. These activities sought to comprehensively explore three strands of evidence (patient, practitioner, research) and surface key stakeholders' multi-faceted (tacit, experiential, and research-based) mindlines. Then we used framework analysis to systematically **combine** and map how these perspectives differed in ways that are important for injured adults' psychological outcomes. This step sought to create a rich form of evidence that, like mindlines, included scientific research and contextually specific, convergent, and/or contradictory narratives. Key themes drawn from this analysis and representative quotes (to aid authenticity) were used to co-produce the script for a play *Altered States* **conveying** diverse evidence about post-injury psychopathology in a 'blended' patient story from just before to 12 months after an accidental injury (with practitioner and research perspectives woven in). The play has eight scenes which conform to stages in the patient journey (as elicited from patient interviews) and were named according to their dominant emotional and experiential flavour, e.g., Scene 3 'Rescue' depicts the arrival of paramedics at the scene, whereas Scene 5: 'Anxious Dependence' shows the uncertainties and insecurities of in-patient care. This step aimed to communicate the complexity and diversity of stakeholder mindlines and their convergence/divergence with the research evidence in an accessible, memorable, and embodied form.

Stage-2 FT workshop delivery

In Stage-2, we delivered two workshops for audiences of the same stakeholder groups (*Workshop 1*: Patients (22), Practitioners (19), Researchers (10) – see Figure 3.2; *Workshop 2*: Patients (12), Carers (3), Practitioners (12), Researchers (6)). These workshops included the play performed by Cardboard Citizens' FT actors and used

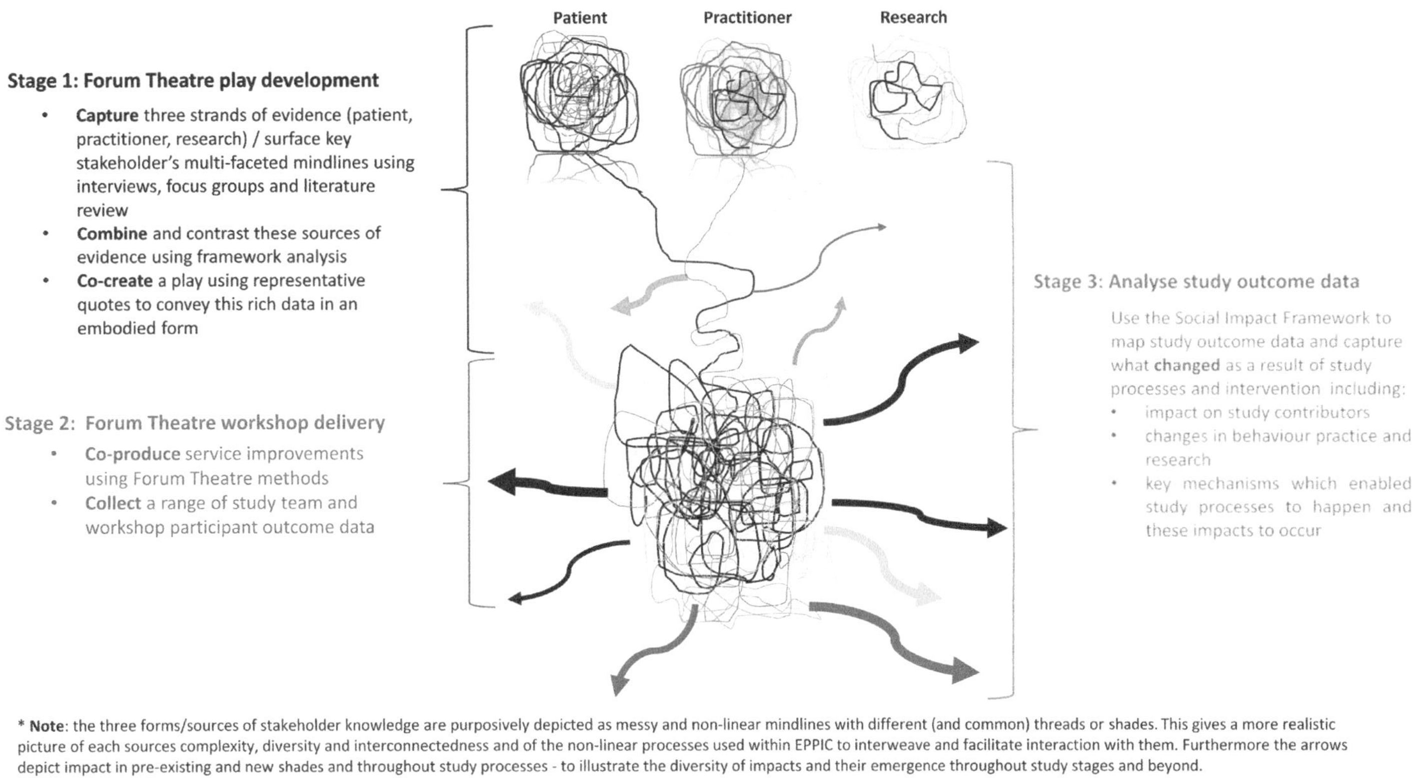

FIGURE 3.1 Showing EPPICs three-stage method for mobilising diverse stakeholder mindlines and research evidence about the psychological impact of injury.

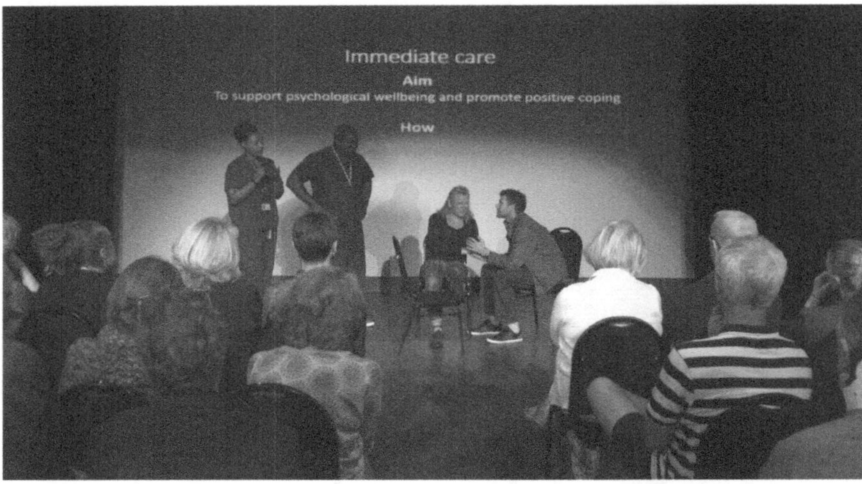
Immediate care
Aim
To support psychological wellbeing and promote positive coping
How

FIGURE 3.2 Workshop 1 – participants watching *Altered States* with scene-relevant research evidence projected behind (included with participant consent).

FT methods to stimulate debate, knowledge sharing, and **co-production** of ideas and recommendations. Interactions between stakeholders helped them to explore similarities and differences between their mindlines and the research evidence, expose gaps and assumptions, and collectively test, reject and/or co-create service improvements.

We also **collected** a range of outcome data, including post-workshop evaluation forms, filmed interviews, follow-up phone calls, three- and six-month practitioner questionnaires, notes on study team debriefing sessions, and individual critical reflections (Figure 3.1).

Stage-3 Analysis of study outcomes

For Stage-3, we used the Social Impact Framework (Beckett, Farr, Kothari et al. 2018) to analyse study outcome data and determine what **changed**, how, when, and why. This framework provides a structured means to capture multi-level (social, relational, tangible, and economic) impacts of co-produced research and mechanisms which give rise to them.

The following excerpts, from **Scene 5** and **Scene 8** of the play, give a flavour of how Stage-1 patient, practitioner, and research evidence was conveyed to Stage-2 workshop audiences. EPPIC's methods can also be viewed in a short film entitled *Altered States; Using Forum Theatre to Mobilise Knowledge and Enhance NHS Care* (https://www.youtube.com/watch?v=QWHAb3Y2eKM), and further Stage-1 and 2 findings can be found in Beckett, Deave, McBride et al. (2022). Powerful emotional components within practitioner mindlines were common, e.g., the personal trauma of caring within resource-strained health services, being unable to provide the care they'd ideally like, and the fear that addressing patients' psychological needs might overwhelm already fragile defence mechanisms.

- ***Scene 5 'Anxious Dependence' (or in-patient care)****: As this scene starts, we see the multi-disciplinary team gathered round a computer, prioritising patients for the days' theatre list. They know orthopaedic trauma outcomes are improved by early surgery, so they're trying to fit patients in. But there are multiple moving/unknown factors, e.g., is the right equipment, surgeon, anaesthetist, and time slot available? Which new emergencies will the day bring? Meanwhile, on the ward, Rachel the patient is immobilised in her bed. She's Nil by Mouth (NBM), hasn't slept much, and is in pain, anxiously waiting for surgery for a complex leg fracture, resulting from a bicycle accident. A confused patient approaches her calling out wildly; he's been doing it all night and Rachel's observed him biting and kicking staff. Theatre porters keep arriving with trolleys, each time she thinks it's her turn, and her anxieties and hopes are aroused, but it's not. She's trying not to be too demanding as she can see staff are busy. By late afternoon she's extremely thirsty, tearful and wound up. A healthcare assistant wonders if she's more upset and agitated than you'd expect. Then a nurse approaches and kindly tells Rachel there's been an emergency so she's off the list, hopefully tomorrow … her husband Steve is sent home disappointed and worried about missing another day's work. Rachel's offered a bowl of cornflakes, which is then hastily removed, and she's NBM again. This cycle is repeated on successive days. Simultaneously, her nurse expresses frustration that ward staff are often the last to hear about list cancellations and have so little control. They're the ones who must break the news to patients. She feels she's become desensitised to the emotional stuff, it's easier "to get your head down, just do the tasks and hope someone down the line will pick it up". She regrets how little time she has for softer skills which make the job worthwhile and that a hard exterior is necessary to survive and function the next day. At the end of the scene, a slide[3] describing the five principles of Psychological First Aid (the most effective means to support resilience and emotional well-being at this stage) is projected on a screen behind the actors. These are ensuring the patient feels safe, hopeful, calm, connected, and has a sense of self and community efficacy.*
- ***Scene 8 Altered States (longer-term rehabilitation: 3–12 months post-injury)****: Rachel's been home for a while, she avoids going out and feels detached from her surroundings and other people. Her leg is physically healing, but she's having flashbacks to her accident and is terrified of falling and ending up in hospital again. Steve, her husband, is frustrated by her fearfulness and inactivity – she's not who she was. He feels burdened by doing everything for her; they're constantly arguing about silly things (e.g., when he hangs trousers on the washing line the 'wrong' way up) and he increasingly stays late at work. Rachel visits her general practitioner (GP) but finds it hard to convey her emotional state. Her GP is somewhat dismissive of her symptoms but offers a prescription for anti-depressants (not counselling – Rachel's treatment of choice). In an aside, the GP explains that counselling waiting lists are six months. Rachel declines and leaves feeling even more alone. Many months later, Rachel realises her drinking is becoming problematic. She visits another GP who again offers anti-depressants – this time Rachel accepts. As the play ends, we see Rachel considering whether to take them and if so, how many. The screen behind reveals that Trauma-Focussed Cognitive Behavioural Therapy is the most effective treatment for individuals with acute traumatic stress symptoms/PTSD and early intervention targeted at clinical presentation, not diagnostic threshold, is recommended.*

The remaining sections focus on what the Stage-3 results tell us about EPPIC's impacts and mechanisms that gave rise to them.

Results

The following sections summarise what the Stage-3 analysis tells us about EPPIC's impact on (a) contributing individuals and groups; (b) how this in turn influenced behaviour, practice, and research; and (c) the mechanisms drawn from KM, mindlines, and FT which gave rise to them.

Impact on contributing individuals and groups

EPPIC's approach had a marked impact on contributing individuals (including workshop audiences and study team members) and on interpersonal relationships between stakeholder groups. Analysis suggested five key areas in which change occurred:

1. **knowledge of the psychological impact of injury** – individuals (all contributor groups) reported they acquired new knowledge and "useful facts and figures" about the risks factors, incidence, symptoms, treatment, and costs of post-injury psychopathology. Their existing tacit and experiential knowledge was also formalised/validated.
2. **confidence in their own knowledge** – individuals (all groups) reported renewed confidence in what they knew and, in the legitimacy, and utility of their individual/collective voices for transforming patient care.
3. **mutual understanding and empathy for each other's lived experience** – they learned what it feels like to be an injured patient, an NHS practitioner, and to conduct research – and gained insight into the challenges and opportunities of each other's worlds. They felt heard, and this increased trust and willingness to work together towards 'common goals'.
4. **attitudes towards KM and research** – contributors found EPPIC's methods new and engaging. They enjoyed "putting their experience to good use" and feeling they could actively change something. They gained insight into creative practices' potential within health research.
5. **inspiring creativity and ideas** – EPPIC's topic/methods also influenced contributors to think more widely about how they could alter their own actions and practice, spread this knowledge, and use FT within clinical practice, education, and research.

Influence on behaviour, practice, and research

The study outcome data contained many examples of changes in behaviour, practice, and research. For example, several patients reported finding the courage to speak to their GP (about their mental health) or self-referred for psychological support. Others revaluated their experience and were finally able to 'move on', swapped contact details, or had more constructive conversations with family members – who, they realised, had also experienced many difficulties. All agreed to further contact and many subsequently became involved as Patient and Public Involvement (PPI) representatives in further research.

Practitioners (including doctors, nurses, paramedics, physiotherapists, and psychologists) reported reflecting on their own practice and reminding themselves of the importance of seemingly little things. They altered how they communicated with patients, revised information leaflets, and inserted questions on emotional well-being into patient assessment forms. Some reported they felt empowered to act as patient advocates, found it easier to "initiate and sustain conversations with senior managers", and that these were in turn more likely to be acted upon (e.g., leading to commissioning of a new practitioner-led liaison service). Practitioners also developed new networks and links, leading to independent spin-off and collaborative research (e.g., *Altered States* is being co-developed into an online training tool for NHS and higher education institution use). Some independently introduced post-injury psychopathology into continuous professional development and master's level clinical training. EPPIC's methods also encouraged clinical teams to "think differently about how we conduct research and quality improvement" and to enhance PPI or use creative methods within more traditional practitioner-led clinical research. The way in which the patient story was told (and felt) also influenced commissioner-provider conversations and the "development and direction" of unrelated services.

Researchers presented the study and its techniques widely, developed mutually beneficial partnerships, were funded for further research, and refined their facilitation techniques (after realising what it feels like to be a research participant). They were reminded of the significance of experiential **and** clinical outcomes and introduced creative methods and 'emotional triggers' into unrelated research. Workshop contributors (patients, practitioners, and researchers) were featured in the study film, which was widely viewed and positively received e.g., "blown away, the possibilities the power of this" (thus adding visibility and value to contributing organisations and to the NIHR). Finally, the FT practitioners introduced what they'd learned into independent work elsewhere, using FT to help homeless people explore and process traumatic experiences.

While these tangible impacts were largely at individual, group, and organisational levels, EPPIC's outputs (workshops, conference presentations, film, publications) also seeded conceptual changes at a macro/societal level. For example, they influenced the methods used in unrelated research, clinical training, quality improvement, and other activities aimed at social change. The study also raised the profile of post-injury psychopathology, mindlines, and the KM field; moreover it showcased a new method of complexity-informed research which had a significant impact on key stakeholders' knowledge, engagement, and capacity for research.

What, in EPPIC's methods, gave rise to these impacts?

That EPPIC's approach impacted on contributing individuals and groups and on their subsequent behaviour (and mindlines) is clear; however, understanding which elements (mechanisms) enabled this research to happen and impact(s) to occur can assist in answering the question, "What can mindlines tell us about improving healthcare by means of research?" Mapping the outcome data onto the Social Impact Framework (Beckett, Farr, Kothari et al. 2018) suggested the following four mechanisms were key: (1) diverse knowledge, (2) drama and storytelling, (3) social interaction, and (4) active co-production and testing of new ideas.

Diverse knowledge

Study team members' diverse knowledge and skills ensured the study design, processes and materials were accessible to its varied audiences and reflected their different narratives, needs, and priorities. Deriving the play from multiple patient and practitioner accounts, and using direct quotes, made it resonant and real for workshop audiences. This helped to foster mutual empathy and mirrored the complexity and tensions within a clinical encounter. It also enhanced the play's perceived legitimacy and made 'uncomfortable knowledge' (Greenhalgh & Papoutsi 2018, p. 3) incontrovertible, e.g., the impact of an elderly confused patient and surgical delays on an immobilised trauma patient (see Scene 5 excerpt).

Drama and storytelling

Study team members' diverse skills resulted in a play that was powerful, absorbing, and believable – yet true to the underlying research. Representing the data through drama made it more memorable, 'colourful', and relatable to the real world. It contextualised the issue, illustrated healthcare's intrinsic complexity, and made the themes real and alive – this triggered "reflection on past (and future) experiences where things could have been/be done differently". Rachel's story was disturbing and visceral, it evoked both an emotional and rational response, which in turn created a potent stimulus for change, e.g., some patients found it 'extremely painful' but ultimately beneficial, while practitioners who had "felt the fearfulness [of hospital patients] … because they have no control" realised that a lot needed "to change to make patients feel safe" and how their practice impacted on patients' "resilience and outcomes".

Social interaction

Interaction between study team members created a diverse pool of knowledge and ideas, enhanced the project's perceived interest and legitimacy, and enabled us to develop wider links and networks – these proved crucial for delivering such a complex and innovative project involving multiple stakeholders. The workshop and audience mix created a 'safe space' in which different experiences and priorities could be aired, understood, and/or challenged and new knowledge and meaning acquired, e.g., revealing a mismatch between hospital practitioners' expectations of community provision and what discharged patients actually got. Meeting other stakeholder groups in a social milieu where "who was who wasn't always clear" and "being in the round with people who are still raw and suffering from injury and with practitioners who wish they could provide better services" made it hard to disengage from the human and contextual realities underpinning this research (as manifest in stakeholders' mindlines).

Active co-production and testing of new ideas

Study team members' diverse knowledge and skills enabled EPPIC to respond to the emerging opportunities and challenges of its varied individual and organisational contributors, e.g., modifying patient and practitioner recruitment methods. FT practitioners' skills were also key in dramatising the evidence and in improvising consequences (expected and unexpected) resulting from audience re-enactments. For workshop contributors, the experimental and participatory feel was "empowering" as was being able to actively try out and collectively discover new ways of doing things.

How were mindlines mechanisms used and enhanced in this research?

EPPIC's methods aimed to mobilise knowledge about the psychological impact of injury by replicating the ways in which mindlines are learned and transmitted. The results in this chapter show that the same mechanisms which enable mindlines to be shared, modified, and applied in the real world (Gabbay & le May 2004, 2011) can also assist in mobilising knowledge generated by research. However, in practice, these essential mechanisms are often constrained or limited. So EPPIC's methods didn't simply replicate but purposively enhanced opportunities for mindlines to be refreshed, challenged, and grounded in research. The following sections explore how this worked.

Enhanced content and reliability of knowledge sources

Patient-practitioner encounters involve a series of negotiations (Gabbay & le May 2011) between diverse, sometimes divergent, narratives to achieve the desired outcomes of care. So mindlines need to contain a rapidly accessible array of knowledge forms and sources, which are regularly refreshed and tested in the context of use. However, in the healthcare environment, opportunities to update knowledge, share ideas or check sources' reliability are increasingly limited, and mindlines are heavily influenced by local factors and organisational demands (Gabbay & le May 2011). Furthermore, despite mindlines' complexity and breadth, practitioner knowledge is generally fragmented by the needs of the clinical setting; insight into the whole patient journey and its outcomes is rare. So mindlines can become stagnated, reinforce suboptimal practices and sustain the status quo, e.g., the neglect of psychopathology in trauma care. EPPIC provided a rich source of diverse evidence which was believable and relatable to the realities of practice yet grounded in systematic research. It provided a summary of key themes in the three data strands, mapped how/where they diverged throughout the trauma pathway, and highlighted experiential and clinical factors impinging on psychological well-being, e.g., how common events such as surgical delays act as secondary stressors and contribute to post-injury psychological morbidity. This furnished workshop participants with contextually situated, reliable, and generalisable evidence, which was ready to be experimented with, spread, and acted upon.

While diverse evidence is key, EPPIC's data also revealed wide consensus on the importance of the topic and alignment between tacit, experiential, and explicit evidence – this fostered shared responsibility and momentum for change – and demonstrated that lack of provision could not simply be attributed to a practitioner knowledge deficit (Wieringa & Greenhalgh 2015).

Widening and diversifying practitioners' social milieu

Social interaction is the primary means by which mindlines are acquired, modified, and shared (Gabbay & le May 2011). However, in practice, space for learning and critical reflection is often scarce or limited to within silos of care. So, while encounters with patients, mentors, and peers may provide rich opportunities for confirming or refuting what works, capacity for prolonged, in-depth, or new exchanges and more formalised training are increasingly rare. So, by purposively constructing a wider social milieu including representatives from diverse stakeholder groups and the whole trauma pathway, EPPIC multiplied opportunities for knowledge sharing, productive interaction, and the emergence of new ideas, e.g., revealing gaps in provision contributing to poorer outcomes of care. Confronting stakeholders with each other's knowledge and realities also enhanced empathy between groups and revealed that the question is not simply "What can clinicians do to improve patient care?", but "What can society expect and how can we collectively make healthcare work?" This was instrumental in the emergence of a new multi-disciplinary community of practice who are still working together to address the issues raised by this research. Research directed towards top-down policy initiatives and universal guidelines often neglects individual citizens and their collective potential to alter their environment – given sufficient knowledge, power, and tools.

Using drama to portray multi-dimensional stories

Within-practice stories, anecdotes, and narratives provide an essential, and memorable, means of making sense of complex information, discerning patterns, communicating ideas, modifying mindlines, and determining action (Gabbay & le May 2011). They also perform a social function by collectively reinforcing self and professional identity and group norms (Gabbay & le May 2011). However, stories shared between practitioners can spread information and misinformation (especially when time to impart and unpack them is constrained). Drama on the other hand enabled us to bring the evidence alive, convey diverse stories (using informants' own words) and highlight their interrelatedness, e.g., how NHS constraints limit patient and practitioner agency and heighten stress, and how these in turn make it hard to act on knowledge from research. Professional actors' portrayal of these narratives also resulted in a richer, more nuanced, and multi-sensory experience. This aroused visceral, emotional, and rational reactions and accurately mirrored the complexity and texture of stakeholder realities.

Theatre-based KM strategies (such as FT) aim to generate an "aesthetic balance" (Bleuer, Chin & Sakamoto 2018) between emotional and cognitive processing. This creates "optimal stress" for learning and transformation – unlike more factual or written content which can induce disinterest or overly emotive or critical content which triggers "defensiveness" (Bleuer, Chin & Sakamoto 2018). In EPPIC FT provided a perfect medium for engaging audiences in each other's lived experiences and in scientific research. Intermingling patient, practitioner, and research/er stories and experiences also challenged some pervasive narratives (e.g., practitioners are uncaring, practice would be exemplary if governed by science, academics are detached from reality, body-mind dualism, and the insignificance of mental health). It reminded individuals of their shared humanity, frustrations, and ambitions and stimulated open, honest, and constructive debate about what the problems are and how they could be solved.

Inviting creativity and experimentation

While deciding on a treatment plan requires assessment of alternative options and a degree of improvisation (Gabbay & le May 2011), opportunities for actively experimenting with patients in real time are understandably limited. Furthermore, in practice, the reflexivity and creativity of this process is bounded by situational and organisational barriers to applying all available knowledge and skills (Gabbay & le May 2011), e.g., in Scene 8, Rachel's GP prescribes anti-depressants to expedite treatment in the knowledge of counselling waiting-list times. Using a simulated situation which actively invited and created a safe space for experimentation and creativity stimulated co-construction of new narratives (Langley, Wolstenholme & Cooke 2018) about post-injury psychopathology and locally actionable solutions for improving care. It did not suggest solutions or provide hard facts (Greenhalgh & Papoutsi 2018) but invited participants to use their own creativity and knowledge to turn complex evidence into action (Langley, Wolstenholme & Cooke 2018).

Conclusion

The mindlines model shows what forms of knowledge are required for effective healthcare practice, and why and how this knowledge is generally transmitted. EPPIC illustrated that these same mechanisms can be used to design and implement contextually situated impactful research and confirmed how co-creative practices can assist that process by putting human experience and realities at the heart of research (Beckett, Deave, McBride et al. 2022; Bleuer, Chin & Sakamoto 2018; Langley, Wolstenholme & Cooke 2018). Such approaches simulate the way in which, in practice, knowledge works and creates the right "conditions for knowledge mobilisation" (Langley, Wolstenholme & Cooke 2018) and for learning and transformation (Bleuer, Chin & Sakamoto 2018).

While the concept of mindlines has been widely shared and used to advance understanding of how, in practice, knowledge works, their implications for developing research methods with practical application and impact in the real world have not been widely explored (Wieringa & Greenhalgh 2015). There is no magic or universal answer (Greenhalgh & Papoutsi 2018), but mindlines can reframe the problem and offer pragmatic and creative solutions for improving practice by means of research.

Summary

- Mindlines containing diverse rapidly accessible evidence are generally transmitted through social means, e.g., anecdotes and storytelling, and require active testing/modification in the context of their use.
- This chapter uses a case study to illustrate how Forum Theatre (FT) – a form of participatory drama using similar mechanisms can mobilise diverse knowledge and catalyse change.
- We used the following three-stage approach to promote improvements in post-injury psychological care: **Stage-1**: FT play (or intervention) development, **Stage-2**: FT workshop (or intervention) delivery, **Stage-3**: analysis of study outcome data to see what changed, how and why.
- We found FT gave rise to multi-level changes in practice, behaviour, and research. Four key mechanisms drawn from KM literature, mindlines, and FT (diverse knowledge, drama and storytelling, social interaction, active co-production) enabled these impacts to occur.
- This case study shows how FT can replicate (and enhance) the way in which mindlines are effectively learned, modified, and transmitted, leading to contextually-situated impactful research.
- It highlights the potential (and need for) co-creative practices, storytelling, and 'emotional triggers' to catalyse change in complex healthcare ecosystems.

Acknowledgements

We would like to thank all the patients, practitioners, and researchers who enabled this innovative research to happen. In particular, these members of the multidisciplinary study team (Toity Deave, Andrée le May, John Gabbay, Urszula Kapoulas, Adele Long, Georgie Warburton, Celia Wogan, Lee Cox, Julian Thompson, Frank Spencer, Denise Kendrick). Also, thanks to Cardboard Citizens and the following five FT actors (Andre Skeet, Denholm Spurr, Jo Galbraith, Kerry Norridge,

Shereena Akoto) who provided essential creative input into the design, implementation, outcomes, and dissemination of this study. We would also like to thank the study sponsors: the University of the West of England, Bristol; University Hospitals Bristol; and Weston NHS Foundation Trust. The study was supported throughout by research teams and practitioners at the following NHS trusts: South Western Ambulance Service NHS Foundation Trust, North Bristol NHS Foundation Trust, North Somerset and South Gloucestershire Clinical Commissioning Group, and by the West of England Clinical Research Network. Finally, we would like to thank the Impact of Injuries Study team and its patient and practitioner contributors without whom this work would not have taken place.

This study was funded by a UK NIHR KMRF awarded to Kate Beckett. This amazing funding stream enabled diverse researchers to experiment with creative means to mobilise knowledge to effect change (KMAlliance.co.uk); it could not have happened without their commitment to it.

Notes

1 Other stakeholders also have mindlines, as Fiona Cowdell shows in Chapter 5.
2 These data were drawn from secondary analysis of IOIS data and primary EPPIC data.
3 In the second workshop, the scientific evidence was presented as a simulated interview between an expert in post-injury psychopathology and an experienced practitioner before the play – to test whether delivering it using a social format made it more memorable and enhanced its assimilation into audience debates and re-enactments.

References

Beckett K, Deave T, McBride T, le May A, Gabbay J, Kapoulas U, Long A, Warburton G, Wogan C, Cox L, Thompson J, Spencer F, Kendrick D. 2022. 'Using Forum Theatre to mobilise knowledge and improve NHS care: the Enhancing Post-Injury Psychological Intervention and Care (EPPIC) study', *Evidence & Policy*, 18(2): 236–264. https://doi.org/10.1332/174426421X16420902769508

Beckett K, Farr M, Kothari A, Wye L, le May A. 2018. 'Embracing complexity and uncertainty to create impact: exploring the processes and transformative potential of co-produced research through development of a social impact model', *Health Res Policy* Sys, 16: 118.

Bleuer J, Chin M, Sakamoto I. 2018. 'Why theatre-based research works? Psychological theories from behind the curtain', *Qual Res Psychol*, 15(2–3): 395–411.

Boal A. 1979. *Theatre of the oppressed*. London: *Pluto Press*, Reprint 2019.

Bryant R, O'Donnell M, Creamer M, McFarlane M, Clark R, Silove D. 2010. 'The psychiatric sequelae to traumatic injury', *Am J Psychiatry*, 167: 312–320.

Gabbay J, le May A. 2004. 'Evidence based guidelines or collectively constructed "mindlines?" Ethnographic study of knowledge management in primary care', *BMJ*, 329(7473): 1013.

Gabbay J, le May A. 2011 *Practice-based evidence for healthcare: clinical mindlines*. Abingdon: Routledge.

Greenhalgh T, Papoutsi C. 2018. 'Studying complexity in health services research: desperately seeking an overdue paradigm shift', *BMC Med*, 16: 95. https://doi.org/10.1186/s12916-018-1089-4

Kellezi B, Baines D, Coupland C, Beckett K, Barnes J, Sleney J, Christie N, Kendrick D. 2016. 'The impact of injuries on health service resource use and costs in primary and secondary care in the English NHS', *J Public Health*, 38(4): 464–471. https://doi.org/10.1093/pubmed/fdv173

Kendrick D, Kelllezi B, Coupland C, Maula A, Beckett K, Morriss R, Joseph S, Barnes J, Sleney J, Christie N. 2017. 'Psychological morbidity, and health-related quality of life after injury: multicentre cohort study', *Qual Life Res*. 26(5): 1233–1250. doi:10.1007/s11136-016-1439-7

Langley J, Wolstenholme D, Cooke J. 2018. '"Collective making" as knowledge mobilisation: the contribution of participatory design in the co-creation of knowledge in healthcare', *BMC Health Serv Res*. 18(1): 585.

Nutley S, Boaz A, Davies H, Fraser, A. 2019. 'New development: what works now? Continuity and change in the use of evidence to improve public policy and service delivery', *Public Money and Management*, 39(4): 310–316.

Oliver K, Boaz A. 2019. 'Transforming evidence for policy and practice: creating space for new conversations', *Palgrave Commun*, 5: 60.

Rycroft-Malone J, Burton C, Bucknall T, Graham I, Hutchinson A, Stacey D. 2016. 'Collaboration and co-production of knowledge in healthcare: opportunities and challenges', *Int J Health Policy Manag*, 5(4): 221–223.

Wieringa S, Greenhalgh T. 2015. '10 years of mindlines: a systematic review and commentary', *Imp Sci*, 10: 45. https://doi.org/10.1186/s13012-015-0229-x

4

MINDLINES IN THE MOMENT

The constant unfolding of complex performance

Dominic Hurst

Introduction

Mindlines guide clinicians' knowledge-in-practice-in-context. How does this unfold in space and time, as people (clinicians, patients, families) come together, each with their own mindlines? How is the practice experienced by each of these actors? And what about material 'things' – such as clinical equipment, computers, furniture? How do they contribute to the unfolding interactions within practices and on the mindlines of those involved?

In this chapter, I will describe research I conducted into the moment-by-moment unfolding of practices in the dental-clinic setting and how mindlines – the knowing possessed by individuals – interact with the knowing that arises in the performance of dental practices.

The detailed description I provide is intended to problematise concepts of practice, not simplify them. By acknowledging complexity, I hope that practitioners, educators, and researchers will be prompted to consider different ways of thinking about how they approach the practices they engage in, induct others into, or analyse and try to improve.

I describe my personal journey from understanding practice naïvely as ordered and relatively simple to an understanding of practices as unfolding, non-linear, unpredictable. In a word, complex.

Throughout my doctoral studies, I was practising in both clinical and educational fields, so towards the end, I reflect on the implications of the mindlines model, as well as my own work, in the clinical educational context.

DOI: 10.4324/9781003158721-4

Professional dental practices and mindlines

Practice is a lot more complex than I used to think. I don't mean that it was complex to do things *per se*, but that I didn't have much of an idea of how practice happens.

I could competently practise as a student, dentist, educator, and researcher. I could go on without knowing how it was that I was going on. I go on largely unaware of what enables me to go on, of the knowing I embody and create in my moment-by-moment interactions with other people and things.

This lack of knowing how it is I do things means much is uncertain and unpredictable. To reduce that uncertainty and unpredictability, I can create ways of knowing that appear more concrete, controllable, and predictable. Plato sought to control uncertainty through the application of general principles, or *episteme*. Intellectuality – the mental activity that creates ideas – helped control the uncertainty inherent in life. Intellectuality was put on a moral and ethical pedestal. Practice – doing stuff – was relegated to a position of inferiority as *techne*.

There is a sense of comfort or security, perhaps, for those of us who want to do things 'right' (whatever that means for each of us) in finding ideas we can, in an uncomplicated way, translate into what we do. The intellectuals generate the ideas, and we apply them as practitioners.

When I began my doctoral degree in evidence-based healthcare, I was engaged in a research field that, to me, largely embraced the intellectual superiority Plato had written about centuries earlier. It appeared to view clinical practices as something wholly different and separate from the knowledge-generative world of clinical research. This perspective assumes that knowledge is produced through research and that all that is left is to translate it into the doing because there is not knowledge in doing.

When the knowledge doesn't get taken up in the doing, there is a so-called implementation, or "know-do", gap. The field includes such terms as "knowledge translation", and there is a "knowledge-to-action" cycle suggesting there is no knowledge *in* action. (Graham, Logan, Harrison et al. 2006) As I engaged with the field through my nascent research practices, I came to feel this intellectual prejudice was ignorant and oppressive. I would later read that Marx stated more than a century ago that intellectual pursuits are themselves, ironically, practices, albeit with different goals from the practices I was involved in as a clinician and educator (Andrew 1975).

Before going further, I think it would be helpful to offer some thoughts about the word 'practice' and how I will use it in this chapter. This is a definition of the noun form of practice from the *Oxford Dictionary*:

> The actual application or use of an idea, belief, or method, as opposed to theories relating to it.

Definitions of practice, such as this, describe activity. Although being a noun the word suggests practice is a "thing", practices are anything but.

This definition separates the intellectual (theories) from the activity (application). It is Cartesian in nature. That is, it splits mind from body, thinking from matter. As I would discover as I read more widely, there were philosophers in the 20th century such as Martin Heidegger and John Dewey who, in contrast, saw theory – the thinking bit – as a continuation of practice (Dreyfus 1991). Dewey called cognition (thinking) a part of our "practical machinery" just like our legs, hands, or mouths. We go on with what we are doing until there is a need to solve a problem. Then we engage the conscious thinking bit to help. We couldn't go on being in this world if we constantly and only engaged the conscious thinking part of our bodies (Blattner 2000). Karl Polanyi stated, "[W]e know more than we can tell" because of our tacit knowledge. Indeed, he argued, we only become aware of the conscious because something tacit precipitates it. As far back as the late 19th to mid-20th century, then, philosophers proposed that ideas come through social interactions in a back-and-forward unfolding of practice. Ideas and action are in a constant dance with each other.

The definition of practice provided earlier, though, was probably how I would have conceived of practice as I engaged with the research norms of the field I found myself in at the start of my doctoral studies.

As time went on, the following definition came to feel more appropriate and is more like the way I defined practice part way through my doctoral studies.

> The customary, habitual, or expected procedure or way of doing something.

This doesn't make ideas or thoughts a necessary precursor to practice. Ideas are not separated from practice. However, as I hope will become clearer later, to me, it suggests procedures or ways of doing things that are predictable, the same, or repetitive. It is more akin to what I will later describe as an 'ostensive' practice – a representation of practice we imagine but not what is performed as people and things interact.

By the end of my studies, I had come to view the unfolding of the interactions between people and things as always new, conditional on the time, place, and human and material actors with which it unfolded. Performed practices are always provisional, ephemeral, and never the same. The practices may seem *familiar* because some of the interactions look like others we have experienced in the past, but we cannot *fully recognise* a given practice because we will never experience the same practice again. (Although there may of course be much in common, each unfolding of practice is unique.) I am not going to posit a different definition of practice here but hope that by the end of the chapter, I will have shown how we might conceive of practices as familiar, though transient and ephemeral, activities. People, guided moment-by-moment by their respective mindlines, interact with each other and with things, all the time generating new knowing that in turn become embodied within their respective mindlines (Lave and Wenger 1991; Schatzki 1997; Gabbay & le May 2011; Hui, Schatzki and Shove 2016).

When I started, the practice I thought we were trying to improve in the field was something more concrete than this, more easily identifiable as a 'thing' to change. Perhaps what I had in mind was something closer to a protocol – an abstract rendition, presented as text and graphics, of the steps a healthcare worker (the patient being passive in this) takes. Practice, from this perspective, *is* some*thing*. It is a product of the work of, directly and indirectly, possibly hundreds of people. We can see or listen to a protocol. Do A, then do B, then C and, if D, then do F, but if E, do G. It is what we call 'ordered'. It could be complicated, involving lots of steps and branches, but would still be linear, controlled, predictable.

There was, though, a bit more than a protocol in my imagination. I could visualise myself doing the steps with the bits and bobs dentists use to do stuff. I might have an image of a generic 'patient', or of a tooth, or of a clinical setting, but they would have been blurred images, lacking any definition. I might have had a bodily sense of the experience of a familiar practice done previously, of some of the difficulties I had faced and might anticipate. I would now call it an ostensive practice – a representation of practice that I consciously and tacitly embody.

Neither proxy nor ostensive practices, though, are the *performed* practices we engage in anew every time we undertake familiar activities, guided by our mindlines, with people and things. There was a difference between what the original mindlines ethnographers observed when general practitioners were interacting with patients and with each other and what they heard when they interviewed participants about what they do. I would describe the former as observing 'performed practices', whereas in the latter they were, in my terms, listening to the participants' description of their 'ostensive practices'. The two are not the same, and this is something I will reflect on in the context of clinical education later in the chapter.

I hadn't developed these nuanced understandings of practice as I started my doctoral research, though. To me, there seemed like a lot to do to fill or bridge the know-do gaps. Knowledge was still the stuff research produced. Practitioners were not following guidance. Lots of barriers were identified to explain why there was a disjunct between the theory of how clinicians should practise and what they practised. There were a lot of theories or frameworks floating around that suggested how practitioners' behaviour could be changed. What evidence there was suggested there was little change even when these theories were used to design interventions.

I struggled with a lot of the theory and became very frustrated at my lack of ability to make sense of it. I have always been someone who needs to know how things are applied to be able to understand them (or at least, think I do), and I found it very difficult to see how I would apply these theories in designing research to improve practice.

I started to lose hope. Given that so many interventions seemed not to lead to discernible changes in the outcomes measured, what hope was there that I would do any better? If there was little chance of success in changing practice, was there any point in starting?

I struggled to reconcile the practices I experienced as a clinician and the linearity of the models of change I read about. Perhaps because of this, I became more sensitive to alternative paradigms of practice. I started to engage more with a different group of theorists and researchers, whose field I was more disposed to, who challenged the privileged position of Plato's *episteme* – intellectual knowledge – over practical and performative knowing, *techne*.

Philosophers such as Aristotle, Marx, Wittgenstein, Heidegger, Dewey, and Bourdieu questioned which sorts of evidence matter and which are needed to practise. More recent authors in the healthcare literature didn't (as I don't) contest the need for research evidence in good practice but, rather, the singular view that this was *all* the evidence that was needed. They showed how healthcare workers generated their own evidence from the social world in which they worked, from their senses (touch, sight, sound, smell), from trial and error as they cared for patients, from shared stories of care and problems solved. The evidence they encountered was much broader than that in research or its products, like guidelines. The knowing that healthcare workers embodied and therefore were able to, in some way, share with others, was a constant to-and-fro, of integrating the practical, social, material, ethical, and moral in the moment-to-moment caring for patients (Carper 1978; Billett 2001; Eisner 1985; Rycroft-Malone, Seers, Titchen et al. 2004; Loftus 2015).

I was intrigued by Anne-Marie Mol's *The Body Multiple* (2002), which described atherosclerosis not as a single disease but multiple diseases depending on who is experiencing it. The patient, medic, surgeon, and pathologist all experience the disease in different ways. The practices that unfold in relation to atherosclerosis are different for each person involved. Why wouldn't all practices be such? The practices unfolding in clinical care are experienced, conceived of, responded to, learned from, made sense of, from each person's (and, I would come to think, thing's) perspective.

How, I wondered, could we ever know if practice conceived of in these ways was evidence-based? Whose practice? Whose evidence?

This field of theory and research had different rules for engaging with the concept of practice from the one I had started in. These rules allowed for practice to be problematised, made more difficult to grasp, to hold onto. As I interpreted it, the norms of this field were to engage with rather than blind-side the disquieting idea that much about the knowing in practices cannot be made explicit, made intellectual and amenable to control of some kind.

It was during this time that I happened across a tweet referencing Gabbay and le May's recently published book. I won't gush too much here for fear of embarrassing them both, but reading *Practice-Based Evidence for Healthcare: Clinical Mindlines* was for me, emotional, liberating, and motivating. It helped me to realise why I was frustrated in not being able to go on with my research using the norms of the field I was in. The concept of mindlines articulated for me, as I know it has for many others, a closer fitting model to my conceptions of how I interacted with clinical practice than any of those assumed in the theories of change I had been trying to make sense of. Gabbay and le May's description of how they thought practice-based evidence informed clinician mindlines legitimised the thoughts and feelings I had had that practice wasn't as simple as some were making out. Mindlines allowed for the full complexity of my practice experience as a clinician and a way into researching that complexity. I could, for the first time in my doctoral journey, imagine how my research might go on.

I stopped thinking about how to change practice because, I realised, I didn't understand what the practice was that I would be trying to change. Indeed, I stopped thinking there is even a thing called practice out there to be discovered and improved, but phenomena created through social (human) and material (things) interaction that we barely had any understanding of. I decided to explore practices that occurred in the dental setting and to theorise how these evolved and how they influenced those involved. Inevitably, given the interaction of mindlines with practice, I would also explore mindlines. Towards the end of Gabbay and le May's book, they describe in largely theoretical terms, the phenomenon of 'co-constructing clinical reality'. This would be like observing and exploring that process in real time.

Through diaries, interviews, and video observation of clinical practices, I explored how dentists, patients, and dental nurses interacted and how their mindlines developed through the moment-by-moment development of unfolding practices. In one study, I asked dentists to record, over a week, the occasions they encountered some information or experienced something confirmatory or new. I asked them to classify the experience according to six domains: What knowledge was shared during the encounter? How was the knowledge encountered? What was the mode of exchange? From whom did the knowledge originate? How many participants were there? Where did the encounter take place? Within a couple of weeks, I interviewed the dentists and used the diary entries as seeds for unstructured interviews. In these, I would simply ask dentists to tell the story around the encounter they recorded. I allowed them to tell this uninterrupted. If there was a pause, then I probed for more reflection or to clarify descriptions. The aim was to explore the meaning that dentists made of their experiences during the encounters and how these experiences influenced what they now knew about how to practise and also how they actually practised – in other words their mindlines and how they interacted with patients.

Each dentist encountered the world from a local, situated perspective. Like Gabbay and le May's observations of medical practices, the dentists' mindlines developed through experiences of interacting with their patients, staff, colleagues, systems, and material things. Their mindlines included perspectives of time in their setting, the properties and potential use of the tools and materials available to them, and the spaces within which they worked and lived.

In describing their ostensive practices, dentists considered each patient as a case that was, consciously or subconsciously, compared against a personal understanding of similar cases. Cases seemed to be an important structuring component within dentists' mindlines. Their case base, we might call it, was built up not merely from their own experience of similar cases but also from the narratives (stories) of cases shared by other dentists, what is sometimes called vicarious experience.

The dentists generally spoke to, texted, or messaged colleagues, either face-to-face or virtually, when they faced a problem about what to do with an individual patient. The dentists sought collective problem-solving about what to do about this patient, now, given these circumstances, rather than seek some form of codified knowledge, for example, a guideline.

Cases were multifaceted, contextualised, and developed around problems. In other words, in their narrative of a case, the dentists might refer to different facets such as the system within which the case presented, personal characteristics of the patient, ethical issues, their emotional responses, the perspectives of colleagues consulted about the case, alternative solutions considered, outcomes of decisions made, and clinical techniques used.

The dentists could sometimes recognise the learning (i.e., the development of their mindlines) in the experiences they shared. But more than this, the way they described their interactions with patients, dental nurses, sales representatives, and the many things in their practices, new learning arose that the dentists seemed unaware of. Development of mindlines was mostly unplanned and, often, occurred by chance. Dentists would be unaware of when, how, or what they would learn from an experience yet to occur.

As I was designing and analysing my next study, I became aware from my reading of other concepts of knowing. In opposition to knowledge being possessed in the bodies of individuals, these other perspectives saw knowing as arising in performance, in the interactions between people and things. Dentists, patients, nurses, and the material objects in the room, would create a performance together, each guided by their respective mindlines (humans) and material properties with potential to be used in some way (things) (Ingold 1996; Cook and Brown 1999; Orlikowski 2002; Feldman 2007; Harris 2007; Marchand 2008; Marchand 2010; Gabbay & le May 2011).

This study suggested how dentists' mindlines might develop based on their accounts of their experiences, their descriptions of *ostensive* practices. To explore how mindlines and *performed* practices interact, I needed to observe practices unfolding rather than rely on the dentists' renditions of them. I placed video cameras in the corner of dental surgeries, left the room, and recorded whatever happened from before a patient arrived to after they left. The videos lasted anything from 15 minutes to an hour, and the camera was placed to maximise the people and things captured. A typical view is shown in Figure 4.1.

With so much visual and acoustic data, I had to develop new methods to find a way that worked for me to analyse all the interactions going on. I initially transposed text alongside stills of the video. Each still captured the moment a physical interaction changed, for example, a dentist or patient turning, the dental chair starting to move. The speech was verbatim, but I also described the actions I saw and my initial interpretations of the actions and interactions. As such, rather than a traditional transcript, what I created was a graphical, interpretive narrative (Figure 4.2).

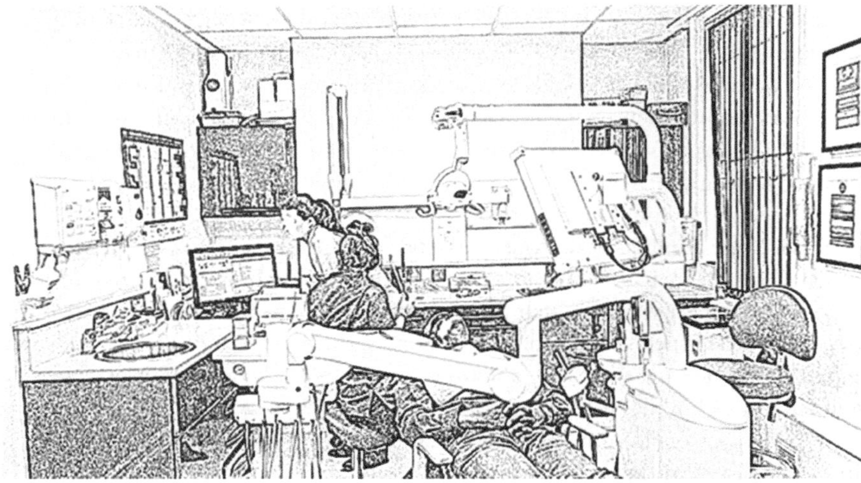

FIGURE 4.1 A typical still from the video of dental surgery (captured as a software-generated line drawing).

This was very important to me as the practice was as much about the bodily doing and the interaction with things as it was about what actors said. The location of a computer, for example, could influence the interactions between patients, dental nurses, and dentists. By making the interaction between the dental equipment, dentist, nurse, and patient amenable to analysis, I could see each actor anticipating the actions of the others.

However, even with the graphic alongside the narrative, this was not a representation of the practices that I felt I needed in order to really appreciate the unfolding practice. I needed to introduce time into the analysis in some way. I needed a format that was somewhere between the mass of data unfolding in a video played at normal speed and the selective data presented in images and text. The latter lacked the time element of practice. The former had too much going on to be able to make sense of it.

One of my first attempts to represent the dynamism and interaction between people and things is shown in Figure 4.3. The concept of knowing in practice as being short-lived is represented by the 'smoke' in which the actions of each person or thing interact and create new actions. The actions and reactions are represented by the arrows. I called each coming together of people and things a conjunction – an episode of unfolding practice that was analytically separable, though in reality not. For example, in the following conjunction, a patient has complained of pain in their gums, and the dentist is beginning to explore this. There would have been other activities in the appointment that were not concerned with the gum pain, which would be outwith this conjunction.

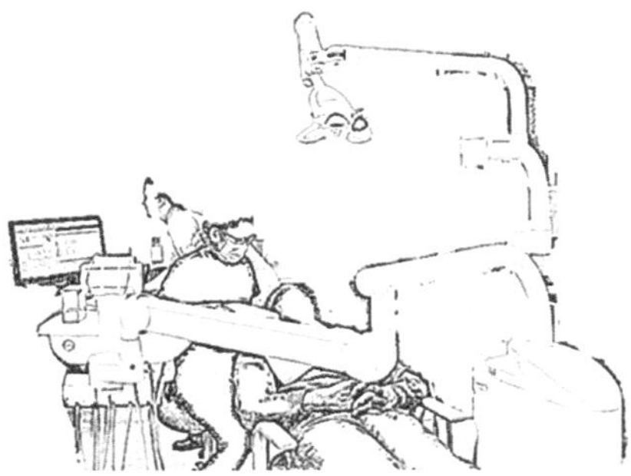 00.05.22	"OK. Brilliant," says the dentist. "Will you just pop your chin up for me?" and reaches up for the dental light, which she swings round and down closer to the patient. The nurse has moved to the computer. The patient lifts his whole head up off the headrest. The dentist notices and says, "ooh no. Head back". The patients says, "sorry" and drops his head back to the headrest. The dentist drops the headrest back a bit as he does. He lifts his head again and the dentist says, "pop your head back." He says, "sorry" as he puts his head back down on the headrest. The dentist says, "pop your chin up" and the patient lifts his chin. "That's it," she says, adjusting the position of the light again and then gently touching the patient's neck behind his chin. "That's perfect." The nurse had turned her head to face the dentist and patient but now leans towards the computer and takes the mouse in her right hand. The dentist passes her right hand under the sensor on the light, which now switches on.
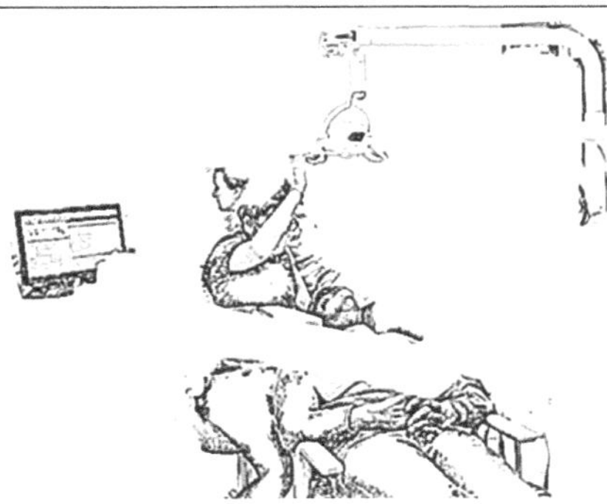 00.05.37	She adjusts the light so that the light falls onto the patient's unopen mouth. "As usual" she says, "I'm going to start by feeling underneath your chin. I'll explain everything at the end. Is that alright?" The patient mutters agreement and the dentist beg ins to palpate under his chin. The nurse is looking intently at the computer screen. The dentist says to the nurse, "extra-oral fine," but the nurse doesn't seem to respond by clicking anything on the computer. The dentist says to the patient after placing her fingers beside his TMJ, "open". The patient opens his mouth. "Close" she says and he does. "Open," she says and he does, as she turns her head toward the bracket table.

FIGURE 4.2 Text graphic analysis.

I would have liked to use a never-ending video of 'smoke' overlaid with the textual and graphical representations of what was going on, but this was beyond my technical skills.

Instead, using video-editing software, I made words spoken and actions observed appear on a screen for the duration they occurred in the videos. The words were in speech bubbles and the actions in pointy circles. As the video played, the speech bubbles and pointy circles would appear and disappear (Figure 4.4).

The phenomena we experience, and which are open to analysis, are actions, including speech. We never know what guides these actions. In qualitative

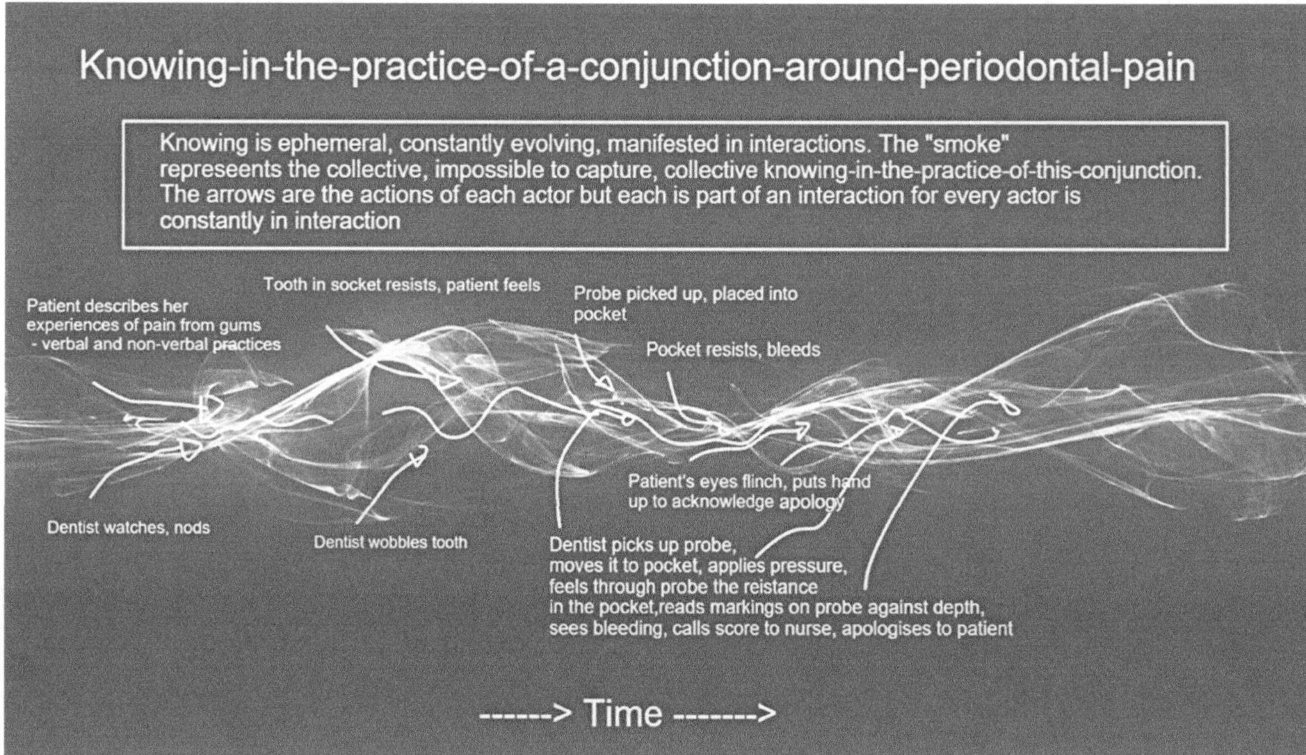

FIGURE 4.3 An early attempt to represent the dynamism and interaction between people and things.

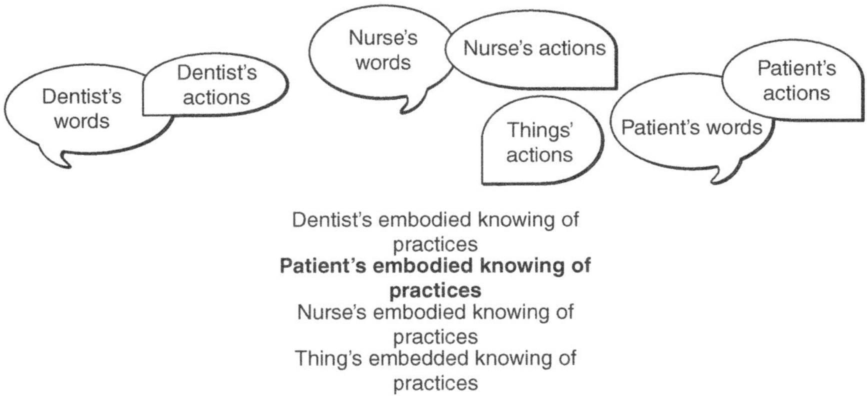

FIGURE 4.4 Representing a conjunction as speech and actions.

research, we infer or interpret what the actors' words and actions might convey. In this study, I wanted to interpret what was being translated into the interaction with others. My understanding of knowing and practice at this time was (and remains) that the knowing we embed in our mindlines is derived from uncountable experiences of historical practices, both professional and not. Reading guidelines and textbooks is practice. Discussing with patients or colleagues is practice. Telling and listening to stories is practice. Enacting clinical techniques is practice. Navigating patient records is practice. Sitting in a dental chair and opening our mouths as a patient (yes, dentists can be patients too!) is practice. All involve us interacting with people and things that, over time, become more or less familiar. Each time we experience the practices, we make sense of them in some way and come to embody a largely tacit understanding of the experience. For me, the experience of historical practices is how we acquire the personal, practice-based evidence that, Gabbay and le May suggested, develops our mindlines.

In the video representations I created, I inferred the historical practices, embedded in mindlines and now guiding the moment-by-moment actions of the people and things in the unfolding practices. The following is a series of stills taken from one of my videos. I included the time in seconds at the bottom to demonstrate the brevity with which actions appeared. The sequence includes everything that was said and done over 19 seconds. At the time of writing, a four-minute section of the original of the video is available to watch online here: https://youtu.be/33zRuOpUJes. (See also some stills from the video in Figure 4.5.)

This method of analysis allowed me to see how unique each unfolding practice was. The actions of each person and thing were contingent on the actions of the other people and things. There was nothing predictable or linear about how the practices unfolded. I could imagine any number of alternative responses to all the

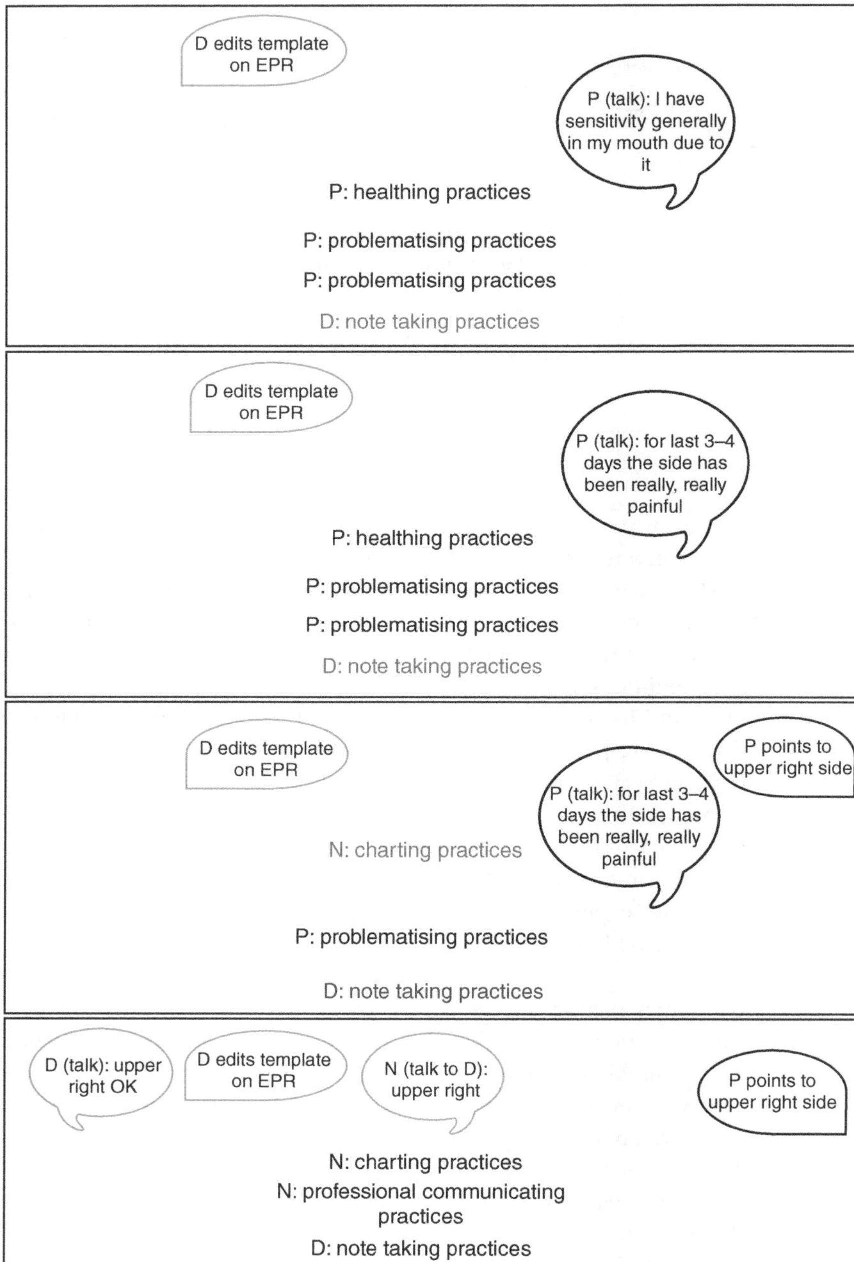

FIGURES 4.5 Speech and actions from the encounter.

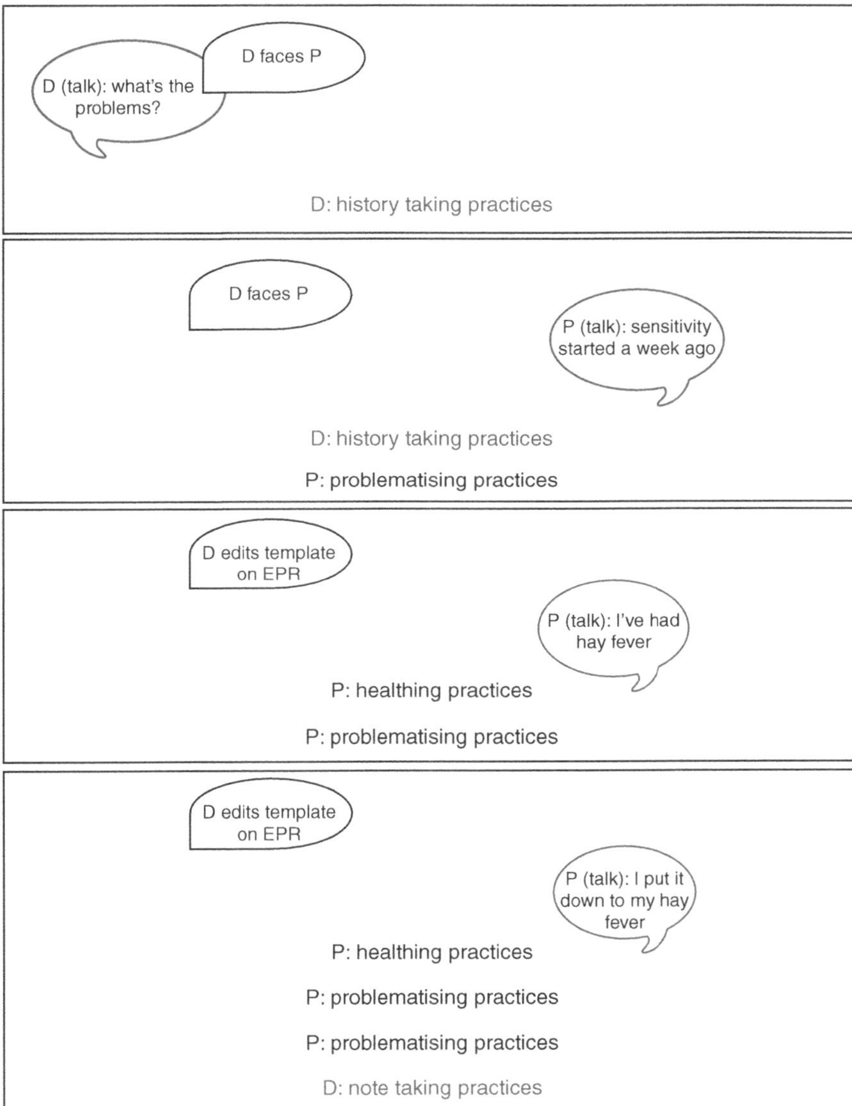

FIGURE 4.5 (Continued)

actions. The dentists, nurses, and patients anticipated the actions of others, but they could not predict them. Indeed, the actions only seemed to occur because the actors anticipated how they thought others would respond, a key element of the mindlines they had formed through personal or vicarious experiences of historical practices. (see Gabbay & le May 2011 p. 168)

In these encounters, relationships between people and things were established as temporary phenomena through discussion and through prodding and probing, reading, writing, seeing, and hearing. That is, as one actor said or did something, the other observed, listened, or felt and, in due course, acted or spoke themselves. This might involve listening to a question and responding, or a patient seeing an instrument orientating towards their mouth and opening it.

In one video, a dentist picked up a dental mirror and probe to check gum health. The dental nurse moved to the computer and readied herself to record the results without the dentist saying anything. The dentist then slid their chair and positioned themselves behind the supine patient's head. The dentist raised the probe and dental mirror over the patient's face, and the patient opened their mouth with no verbal prompting. The dentist, nurse, and patient all appeared to be anticipating the other's – and the things' (computer, probe, chairs) – actions and reactions.

This is not to say that all the reactions were correctly anticipated. In another interaction, a dentist had asked a patient to lift their chin and the patient lifted his whole head forward, tilting his chin into his chest, the opposite of what the dentist had anticipated. Nonetheless, the dentist had anticipated an action; the patient had acted and, in turn, anticipated a reaction from the dentist.

The anticipation of others' actions suggested to me that the actors had embodied understandings of how people and things had reacted in their experience of historical practices. That is, they expected that something would happen, if they did something, because they had an embodied knowing of historical practices maybe with familiar interactions to this one but, also, unfamiliar ones. The anticipation of actions is a way in which each actor's mindlines could translate into the action of the here-and-now practice.

In such hands-on practices as occur in the dental setting, mindlines necessarily incorporate motoric representations that guide what the dentists, nurses, and patients do as part of the unfolding practice. That is, all the actors arrive with and develop representations of the motion in their respective ostensive practice. This preparedness to act bodily beyond the organs of speech, allows people to imagine solutions as they anticipate how the other people and things will respond when they interact physically with them, for example, to manipulate dental equipment and computers, palpate parts of a patient's mouth, orientate the head, apply force.

Practices are suffused with power or influence as the different actors attempt to translate their respective knowing of the unfolding situation into the ongoing practice. Power, or lack of it, enables or constrains the ability of different actors to translate their mindlines into the practice. This is partly why ostensive practices are so different from those that are performed, why practices are complex rather than linear.

Influence is in the direct actions and reactions between one person and another, but is also mediated through things. Power was mediated, for example, through the payment system on the computer or through regulations and good practice and professional standards embedded in the templates the dentists used on the electronic patient record. Power was mediated through the allotted time available for appointments determined, perhaps, by a practice manager or owner. There was frequently a tussle with the remote forces as dentists, patients, and nurses sought to bypass the rules, pay lip service to them, or grudgingly accept them.

Practices unfold through the adaptive translation of mindlines from the different people and things they interacted with. People and things did what they could, given the interactions between them, and generated actions (for example, creating a problem, creating a solution) for the practice to go on, to end, and for these actors to disperse. Like the bricoleur who, with their limited skill set and tools, solves problems as best they can, together people and things generated and solved problems in a *collective* bricolage. Patients used the words they knew from non-dental experiences, for example, to describe their dental experiences (see the stills of the video in Figure 4.5). They offered focused reflections on experiences they had, such as taking medication when they should not because of a medical diagnosis. They offered up proposals of what could be wrong, of what prior treatment they had received that might be relevant, of their habits and their symptoms. Dentists watched and listened, made suggestions of diagnoses and treatment approaches, used the instruments and materials at hand in different ways. All of them, working together, guided by their respective mindlines, created the practice in that moment.

In the image in Figure 4.6, taken from one of the videos, is a moment in the practice achieved with barely a word spoken. The dentist, patient, nurse, camera, and computer are all poised to capture an image of a broken tooth. This is an example of a moment in which each person and thing, translating their respective mindlines into practice, create the collaborative knowing of practice.

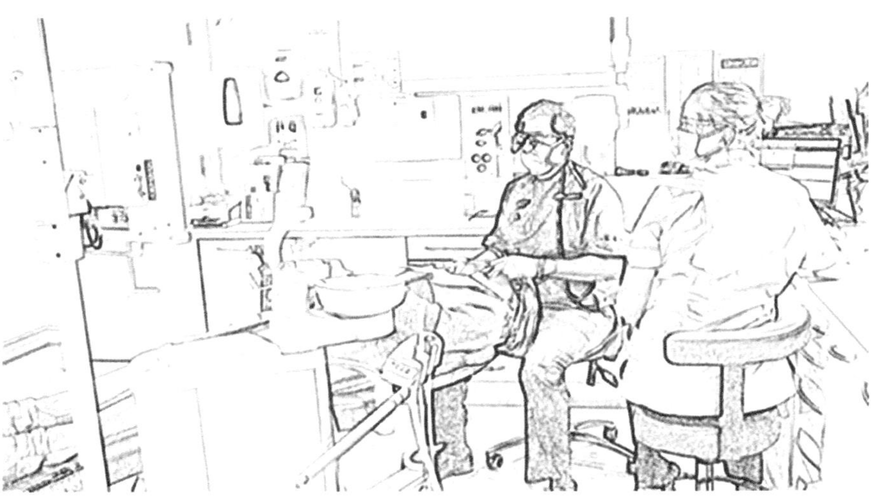

FIGURE 4.6 A quiet moment before taking the image of the broken tooth.

Implications for clinical educational practices

Theorising about practices and how mindlines interact with actions is all well and good for a doctoral thesis. But what does it matter in the "real world" of clinical and educational practices that I am engaged in? Here are a few considerations.

We need to be clear that practices and the actions clinicians and student-clinicians enact within them are not ordered, not linear, and not predictable. Thinking about practices as proxy, ostensive and performative, whilst conceptual rather than real, can help us to help ourselves and our students or, as I sometimes think of them, apprentice clinicians, to develop mindlines that might guide more useful, effective, and ethical practices.

As educators of apprentice clinicians, when we describe protocols or instructions in verbal or written forms, we are describing generalised, ostensive, proxy practices. Whilst important and necessary (like research evidence in guidelines), we must appreciate that these proxy practices are just one source of evidence that will be made sense of and incorporated in some way into apprentice clinicians' respective mindlines.

Videos and demonstrations of how experienced clinicians act, whether at the technical level of manipulating a dental drill when cutting a plastic tooth or the social level of exploring a problem with a patient in a clinic, enable apprentice clinicians to form motoric, social, ethical, and moral representations of the practice too. These are their nascent ostensive practices – their representations of what they might do in a situation like this. However articulate we think our verbal and written instructions, and our demonstrations and videos are, the ostensive practice an apprentice clinician is developing is also being influenced by the many other experiences they have with peers, with other educators in and outside our institutions, with patients, and with things. As the apprentice clinicians perform practices, they do so with patients and their families, with dental nurses, with clinical tutors of some kind and with material things such as the instruments, charts, software that they have to learn to use. Each of the human actors translates their mindlines into the practice and the material things have a readiness (or not, sometimes) to be used in some way.

As with any clinical practices, the outcomes of the collective bricolage we are all engaged in as we supervise students in their practices are problematic to define, *let alone* the actions that allowed them to occur. Because they are available to us to hear, see, and feel, I think we tend to focus on the explicit verbal or textual and technical accomplishments of students, for example, a verbal presentation of a patient's complaint, a completed medical history form, a well-prepared dental cavity. However, there are always multiple, sometimes contradictory, outcomes. Most of them are not immediately available to us for evaluation, given the largely tacit development of mindlines. What was the emotional outcome for the patient and for the student, for example, and how did that influence how each acted? How did unfolding of the practice correlate with how the student imagined the practice would unfold? What bodily, ethical, or moral learning occurred? How do we all feel about the guidance to do this practice now that we have had a go?

As educators, if we feedback on socio-material practices, we need to help students develop an awareness of their actions within it, and those of the other people and things who take part. What is the context in terms of time and space, and what is going on emotionally and imaginarily as well as conceptually and practically as they perform in this context? Most of this we cannot articulate. Thus, we must recognise that we, as educators, need to find ways to help students relive their bodily experiences as they acted and reacted, and to help them develop their own embodied sense of what is more likely to result in a recognisable set of actions we call competent. Maybe the aforementioned techniques that I developed could help us to do that.

Important in the development of mindlines, as reported in this chapter, is vicarious experience shared in narratives and case-based discussions. To perform practices – with all the complexity inherent within them – in a more competent manner, apprentice clinicians need to develop nuanced representations of practice in their mindlines. We cannot, as educators, determine those representations of practice directly. They will develop as the apprentice experiences practices themselves in unknowable ways. To maximise the opportunity to develop the nuanced understandings, though, they need to have the opportunity to develop them through shared experiences of others' performed practices too. We need to be encouraging activities that enable experts and apprentices alike to share their experiences of practices, not as a sanitised, procedural rendition of ostensive practice but as complex narratives of performed practice, replete with the moral and ethical; tips and tricks; physical demonstrations, as well as verbal descriptions; and tacit knowing expressed in metaphors. Helping students to develop their clinical mindlines is as much about how we act as what we say and that this goes beyond the technical. As clinical educators, we need to develop a mindful awareness of the clinical educational practices we are engaged with. We need to be aware of what is unfolding and find ways to explore how what we do and say influences how students develop mindlines.

It may be that educators could use methods such as those described here to uncover the way the many strands that go on in any given encounter unfold; they could then work with students – and with each other – to analyse short passages of activity to uncover how their performed practice evolves, how it differs from their ostensive practice and why. Doing so would also help educators to recognise how their students – and, using this as a reflective tool, they themselves – are learning and how to learn better in future.

Summary

- I have explored concepts of practice and suggested that performed practices are those, guided by our mindlines, in which we interact with people and things, moment to moment.
- They unfold in unpredictable, un-replicable ways that somehow need to be generalised and packaged if they are to be represented to others.

- In contrast, *ostensive* practices are the representations we have of these complex practices, bound up in our mindlines.
- Ostensive practices are derived through our personal and vicarious experiences of historical practices – not only our own clinical practice, but listening to the experiences of others, reading guidelines, following protocols, teaching, perusing journals, and so on.
- Ostensive practices, which are the ones we teach, are how we imagine practices might unfold. They help us anticipate others' actions and, in this way, guide our performed practices moment-by-moment.
- I have suggested that complex practices are intimately bound up with the influence and development of mindlines that go beyond ostensive practices.
- This opens up the possibility of finding ways to explore other, less immediately accessible, ways to develop mindlines and learn practice as it is actually performed, rather than relying on the ordered, linear models of ostensive practice.
- I have proposed a method by which we could explore actual performed practice, which might enable us to find new ways to help learn how to practise.

Acknowledgements

I would like to acknowledge my primary supervisor, Trisha Greenhalgh; secondary supervisors, Sharon Mickan and Derek Richards; and the dentists, nurses, and patients who participated in my research.

Bibliography

Andrew E. 1975. 'A note on the unity of theory and practice in Marx and Nietzsche'. *Political Theory*, 3(3):305–316.

Billett S. 2001. 'Knowing in practice: re-conceptualising vocational expertise'. *Learning and Instruction*, 11(6):431–452.

Blattner WD. 2000. 'The primacy of practice and assertoric truth: Dewey and Heidegger', in JE Malpas, MA Wrathall, HL Dreyfus (Eds.) *Heidegger, authenticity, and modernity: Essays in honor of Hubert L Dreyfus*. Cambridge, MA: MIT Press, pp. 231–249.

Bourdieu P. 1990. *The logic of practice*. Cambridge, UK: Polity.

Callinicos A. 1985. 'Anthony Giddens: a contemporary critique'. *Theory and Society*, 14(2):133–166.

Carper B. 1978. 'Fundamental patterns of knowing in nursing'. *Advances in Nursing Science*, 1(1):13–23.

Cook SD, Brown JS. 1999. 'Bridging epistemologies: the generative dance between organizational knowledge and organizational knowing'. *Organization Science*, 10(4):381–400.

Costall A, Leudar I. 1996. 'Situating action I: truth in the situation'. *Ecological Psychology*, 8(2):101–110.

Dreyfus HL. 1991. *Being-in-the-world: a commentary on Heidegger's being and time, division I*. Cambridge, MA: MIT Press.

Dreyfus HL, Wrathall MA, Malpas JE. 2000. *Heidegger, authenticity, and modernity: essays in honor of Hubert. DreyfusL*. Cambridge, MA; London: MIT Press.

Eisner E. 1985. 'Aesthetic modes of knowing', in E Eisner (Ed.) *Learning and teaching the ways of knowing*. Chicago: University of Chicago Press.
Eraut M. 2000. 'Non-formal learning and tacit knowledge in professional work', *British Journal of Educational Psychology*, 70:113–136.
Estabrooks CA, Rutakumwa W, O'Leary KA, Profetto-McGrath J, Milner M, Levers MJ, Scott-Findlay S. 2005. 'Sources of practice knowledge among nurses'. *Qualitative Health Research*, 15(4):460–476.
Feldman MS, Orlikowski WJ. 2011. 'Theorizing practice and practicing theory'. *Organization Science*, 22(5):1240–1253.
Gabbay J, le May A. 2004. 'Evidence based guidelines or collectively constructed "mindlines?" Ethnographic study of knowledge management in primary care'. *British Medical Journal*, 329:1013–1016.
Gabbay J, le May A. 2011. *Practice-based evidence for healthcare: clinical mindlines*. London; New York: Routledge.
Giddens A. 1984. *Elements of the theory of structuration. The constitution of society: outline of the theory of structuration*. Cambridge, UK: Polity, pp. 1–40.
Graham ID, Logan J, Harrison MB, Straus SE, Tetroe J, Caswell W, Robinson N. 2006. 'Lost in knowledge translation: time for a map?' *Journal of Continuing Education in the Health Professions*, 26(1):13–24.
Grenfell M. 2014. *Pierre Bourdieu: key concepts*. Abingdon, UK: Routledge, pp. 48–64.
Harris M. 2007. *Ways of knowing: anthropological approaches to crafting experience and knowledge*. Oxford, UK: Berghahn Books, pp. 1–24.
Heidegger M. 1962. *Being and time*. Translated by J Macquarrie & E Robinson. Oxford, UK: Blackwell. Reprinted 2001.
Higgs J, Jones MA. 1995. *Clinical reasoning in the health professions*. Oxford: Butterworth-Heinermann.
Hui A, Schatzki T, Shove E. 2016. *The nexus of practices: connections, constellations, practitioners*. London, UK: Routledge.
Hunter K. 1996. 'Don't think zebras': uncertainty, interpretation, and the place of paradox in clinical education'. *Theoretical Medicine*, 17(3):225–241.
Hurst D. 2019. General dental practitioners' knowledge encounters: how do dentists build their knowledge in practice? Doctoral thesis, University of Oxford.
Ingold T. 1996. 'Situating action VI: a comment on the distinction between the material and the social'. *Ecological Psychology*, 8(2):183–187.
Johannessen KS. 1988. 'The concept of practice in Wittgenstein's later philosophy'. *Inquiry*, 31(3):357–369.
Kemmis S. 2005. 'Knowing practice: searching for saliences'. *Pedagogy, Culture and Society*, 13(3):391–426.
Lave J, Wenger E. 1991. *Situated learning: legitimate peripheral participation*. London and NY: Cambridge University Press.
Loftus S. 2015. 'Embodiment in the practice and education of health professionals', in B Green, N Hopwood (Eds.), *The body in professional practice, learning and education: body/practice*. Cham, Switzerland: Springer International Publishing pp. 139–156.
Marchand THJ. 2008. Muscles, morals and mind: craft apprenticeship and the formation of person. *British Journal of Educational Studies*, 56(3):245–271.
Marchand THJ. 2010. *Making knowledge: explorations of the indissoluble relation between mind, body and environment*. Oxford, UK: Wiley-Blackwell.
Marx K, Engels F. 1978. *The Marx-Engels reader*. Edited by RC Tucker. New York, NY: W.W. Norton.
Mol A. 2002. *The body multiple: ontology in medical practice*. Durham, NC: Duke University Press.

Montgomery K. 2006. *How doctors think: clinical judgment and the practice of medicine*. Oxford, UK: Oxford University Press.

Montgomery-Hunter K. 1989. 'A science of individuals: medicine and casuistry'. *Journal of Medicine and Philosophy*, 14(2):193–212.

Nicolini D. 2013. *Practice theory, work, and organization: an introduction*. Oxford, UK: Oxford University Press.

Nicolini D, Gherardi S, Yanow D. 2015. *Knowing in organizations: a practice-based approach*. Abingdon, UK: Routledge.

Orlikowski WJ. 2002. 'Knowing in practice: enacting a collective capability in distributed organizing'. *Organization Science*, 13(3):249–273.

Polanyi M. 1958. *Personal knowledge. Towards a post-critical philosophy*. London, UK: Routledge & Kegan Paul.

Polanyi M. 2009. *The tacit dimension*. London, UK: University of Chicago Press.

Schatzki TR, Knorr-Cetina KD, von Savigny E. 2001. *The practice turn in contemporary theory*. London: Routledge.

Rycroft-Malone J, Seers K, Titchen A, Harvey G, Kitson A, McCormack B. 2004. What counts as evidence in evidence-based practice? *Journal of Advanced Nursing*, 47(1):81–90.

Schatzki TR. 1997. 'Practices and actions: a Wittgensteinian critique of Bourdieu and Giddens'. *Philosophy of the Social Sciences*, 27(3):283–308.

Todres L. 2008. 'Being with that: the relevance of embodied understanding for practice'. *Qualitative Health Research*, 18(11):1566–1573.

5

USING CO-CREATION TO MODIFY MINDLINES AND IMPROVE CHILDHOOD ECZEMA CARE

Fiona Cowdell

Introduction

> *I'm red. I spread hate.*
> *What's my name? It's eczema.*
> *I am powerful.*

Childhood atopic eczema impacts well-being and has a high self or parent-management demand requiring regular and consistent application of topical medication. National evidence-based guidance for childhood eczema exists. However, in common with much research-based evidence, application of this guidance is limited. We know that disseminating information and/or telling people what to do does not change practice.

Knowledge mobilisation (KM) seeks to get evidence into everyday practice, in essence, KM is about sharing *knowledge* between different *communities* to catalyse *change* (Wye, Cramer, Beckett et al. 2020). In an extensive search of KM techniques, I discovered mindlines, a concept that intuitively made sense to me as a nurse and fitted with my real-world experiences. In this chapter, I recount how I used traditional and creative approaches to investigate lay and practitioner eczema mindlines and to co-create and implement strategies to alter and enhance these mindlines across lay-practitioner-wider-society boundaries. My aims were to, (i) use diverse and creative means to bring this evidence alive; (ii) share simple, consistent, evidence-based messages, to instil shared language and understanding; (iii) integrate reliable and useful knowledge and erase outdated or inaccurate information; and (iv) ultimately, improve self-management practices and consultation experiences (see, for example, the "Dragon" animation https://www.bcu.ac.uk/health-sciences/research/centre-for-social-care-health-and-related-research/research-projects/

DOI: 10.4324/9781003158721-5

BOX 5.1 KEY CHALLENGES OF CHILDHOOD ECZEMA

- Mainly treated by non-specialists in primary care
- Consultations often unsatisfactory for both parties
- High self/parent-management demand
- Treatment failure is common
- Concern about topical steroid use is widespread
- Information quality is variable and overload commonplace

eczema-mindlines/the-dragon-in-my-skin). This chapter illustrates how mindlines principles can inform effective KM strategies with wider application for other long-term conditions.

The challenge of childhood eczema

Atopic eczema affects around 20% of young children; it is a long-term relapsing condition which affects well-being and quality of life for children and their families. Key challenges are summarised in Box 5.1.The fundamentals of caring for childhood eczema are straightforward but often, for a whole raft of reasons, not enacted as effectively as possible by healthcare practitioners (HCPs) or parents and children. Although high-quality evidence exists (https://www.nice.org.uk/guidance/cg57), this does not take into account the complexity and constraints of everyday practice and self-care which are at the core of mindlines theory. Pragmatic guidance on eczema management is provided by clinical experts who speak of "two things done well[1]", referring to regular and consistent application of emollients and using topical steroids at times of flare, and "get control, keep control" referring to using topical steroids to reduce inflammation and regular and consistent application of emollients (Williams 2011).

The aims of my work were to:

- understand existing lay and HCP eczema mindlines;
- work with laypeople and HCPs to co-create affordable, practical, cost-effective, acceptable, safe, and equitable (Michie, Atkins and West 2014) strategies to alter and enhance existing mindlines;
- deliver new 'interventions' to support changes in practice/health behaviours to enhance self-management practices and consultations experiences.

My approach was informed by the Socialisation, Externalisation, Combination, and Internalisation (SECI) spiral (Nonaka, Toyama and Konno 2000) as also explained by Gabbay and le May (2011) (See Box 5.2).

BOX 5.2 THE SECI SPIRAL

- **Socialisation**: transfer of knowledge between people, often an implicit process that conveys day-to-day norms in a specific group or situation.
- **Externalisation**: tacit knowledge is made more explicit, and people make collective sense of their own and others' knowledge, often resulting in more widely comprehensible explicit knowledge.
- **Combination**: other sources of knowledge (for example, clinical guidelines) are melded with the explicit constructs from the original tacit knowledge.
- **Internalisation**: the individual transforms this combined knowledge into understanding that fits with their own knowledge and experience.

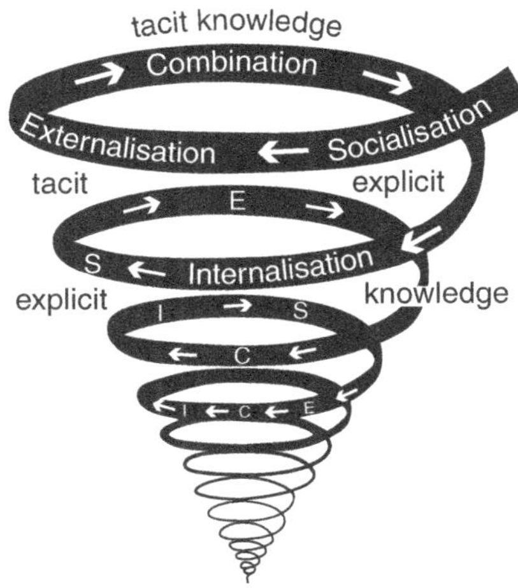

SECI spiral (Nonaka, Toyama and Konno 2000)

Understanding eczema mindlines

To understand ***socialisation*** processes and uncover the complexity of how and why HCP and parent-child lay eczema mindlines develop, evolve, and are transmitted, I used ethnographic observation, informal conversations, interviews, and documentary review to build up a rich picture of day-to-day practice. I spent several months working alongside general practitioners (GPs), including trainees and locums, nurses and health visitors, receptionists, and community pharmacy staff, observing numerous interactions. The essence of lay and HCP eczema mindlines is illustrated in Boxes 5.3 and 5.4:

Laypeople and HCPs alike struggled to ***externalise*** their tacit knowledge to make it explicit; the interview process provoked deep thinking about where knowledge and beliefs had come from and whether they were valid. Surfacing eczema mindlines exemplified the key role tacit knowledge plays in guiding decision-making and actions for laypeople and HCPs alike. Nonaka and Takeuchi (1995) point to two types of tacit knowledge, (i) technical know-how an "informal craft-based

BOX 5.3 THE ESSENCE OF LAY ECZEMA MINDLINES

- *Care informed by "trial and error", "I've tried everything. ... I know what works for me".*
- *Family, friends, and wider-society influential, offering sometimes unsolicited advice.*
- *"Old wive's tales" assimilated, "just knowing", "steroids ... back of your mind, bad for the skin, thins it, don't know where from".*
- *New knowledge from NHS Choices and patient.co.uk trusted but too generic and not applicable for their circumstances and needs.*
- *"Googling" frequent, ability to judge the value of information varied, degrees of caution, and all had a line which they would not cross in terms of acting on information.*
- *Poor consultation experiences, "not worth consulting".*

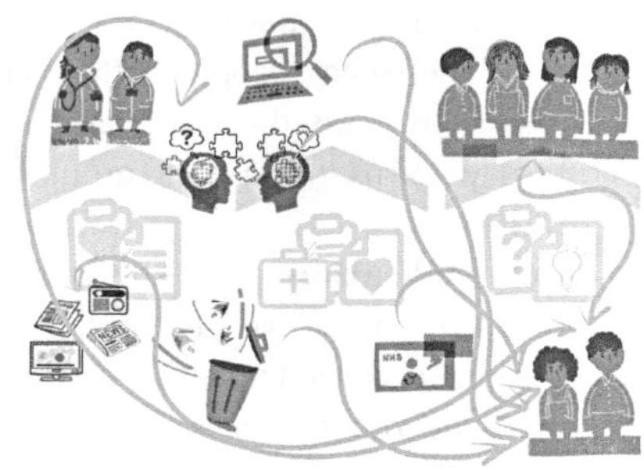

Source: (Cowdell 2018)

skill" that cannot readily be articulated, and unconscious schemata "the schemata, mental models, beliefs and perceptions so ingrained that we take them for granted" (Gabbay and le May 2011, p. 99). The patients and HCPs in my study illustrated how this informal knowledge is far more influential than formal codified guidance.

Eczema mindlines were relatively static; people had tacit knowledge that informed brief and often unhelpful interactions. One powerful influencer was the low priority afforded to eczema by many HCPs and the impact this had on laypeople who often chose to stop consulting or bring eczema as a secondary complaint in a consultation. Eczema knowledge is deeply embedded in social norms and so is rarely externalised. HCPs in particular had limited motivation to combine their existing tacit knowledge with external, codified knowledge sources such as clinical guidelines and thus internalisation (with improvement in practice) was infrequent. Understanding mindlines, and importantly the relationships of mindlines between stakeholders, offers the promise of opportunity for people to engage in the type of social processes which are far more likely to change practice than the production of yet more codified information (Gabbay and le May 2011).

BOX 5.4 THE ESSENCE OF HCP ECZEMA MINDLINES

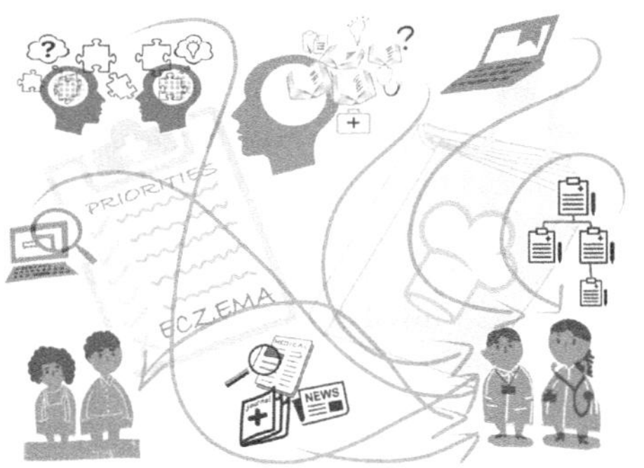

- *Low-priority condition which is simple to manage, "eczema is simple to treat, nothing much has changed over the years", "the recipe doesn't change".*
- *Prescribing limited by local formularies.*
- *Limited motivation to change current practice.*
- *Management as a long-term condition rare.*
- *Approach automatic, often unthinking, likened to a "satnav ... you stop thinking, the little NHS boxes [on the computer] tell you what to prescribe".*
- *Value given to patient experience varied: "listen and learn", "actually taking notice of what they're telling me" to "patient experience stuff can be counterproductive".*

Source: (Cowdell 2018)

In summary, parents and children acquire knowledge and beliefs from many sources, including personal experience, family, friends and wider society, trial and error, online, and from practitioners. Quality of HCP advice is variable, with the most trusted, useful, and personalised advice being given by dermatology specialist nurses (although few participants had benefited from such consultations). HCPs' actions are built on the belief that eczema is simple to treat and prescribing options limited. Knowledge is based on early education, interactions with colleagues, practical experience, and patients. Therefore, efforts to alter and enhance mindlines need to be a mutual endeavour which transcends lay-practitioner-wider-society boundaries to develop shared and consistent language and understanding; this required a co-creation approach.

Combination through co-creation

Co-creation in healthcare is increasingly seen as a 'good thing' and, more importantly, is essential in moving beyond socialisation and through ***externalisation*** to ***combination***.

Co-creation is a logical approach to finding strategies to alter and enhance mindlines, given the complexity, context specificity, and intertwined nature of lay-practitioner mindlines and the need to consider the wider social milieu. The goal in co-creation was to (i) find strategies to help others internalise reliable, useful, and contextually appropriate knowledge and erase outdated or inaccurate information and (ii) to offer shared language and understanding across boundaries. Although language and definitions of co-creation vary, the idea that it should involve laypeople and professionals working as equals at each stage of the research process is consistent (Co-create 2021; NIHR 2021). Fundamental questions in preparation for co-creation include: who is participating, in what, and for whose benefit (Cornwall 2008)?

Co-creation workshops

Co-creation work was guided by eight principles of the 'Gold Standard' Coproduction Matrix (Co-create 2021); all activities should be holistic, resourced, transparent, inclusive, iterative, positive, equal, and sustainable. The co-creation group comprised laypeople with, and parents of children with, atopic eczema, HCPs, a researcher, and a facilitator (n = 22). We met face-to-face three times with iterative email communication before, between, and after sessions. Before the workshop, one co-creator received the original mindline publication of Gabbay and le May (2004) with illustrations and explanations of lay and HCP practitioner eczema mindlines. Each workshop started with a discussion about mindlines, which intuitively "made sense" to all. Data included facilitator notes, flip charts documenting individual and group presentations, and artefacts. Data collection and analysis were iterative. Between workshops, data summaries were sent to all participants for comment, amendment, and supplementation.

Workshops one and two

HCPs attended workshop one and laypeople workshop two where the purpose was to externalise existing tacit knowledge, allowing participants to make collective sense of their own and others' knowledge, thus increasing understanding. To remain close to context and give participants a familiar and comfortable starting point, two core questions were posed to generate rich discussion: (i) what makes a good eczema consultation in primary care[2] and (ii) what should laypeople and practitioners start, stop, and continue if they are to improve eczema consultations and self-management? Question two elicited the interactions and approaches to treatment that work well and should be continued, what new ones should be initiated, and which are unhelpful and should be stopped. A summary of co-creators' thoughts is provided in Boxes 5.5 and 5.6.

Data from workshops one and two and subsequent email exchanges were collated and analysed to identify priority areas to alter and enhance lay and HCP eczema mindlines. These were (i) prioritise eczema, (ii) manage eczema as a long-term condition, (iii) prepare for each consultation, (iv) be consistent with treatment, (v) work together, (vi) get the right emollient, and (vii) use steroids appropriately.

BOX 5.5 SUMMARY OF THOUGHTS ON Q1, WHAT MAKES A GOOD ECZEMA CONSULTATION IN PRIMARY CARE?

Laypeople

- *HCP who empathised with the impact that eczema had on quality of life and made time to talk.*
- *HCPs being open about their knowledge and its limitations, provided they could signpost to required information.*
- *HCPs to value their expertise.*
- *"Help manage long-term rather than short-term solutions for flares".*
- *Working in partnership with HCPs to "come to an understanding, work together" to self-manage as effectively as possible.*

HCPs

- *Based on empathy.*
- *Involving a reciprocal conversation between "equals" to generate shared understanding of eczema and treatment history so that both parties understand and "play the same tune, be on the same page".*
- *Delivering consistent messages to reduce misunderstandings and enhance patients' confidence.*
- *Agreeing on goals to "get control and keep control".*
- *Accommodating patient and family preferences for treatments, whilst acknowledging this could be challenging within the confines of local prescribing guidelines.*

BOX 5.6 SUMMARY OF THOUGHTS ON Q2, WHAT SHOULD LAYPEOPLE AND PRACTITIONERS START, STOP, AND CONTINUE TO IMPROVE ECZEMA CONSULTATIONS AND SELF-MANAGEMENT?

Laypeople and HCPs

- *Treat eczema as a long-term condition*
- *Be prepared for the appointment*
- *Prioritise eczema*
- *Engage in shared decision-making*
- *Use topical treatments consistently*

Workshop three

In workshop three, co-creators came together to consider ***combination*** of tacit and codified knowledge. They emphasised the core challenges of eczema being a low-priority condition, views about treatment being deeply entrenched, and some reluctance to engage in shared decision-making. Commonalities in thinking included the following:

- Interventions to alter and enhance the mindlines of either group in isolation would not be effective as they are intertwined and co-dependent and so must be addressed in parallel.
- Eczema mindlines are influenced by a wider social milieu, this may reinforce powerful messages, such as children "grow out of eczema" and the myth that topical steroid preparations are necessarily "dangerous".

Changes in mindlines would only occur in the context of trust and 'realness' for lay-people and practical, locally relevant, hints and tips, tailored, 'no faff' approaches for HCPs (Cowdell 2019). Simply providing more information would not influence mindlines; information overload was already problematic. We revisited existing evidence (https://www.nice.org.uk/guidance/cg57) and consulted with the National Eczema Society to ensure that when ***combination*** occurred it integrated reliable evidence in user-friendly language. To meet identified need, we developed five key, consistent, evidence-based messages to become the bedrock of eczema mindlines alteration and enhancement:

i. Eczema is more than just dry skin.
ii. Eczema does not just go away.
iii. Moisturisers are for everyday.
iv. Steroid creams are okay when you need them, and
v. You know your child's eczema best.

Creating this firm foundation could enable shared language and understandings and support more equal interactions between laypeople and HCPs. Each priority was underpinned by a set of simple, illustrated messages. Potential approaches to alter and enhance mindlines included, for example, 'pop up' events in public arenas, sharing the messages in skincare sections of supermarkets, targeting information in 'Healthy Living Pharmacies', using 'Steroid Sam the emoji' in information to illustrate benefits of topical steroids when needed, and using the Patient-Oriented Eczema Measure/Children's and Dermatology Life Quality Index to improve confidence in 'proving' impact of eczema during consultations. As each idea was discussed, the strengths and weaknesses were identified. Many were abandoned as not being feasible due to lack of time and funding.

In summary, co-creators agreed five key, consistent eczema messages should be shared across lay-practitioner-wider-society boundaries using accessible, engaging, easy-to-understand formats to promote shared language and understanding. Co-creation work was necessarily time limited, I left the sessions with a set of key messages and ideas about how these may best be shared.

Internalisation: altering and enhancing mindlines

To date, relatively little has been written about strategies to alter and enhance mindlines, particularly approaches that attempt to bridge lay-practitioner-wider-society boundaries. In the course of the workshops, co-creators combined their eczema knowledge; the challenge here was to find ways to support ***combination*** and ***internalisation*** at a wider level. Co-creators' thinking aligned closely with Gabbay and le May's (2011) analysis of the uptake of new evidence. They point to the inherent messiness of the adoption of new evidence, demonstrating the chasm between the orderly, linear, and rational route sometimes espoused in evidence-based practice and the reality of day-to-day practice. Equally, whilst valuing the SECI spiral, Gabbay and le May (2011) emphasise that mindlines take into account a more complex view of how internalisation occurs and offer valuable pointers:

i. Certain types of evidence and the way in which this evidence is presented are better accepted than others. Personal experiences and views of locally respected experts, often shared through stories and anecdotes, are powerful currency. Immediate credibility and relevance trump perceived scientific validity. Information that can be transformed and linked to existing knowledge supports reformulation of new information in a way that makes sense to individuals.
ii. People need to surface and communicate existing tacit knowledge and combine and internalise (or reject) new information and assess this for relevance and fit with their situation.
iii. The fate of information is influenced by negotiation, how accessible and plausible it is to all involved, and the credibility of the bearer.
iv. The desirability and possibility of putting new knowledge into practice depends on roles, power differentials, and individuals' credibility, all of which are in a state of perpetual flux.

Strategies to alter and enhance eczema mindlines were informed by four elements: (i) knowledge brokering, (ii) social marketing, (iii) 'Ba', and (iv) the ripple-effect model. Each is described briefly in the following sections.

Knowledge brokering

My role was as a knowledge broker, "one who connects science and society by building networks and facilitating opportunities among knowledge producers and knowledge users" (Thompson & Schwartz Barcott 2019, p. 26). Activity is based on five elements: (i) establish – identifies potential stakeholders, (ii) engage – recognises stakeholders' cultural norms and practices, (iii) educate – facilitates multidirectional knowledge exchanges, (iv) empower – builds capacity for shared decision-making, and (v) evaluate – considers processes, outcomes, and impacts.

Social marketing

Social marketing (SM), used internationally in healthcare since the mid-1970s, melds concepts from commercial marketing and social sciences (Walsh, Rudd, Moeykens et al. 1993). SM goes beyond providing information, encompassing health communication techniques based on mass media. Messages can be mediated through other sources, in our case potentially practitioners and lay influencers. Communication approaches are varied and may include targeted message placement, health promotion, dissemination, and community outreach (Evans 2006). SM works here given the high prevalence of childhood eczema, the aim of changing practices, and the need to get simple, consistent messages to a diverse range of people who may influence treatment, including those living with eczema, HCPs, and members of the wider community, for example, grandparents, friends and influencers such as community leaders.

'Ba'

Mindlines build on the work of Polanyi (2009) and Nonaka and Takeuchi (2007), in particular, the SECI spiral in which knowledge is perpetually produced and transformed as users interact, collaborate, and learn. Gabbay and le May (2011) emphasise knowledge-in-practice-in-context, recognising that in each context new knowledge is transformed by complex social processes. The work of Nonaka and colleagues offers new insights into altering mindlines, drawing on the relationship between the SECI spiral and *Ba*. *Ba* originates from philosophers Nishida and Dilworth (1970) and was advanced by Shimizu (1995); it is a shared space for knowledge creation and sharing. *Ba* is not about the space itself (Bartolacci, Cristalli, Isidori et al. 2016) but instead is a shared context-in-motion which progresses over time and has no firm boundaries or membership. It is about the here-and-now and flourishes with people who contribute diverse viewpoints (Nonaka and Toyama 2003). *Ba* space occurs naturally, is not preordained; relationships change over time (Nonaka and Konno 2003). Communication flows iteratively back and forth between *Ba* members and can be face-to-face or virtual, involving individuals or groups according to need and opportunity (Krahe, Lalley and Solomons 2014). Given the need to alter and enhance mindlines, both lay and HCP, across communities the notion of deliberatively creating *Ba* and integrating innovative approaches to communication offers new opportunities.

Ripple-effect model

Language of the ripple effect is varied but in essence refers to the spreading effect or series of consequences caused by a single action or event (Newman 2003), akin to a series of waves. Although mainly referenced in supply-chain literature, the ripple effect is documented in healthcare, for example in the diffusion of health education messages from nursing students via primary school children to their parents and onward to neighbours (Nambozi 2014). The ripple effect may also have a reciprocity characterised by mutual sharing of expertise, experience, attitudes, beliefs, and skills. An example many will relate to is the reciprocity we use when driving, if another driver helps us, we are more likely to help others and vice versa (Tennant 2016). Just as considerate driving can generate a ripple effect of safer journeys (Tennant 2016), so clear, consistent messages, and shared understandings may support better eczema care.

Mindline alteration and enhancement

Initially, my focus was on the small, deprived, multicultural area of an East Midlands city in the UK where I collected early data. Box 5.7 provides exemplars of activity and illustrations of the five key messages which were used in advertising for events and illustrated and printed on postcards with supplementary information on the back.

Later I expanded the reach of activity with a focus on continuing to share key messages and sharing with the wider community to normalise eczema amongst children aged 5–7 years and their teachers. The latter was influenced by lay feedback about the need to educate the educators and help others understand the impact of living with eczema and promote empathy.

An author and illustrator embedded the five key messages in a children's book *The Dragon in My Skin*. We then ran a series of co-creation workshops with children living with eczema aged 4–10 years and their parents. The children, alongside the team, developed words and sounds for a Dragon song. Children recorded themselves reading the book and singing the song, this was merged with professional vocals and backed by an orchestra to create the Dragon animation. The film premiered at an online event in March 2021 and is now freely available online (see the Introduction to this chapter). Taking this content as a starting point a group of education academics developed a series of illustrated, curriculum-linked activities relating to each primary-school subject area: English, maths, science, physical education and dance, music and personal, social, health, and economic education, each at three graduated levels of complexity, which we have called 'hatch, grow, and fly' in keeping with the Dragon theme.

BOX 5.7 EXEMPLARS OF ACTIVITY AND ILLUSTRATIONS OF THE FIVE KEY MESSAGES

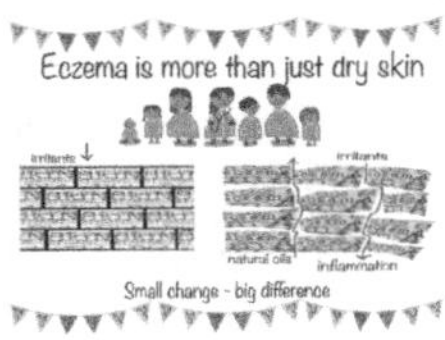

Eczema is more than just dry skin

Venue: community pharmacies
Target group: customers and pharmacy staff
Intervention: posters and postcards
Evaluation method: feedback from staff

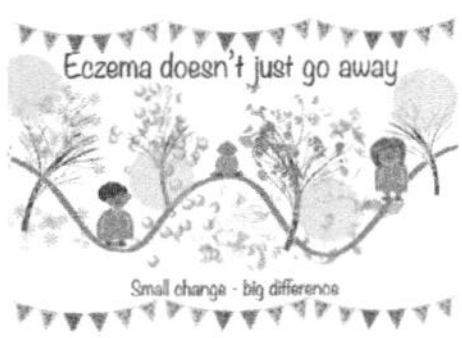

Eczema doesn't go away

Venue: shopping centre
Target group: passing shoppers and staff
Intervention: brief consultation with expert dermatology nurses, trying emollient products, and postcards
Evaluation method: footfall, observation of responses, and nature of interaction with nurses

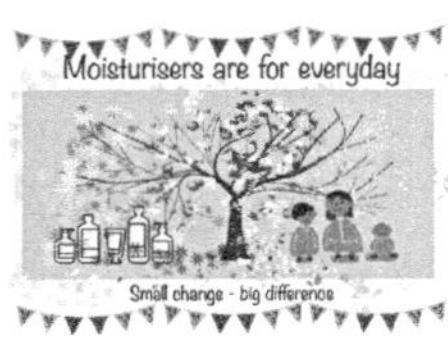

Moisturisers are for everyday

Venue: primary school
Target group: children aged 5–6 years, teachers and parents
Intervention: story reading, drawing activity, and conversations. Information for parents
Evaluation method: response from children, feedback from staff

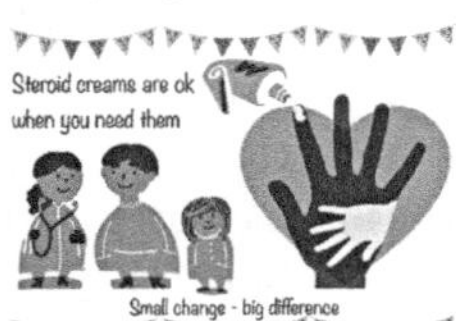

Steroid creams are ok when you need them

Venue: healthcare facilities
Target group: health visitors, community public health nurses, GPs, and other HCPs
Intervention: workplace-based, mindline-informed, case study–based interactive sessions
Evaluation method: informal conversations, qualitative interviews, and post-session questionnaire

Venue: online
Target group: people seeking further information
Intervention: website with further information and animation
Evaluation method: visits to site and views of animation

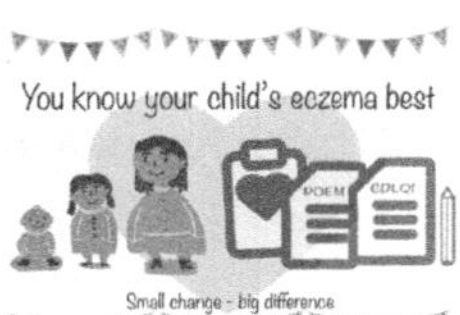

You know your child's eczema best

Venue: place of worship
Target group: children and their parents
Intervention: storytelling and conversations with children and parents
Evaluation method: feedback from children and parents

Impact

Assessing the impact of using KM techniques to alter and enhance eczema mindlines is inevitably messy and multi-factorial. To aid clarity, I have drawn on two schools of thought. Firstly, the contributions approach, which accepts this work as being just one of many factors that contribute to change (as opposed to attribution, which claims change is due to the intervention alone) (Morton 2015). Secondly the Social Impact Framework, which promotes a broad and inclusive notion of impact across the domains of individual, group and interpersonal, organisation, society and infrastructure, and paradigm (Beckett, Farr, Kothari et al. 2018). Proving change is limited as it may be subtle and go unseen. At the time of writing, indications of impact are promising. Practitioners, parents, and children have given concrete examples of changes in thinking and/or action. Over 500 trainee teachers are using the teacher resource pack, and a copy of the book with links to resources has been sent to over 800 schools. Online resources have been shared across national and international teaching communities via existing extensive online networks. Through a web of connectivity, largely word of mouth, resources have been requested by healthcare colleagues at individual, departmental, and organisational levels. Likewise, resources have been sent to educators, particularly those with a focus on mental health and well-being. Additionally, we are translating resources to French and Portuguese. Engagement with project-specific social media was modest, but web pages had good view quality, users engaged with the content and spent time reading it, as indicated by an average time of five minutes compared with the norm of 35 seconds to one minute. Box 5.8 presents exemplars of feedback and indicators of mindline changes.

BOX 5.8 EXEMPLARS OF FEEDBACK AND INDICATORS OF MINDLINE CHANGES

- *"I use the postcards in practice and in teaching my students about care of the skin on a regular basis" (Health visitor)*
- *"Evie wanted me to tell you that she has put her spray on all over to look after her dragon" (Mother with daughter aged 5 years)*
- *"Main things I took away … using one application of steroids is just as good as two. Go big, go early with the steroid" (GP)*
- *"I am so glad that this will now be shared in schools to raise awareness amongst children of what some of their friends are going through and to hopefully encourage more parents to talk about this and share experiences of what treatments have worked for their children" (Mother)*
- *"It's certainly made me more confident in prescribing" (Nurse practitioner)*
- *"I've double checked that they've got enough of the emollients" (GP)*

- *"My daughter is a primary teacher and I was telling her about it last night. Her response was, 'that sounds great – I'll definitely use it. It would have made me feel so much better in school if we'd had something like that'" (Mother and teacher)*
- *"We shared the information with parents via our weekly Newsletter last week and have included the book in our family information 'lending library'. We have already had a request from a parent to 'borrow' the book and I have forwarded details of the website" (Teacher)*
- *"Your film and music are absolutely fab! You've taken a debilitating but common and overlooked problem and made it come alive! I loved it all and found it very moving" (Nurse)*
- *"I have attached some posters the children in my year 1 class did today leading on from our 'Dragon in My Skin' lesson last week. They really enjoyed the lesson and loved the song!*

  We had a lot of discussion around the topic of eczema and we then went on to talk about feelings and how things such as eczema can affect our moods" (Teacher)

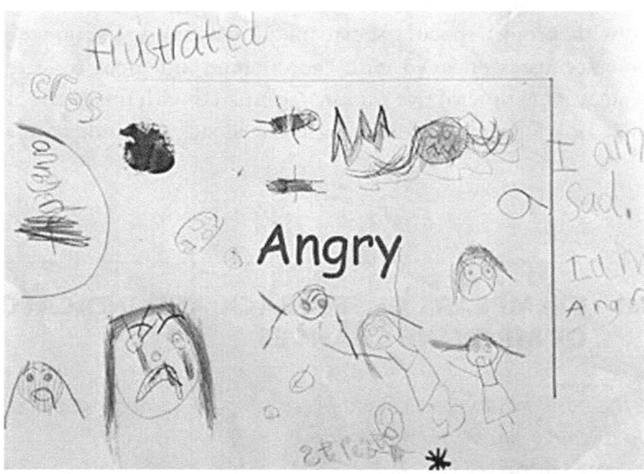

How things such as eczema can affect our moods

- *"The children had some really mature discussion during this lesson, and I have to say I was impressed, a couple of children with eczema were heavily involved in this and told other pupils some of their experiences (without being prompted or pressured to do so)" (Teacher)*

Reflections on altering and enhancing eczema mindlines

Uncovering eczema mindlines exposed some dispiriting facts. In particular: the burgeoning amount of variable quality information available, a sense that practitioners had limited motivation to change practice, the micro-level 'gloom à deux' with laypeople, HCPs sharing a perception of hopelessness (Dodd n.d.), and a wider view that eczema is a "health problem which is not an illness" (Cornwell 1984) and therefore perceived as low priority and open to treatment suggestions from anyone.

At the core of this KM activity is ***connectivity***, a complex spider's web, between people and across organisations and wider society. People are at the heart of this work. Of note were the time, determination, interpersonal skills, belief, and creativity required to be an effective knowledge broker. Not all areas were receptive to my offer, and in some cases, it took persistence and negotiation to be allowed in. Reasons to decline included, from schools "the curriculum allows no space for extras", from supermarkets "we only support one charity each year" (highlighting a fundamental misunderstanding of this work despite several conversations and emails), and suspicion from some gatekeepers of the message that steroid creams are okay when you need them. The most effective approach was to personally visit leaders in my capacity as a nurse (and so presumably viewed as trustworthy). Personal connections were pivotal, starting with my need to connect with a person rather than an organisation to deliver events. As I met people, they introduced me to their networks; for example, a GP invited me to his Mosque where I met a community pharmacist, and so it went on by word of mouth, allowing me to create a density of coverage in the small geographical area. Similarly, the spreading of the teacher resource pack was through a web of contacts. Once access was secured, the sessions were of value. In the shopping centre, 94 people had brief nurse consultations about their own, their child's, or wider family or friend's eczema. Over 60 HCPs attended mindline-informed sessions, a significant number given the low priority of eczema and work pressures.

Alongside face-to-face events, Twitter and Facebook accounts were started and a website set up. After an initial flurry of interest, these were of limited value, although people enjoyed the series of Haiku (see top of chapter). Information overload is a common phenomenon; in the early 2000s, information production was increasing at 50% per year but consumption at less than 2% (Brown and Dugiud 2002). Two decades on, production continues apace, and volume is overwhelming us. Globally, there are well over three billion internet users with an estimated two billion using social media (SoMe). Whilst being free and easy to use, these media can also lead to rapid, widespread transmission of misinformation (Welch, Petkovic, Simeon et al. 2018). The value of SoMe in this work was in raising the profile of eczema and starting conversations. Links between people spiralled; people are good at identifying others, and whilst systems offer generalities, people address particularities (Brown and Dugiud 2002) and can adapt engagement to individuals and context. That is not to say SoMe cannot also contribute directly to mindline alteration;

judicious use has supported development of innovative and creative ways to share the five key messages. This more widespread distribution, particularly the teacher resource pack, plays to the strengths of SoMe in creating interactive, collaborative networks which are dynamic and embedded in social contexts (Luca, Hibbert and McDonald 2016). These networks have been built by individuals in the core team and have rippled out more widely than anticipated; for example, resources are in the process of being translated into other languages.

A core feature of eczema mindlines was emotion, also a central factor in *Ba* in terms of both shared experiential knowledge and as context for socialisation processes (Nonaka, Toyama and Konno 2000). Efforts to alter eczema mindlines have invoked positive emotion, for example, through valuing each and every person's contribution, bringing together groups of people to better understand each other's worlds and by working together to develop creative ways to share simple messages and sharing these messages using accessible and attractive media. Using mindline-informed sessions for HCPs allowed us not only to work with them to uncover their tacit knowledge and link new nuggets to this but also privileged and respected their expertise and created an atmosphere of positive emotion. There are suggestions that positive emotion inspires resourcefulness and innovation (Hodgins and Dadich 2017; see also Chapter 6), influences how knowledge is assimilated (Forgas and Smith 2007), shapes sense-making (Steigenberger 2015), and provides a powerful stimulus to action (Sebrant 2014). The mindline-alteration strategies used here promoted positive emotion whilst offering digestible nuggets of knowledge which early evaluation suggests have been integrated into eczema mindlines. Ultimately securing shared language and understanding through integration of the five key messages has the potential to improve consultation experience and self-management practice in childhood eczema. In healthcare, emphasis is placed on self-management of long-term conditions (DH 2014) and shared decision-making (Légaré, Adekpedjou, Stacey et al. 2018). Both benefit from shared language and understanding between laypeople and HCPs. Although this work focuses on altering and enhancing eczema mindlines, the approach could equally be applied to other long-term health conditions.

Summary

- Effective self or parent-management of childhood eczema requires shared language and understanding between child, parent, and healthcare practitioner.
- Entrenched beliefs, such as steroid preparations being harmful, are powerful and can lead to sub-optimal healthcare practices.
- Changing practice requires externalisation *and* reflection on these tacit beliefs.
- New and already available codified information needs to be linked with existing knowledge and experience and adapted to the local context to be combined, internalised, and used to change mindlines.
- Multiple, low-cost approaches have been successful in altering and amending eczema mindlines across lay-practitioner-wider-society boundaries.
- These approaches may equally be applied to other long-term conditions.

Acknowledgements

Thanks to all research participants and to colleagues in the Darwin Mindlines Group for their help in making this study and chapter possible. Also thanks to Jay Nolan Latchford for the illustrations https://www.jnl-art.com/.

I was funded by a National Institute for Health Research Knowledge Mobilisation Research Fellowship (KMRF-2015-04-004). This chapter presents independent research funded by the National Institute for Health Research (NIHR). The views expressed are those of the author and not necessarily those of the NHS, the NIHR, or the Department of Health and Social Care.

Notes

1 Provenance of this phrase is uncertain. I associate it with Professor Hywel Williams, consultant dermatologist, and Sandra Lawton, consultant dermatology nurse.
2 Thoughts here were primarily around GP consultations but also included interactions with other HCPs in particular community pharmacists, pharmacy counter asssssistants, nurses, and health visitors who, many suggested, may be better placed to provide eczema care.

References

Bartolacci C, Cristalli C, Isidori D, Niccolini F. 2016. 'Ba virtual and inter-organizational evolution: a case study from an EU research project'. *Journal of Knowledge Management*, 20: 793–811.

Beckett K, Farr M, Kothari A, Wye L, le May A. 2018. 'Embracing complexity and uncertainty to create impact: Exploring the processes and transformative potential of co-produced research through development of a social impact model'. *Health Research Policy and Systems*, 16:1–8.

Brown JS, Dugiud P. 2002. *The social life of information*. Boston: Harvard Business School Publishing.

Co-create. 2021. Core values. https://www.wearecocreate.com/about (accessed 18 May 2021).

Cornwall A. 2008. 'Unpacking 'participation': models, meanings and practices'. *Community Development Journal*, 43:269–283.

Cornwell J. 1984. *Hard-earned lives: accounts of health and illness from East London*, London: Routledge & Kegan Paul.

Cowdell F. 2018. 'Knowledge mobilisation: an ethnographic study of the influence of lay mindlines on eczema self-management in primary care in the UK'. *BMJ Open*, 8(8):e021498.

Cowdell F. 2019. 'Knowledge mobilisation: an ethnographic study of the influence of practitioner mindlines on atopic eczema self-management in primary care in the UK'. *BMJ Open*, 9(7):e025220.

Department of Health. 2014. A mandate from the government to NHS England. https://assets.publishing.service.gov.uk/government/uploads/system/uploads/attachment_data/file/256497/13-15_mandate.pdf (accessed 18 May 2021).

Dodd M. n.d. Motivational interviewing ideas for peer mentors. https://chess.wisc.edu/niatx/toolkits/system/IA_MIforPeerMentors.pdf (accessed 18 May 2021).

Evans WD. 2006. 'How social marketing works in health care'. *British Medical Journal*, 332: 2–10.

Forgas JP, Smith CA. 2007. 'Affect and emotion'. In M Hogg, J Cooper (Eds.) *Sage handbook of social psychology*. Thousand Oaks: Sage Publications, pp. 146–175.

Gabbay J, le May A. 2004. 'Evidence based guidelines or collectively constructed "mindlines?" Ethnographic study of knowledge management in primary care'. *British Medical Journal*, 329:1013–1016.

Gabbay J, le May A. 2011. *Practice-based evidence for healthcare: clinical mindlines*. London: Routledge.

Hodgins M, Dadich A. 2017. 'Positive emotion in knowledge creation'. *Journal of Health Organization and Management*, 31:162–174.

Krahe JA, Lalley C, Solomons NM. 2014. 'Beyond survival: fostering growth and innovation in doctoral study–a concept analysis of the Ba space'. *International Journal of Nursing Education Scholarship*, 11:11–18.

Légaré F, Adekpedjou R, Stacey D, Turcotte S, Kryworuchko J, Graham ID, Lyddiatt A, Politi M, Thomson R, Elwyn G, Donner-Banzhoff N. 2018. 'Interventions for increasing the use of shared decision making by healthcare professionals'. *Cochrane Database of Systematic Reviews*, 7. Art. No.: CD006732. DOI: 10.1002/14651858.CD006732.pub4

Luca NR, Hibbert S, McDonald R. 2016. 'Towards a service-dominant approach to social marketing'. *Marketing Theory*, 16:194–218.

Michie S, Atkins L, West R. 2014. *The behaviour change wheel. A guide to designing interventions*. 1st ed. Great Britain: Silverback Publishing. 1003–1010.

Morton S. 2015. 'Progressing research impact assessment: a "contributions" approach'. *Research Evaluation*, 24:405–419.

Nambozi G. 2014. An evaluation of community based university nursing education programme and stakeholders' experiences. https://hydra.hull.ac.uk/assets/hull:14394a/content (accessed 18 May 2021).

National Institute for Health Research. 2021. Co-production in action. https://www.learningforinvolvement.org.uk/wp-content/uploads/2021/04/NIHR-Co-production-in-Action-Number-One-April-2021.pdf (accessed 18 May 2021).

Newman ME. 2003. 'Ego-centered networks and the ripple effect'. *Social Networks*, 25(1):83–95.

Nishida K, Dilworth DA. 1970. *Fundamental problems of philosophy the world of action and the dialectical world*. Tokyo: Sophia University.

Nonaka I, Konno N. 2003. *Methodology of knowledge creation*. Tokyo: Toyo Keizai.

Nonaka I, Takeuchi H. 1995. *The knowledge creating company: How Japanese companies create the dynamics of innovation*. New York: Oxford University Press.

Nonaka I, Takeuchi H. 2007. 'The knowledge-creating company'. *Harvard Business Review*, Jul 1;85(7/8):162.

Nonaka I, Toyama R. 2003. 'The knowledge-creating theory revisited: knowledge creation as a synthesizing process'. *Knowledge Management Research & Practice*, 1:2–10.

Nonaka I, Toyama R, Konno N. 2000. 'SECI, Ba and leadership: a unified model of dynamic knowledge creation'. *Long Range Planning*, 33:5–34.

Polanyi M. 2009. *The tacit dimension*. Chicago: University of Chicago Press.

Sebrant U. 2014. 'Emotion, power and identity. Emotional display of envy when taking on management roles in a professional hierarchy'. *Journal of Health Organization and Management*, 28:548–561.

Shimizu H. 1995. 'Ba-principle: new logic for the real-time emergence of information'. *Holonics*, 5:67–79.

Steigenberger N. 2015. 'Emotions in sensemaking: a change management perspective'. *Journal of Organizational Change Management*, 28:432–451.

Tennant C. 2016. 'The "ripple effect" of driving behaviour'. https://blogs.lse.ac.uk/psychologylse/2016/01/25/the-ripple-effect-of-driving-behaviour/ (accessed 18 May 2021).

Thompson MR, Schwartz Barcott D. 2019. 'The role of the nurse scientist as a knowledge broker'. *Journal of Nursing Scholarship*, 51(1):26–39.

Walsh DC, Rudd RE, Moeykens BA, Moloney TW. 1993. 'Social marketing for public health'. *Health Affairs*, 12:104–19.

Welch V, Petkovic J, Simeon R, Presseau J, Gagnon D, Hossain A, Pardo JP, Pottie K, Rader T, Sokolovski A, Yoganathan M, Tugwell P, DesMeules M. 2018. 'Interactive social media interventions for health behaviour change, health outcomes, and health equity in the adult population'. *Cochrane Database of Systematic Reviews*, 2. Art. No.: CD012932. DOI: 10.1002/14651858.CD012932.

Williams HC. 2011. 'Preventing eczema flares with topical corticosteroids or tacrolimus: which is best?' *British Journal of Dermatology*, 164:231–233.

Wye L, Cramer H, Beckett K, Farr M, le May A, Carey J, Robinson R, Anthwal R, Rooney J, Baxter H. 2020. 'Collective knowledge brokering: the model and impact of an embedded team'. *Evidence & Policy: A Journal of Research, Debate and Practice*, 16:429–452.

6

THE CONFLUENCE OF MINDLINES AND EMOTION IN COMMUNITY-BASED PALLIATIVE CARE

Michael Hodgins, Ann Dadich and Jane Bye

Introduction

Emotions are inherently part of the healthcare of patients and families navigating trajectories of pain, suffering, loss, and recovery. Clinicians are in no way exempt from the emotionality of healthcare. However, the prevailing sentiments of professionalism and stoicism as part of the clinical identity, bound with the rational institution of evidence-based healthcare, has marginalised emotion within clinical practice. Our research suggests that when emotion and evidence-based healthcare (conceptualised as mindlines) are brought into proximity, they often allow for creative and productive ways of caring. We specifically explore the speciality of community-based palliative care, which involves a great deal of emotional complexity due to the existential and physical suffering occurring within the 'messy' space of a patient's home.

Emotion was often foregrounded in our research, as clinicians frequently indicated how emotions enabled effective palliative care:

> When you are more sensitive to what your patients' needs are… [and] able to plan for palliative care, I think emotions help a lot. You cannot do your job without emotions.
>
> (*Palliative-care nurse*)

Yet emotion also hindered palliative care, clouding clinical judgement, and obscuring a 'bigger picture', as that same nurse described:

> Having that guilt in relation to a patient's death can be very debilitating. You ask yourself, "Could I have done something differently to prolong their life?" rather than learn from that experience and move on.
>
> (*Palliative-care nurse*)

DOI: 10.4324/9781003158721-6

Emotion – in this case guilt – was "debilitating", and its suppression was important for self-preservation. Our research explored the complex relationship that emotion has to the patterns of meaning and threads of collectively shaped 'reality' that become practice in community-based palliative care.

Emotion and mindlines

The role of emotion has typically been understated or marginalised in research on formal and informal learning. Benozzo and Colley (2012) noted that scholars have generally "conceive(d) the... construction and acquisition of knowledge as separated from emotive processes" (p. 306). Similarly, Hökkä and colleagues (2020) found very few studies that explored the relationship between emotions and learning at work. Complicating research on emotions and workplace learning are the varied understandings of emotion, which is sometimes confused with affect (Hochschild 1983; Kemper 1981; Thrift 2004). Emotions are often described as internal, biological feelings experienced in relation to external stimuli (Parkinson 1995). To counter this understanding, others have situated emotion within and dependent on relationships and culture (Hochschild 1983; Zembylas 2007). Both approaches are limited. The former neglects cultural, political, and other social forces that shape emotion – yet the latter often ignores the importance of individual experiences of emotion (Zembylas 2007). Some research (including that presented here) offers a middle ground of emotion, sometimes termed the 'interactionist' approach (Savage 2004). Vital to this approach is the socially embedded nature of feeling and experience, which are localised in the body and relationships between bodies (Pile 2010).

To improve health services, we need to investigate more deeply the relationship between emotions and workplace learning, to understand how emotions can enhance or hinder the processes of formal and informal learning. The prevailing view of knowledge in health-service delivery, and evidence-based healthcare, often struggles to account for the application of evidence in messy, emotionally, or politically charged contexts (Greenhalgh 2013; Wieringa, Engebretsen, Heggen et al. 2018). Although Gabbay and le May (2011) recognised that clinical practices are socially (re)constructed by and among different clinicians, they paid little attention to the role of emotion in this process. Our chapter explicates how emotions and mindlines are assembled in practice. Using the example of palliative care, we argue that mindlines can be understood as 'assemblages' based on Deleuze and Guattari's (1987, 1984) work, comprising varied dimensions that form different ways to deliver palliative care. These include ideas, practices, identities, and emotions. With this understanding, emotion coexists within mindlines along with clinicians' "skills, norms, attitudes, and infrastructural demands" (Gabbay and le May 2011, p. 193). We suggest that emotion is implicated in how clinicians develop their capacity to deliver palliative care, and in doing so, we demonstrate that emotion is integral to the ways that palliative-care clinicians make sense of the care they deliver and the decisions they make.

Study details

Our research took place in a community health centre, located in the most populous Australian state, New South Wales. Within the district, community-based palliative care involved specialist nurses whose consultancy role supported generalist community health nurses who case-managed palliative-care patients residing at home. The palliative-care team was also supported by palliative-care doctors, based at the local hospital, who attended both regular case-review meetings at the centre and home visits, when required. Seventeen primary participants from the community health centre were involved in the study, including nine generalist nurses, five specialist nurses, and three specialist doctors. The study also involved approximately 50 secondary participants – namely, patients and carers who were observed or who participated in conversations.

We collected data by shadowing primary participants as they worked, documenting our observations, and interviewing them. Through this work, we wanted to clarify how emotions were constituted with other parts of community-based palliative-care knowledge, and explore how emotion stabilised and transformed mindlines. To do this, we drew from Deleuze and Guattari's (1987, 1984) notion of the assemblage. For our purposes, the assemblage was a conceptual framing that dictates reality as comprised of constantly changing arrangements of diverse things. These arrangements are pulled together and fall apart, based on whether they work. Mindlines can be neatly conceptualised as assemblages because they are representations of the way things ought to work. Clinicians understand and express them through their description of diverse things; for instance, actions, emotions, human and non-human actors, and the identities or 'subjects' they constitute. Also, mindlines, like the way Deleuze and Guattari described assemblages, are constantly in flux. They move according to their usefulness to the situation at hand.

Drawing on the assemblage helped us to map the diverse elements that make up mindlines – helping us to consider the conceptual (ideas formed from evidence, knowledge of guidelines, experiential knowledge, emotions) and material elements of specific mindlines (identities, practices, emotions). Examining the emotions the clinicians discussed or experienced with reference to a central idea or practice (e.g., an evidence-based practice) helped to create a taxonomy of mindline-emotion assemblages. This chapter explores how these mindline assemblages informed learning – in particular, it demonstrates how emotions and mindlines were assembled in proximity to direct peers' attention, exemplify good practices, and establish the limits of care.

Partitioning emotion during clinical interactions

During clinician interactions, emotional performances[1] helped to share knowledge around the appropriate mindline assemblages for specific situations. The manifestation or absence of emotion aligned with how some mindline assemblages were privileged in clinical interactions, influencing how palliative care was demonstrated.

Case review discussions were predominantly formal, stemming from a general concern for a patient's physiological concerns. Nurses presented patients in terms of disease, along with significant symptoms, such as pain, constipation, nausea, and social issues, including those involving carers. By directing their attention to diagnosis, the clinicians indicated that case review was primarily a space for mindline assemblages associated with the body. Specialist nurses would wait patiently while someone 'looked up' a diagnosis on a laptop. The presence of a specialist palliative-care doctor added to the formality – they provided additional medical advice and helped to formulate care plans.

By discussing the patient in a case review with reference to their primary diagnosis, the nurses prioritised this aspect of palliative care. This downplayed the emotive aspect of palliative care, which they often revealed after the primary diagnosis, symptoms, and treatments were presented:

GENERALIST NURSE 1: He's lung [cancer]. He has [metastases] in brain and bone. Currently on active treatment at [the hospital]. He lives with his wife and daughter. He was initially visited by [the nurse]. He was actually referred twice and refused the service. They recently changed their minds and want support. They're an ESL [English second language] family so, when I've been out, I've been getting the daughters to interpret. The thing is, the daughter also has brain cancer. The last time I was there, the patient's wife was laughing at the daughter because she doesn't understand what is going on.

SPECIALIST NURSE 1: I think her prognosis is that she's likely going to die before the dad.

SPECIALIST NURSE 2: Geez.

GENERALIST NURSE 1: The family want mobility support and equipment at the moment.

SPECIALIST NURSE 2: Have you thought about a social worker? It sounds like they need financial and emotional support more than anything.

Nurses' references to illness, symptoms, and treatment were usually followed by the most pertinent symptoms and/or social issues that need to be addressed, which were not documented. The initial discussion and its documentation were emotionally detached, with nurses monotonously listing symptoms and disease variables like they were recalling items for a shopping list. This period of the case discussion moved quickly, without the notable performative flourishes of later periods of the discussion.

Through our research, we came to understand this as the main emotional timbre of physiological and professional mindline assemblages; for instance, the objectification of patient bodies as a set of systems to be treated, and implicit imperatives to remain objective when engaging with patients. Palliative-care clinicians prided themselves on their holistic care, suggesting a conceptualisation of health as more than the traditional notion of 'normal functioning' or the absence of disease. However, to care for the whole patient required care of the body, addressing the physiological symptoms of a life-limiting illness. Patient comfort as a goal of palliative care and a good death was contingent on alleviating the symptoms that caused discomfort. This largely revolved around managing different types of physical pain or discomfort through pharmacological intervention. Despite the exhortations of holistic care within the community health centre, physiological care was given high priority, and the absence of emotion within clinical interactions in relation to this goal represents the reverence clinicians afforded it.

Using emotion to prioritise care

Clinicians attempted to remain unemotional and objective when prioritising the body or diagnosis during the case review, but conversely, they implicated emotion during the discussion of other concerns, enabling the clinicians to create flashpoints of care. These flashpoints shone during clinical interactions brimming with heightened emotions, fostering in-depth conversation, and informal learning, reverberating into ongoing practice. Consider, for instance, the moment the generalist nurse in the aforesaid excerpt identified the patient's daughter as living with brain cancer and specialist nurse 2's reaction. This moment prompted conversation between all three nurses about the benefits of a social worker. Emotions assembled with clinical concerns heightened conversation about the issue at hand.

In these contexts, nurses often seemed to purposefully perform emotions to focus colleagues' attention on areas of concern requiring novel and complex solutions. For example, clinicians often expressed sadness to accentuate features of care – be it the care of the patient, a family member, the self, or a colleague. This demonstrated the purposefulness of sadness within mindline assemblages related to carer stress, social concerns, or pain management. For instance, in describing a patient as "someone [who makes] you feel sad when you leave", one specialist nurse vented her compassion to colleagues. This influenced how they perceived the patient and planned her care to accommodate the patient's needs. Similarly, consider how a junior generalist nurse advocated for this patient by pleading for resources to moderate the patient's loneliness:

> I'm not going to discharge her because we are the only people she sees.
> (*Generalist nurse 2*)

During case reviews, nurses referred to established emotion scripts or norms. For example, the discussion of children, either as a patient or a patient's family member, became a powerful marker. In one interaction, a nurse used the opportunity to review a patient to highlight family trauma:

GENERALIST NURSE 3: [The patient] get[s] respite [through] My Aged Care [a government initiative] starting early next week so she can take [the patient's grandson] for some therapy. He can't talk; he just says "Uh oh. Uh oh". That's the only word he uses…

GENERALIST NURSE 4: He's developmentally delayed.

SPECIALIST NURSE 1: Oh, is he?

GENERALIST NURSE 4: Yeah. ... [The carer] said to me that it's going to be traumatic for [the patient's grandson] if [the patient] passes away...

SPECIALIST NURSE 1: He's in a pressing gap. He's in limbo, isn't he?...

SPECIALIST NURSE 2: I was just thinking about ... [a] clinical psych or something; maybe talking to [a clinical psych] about it and seeing what she can suggest.

The distress imbued within the reference to the child's disability, the child's potential trauma, his connection to the patient, and the potential absence of support for the child heightened the patient's needs. During the case review, this attention to the emotive aspects of the patient's situation by generalist nurses ensured the specialist nurses considered and attended to these needs. Detail on the distress helped to invoke empathy and inform care. This detail shifted emotions and in turn shifted the case review. When clinicians went 'off script' by alluding to patient sadness or suffering, their persona changed. They used words that were more personal and colloquial. Generalist nurse 3's observation that the patient and his grandson "talk to each other" was not pressing clinical information; nevertheless, it fostered connection with the patient. Foreshadowing the potential suffering after the patient's death established a collective fear of a bad death. Clinicians' voices took on a different timbre. When compared with the detached discussion of the patient's primary diagnosis and symptoms, the clinicians engaged in an enlivened discussion – they connected with and showed greater investment in the situation.

Case review was also filled with humour and joy as clinicians celebrated palliative care. This included shared 'victories'. During one case review, a nurse stated that her patient had been taking less pain medication, suggesting his pain was well controlled with the dosage prescribed. The specialist doctor exclaimed with joy, "Yes! That's fantastic", accompanied by a fist pump in the air. The doctor then told the story of the patient's pain; while the disease had improved, the patient's neuropathic pain had not. After struggling to identify the reason, she had discovered the cause – she was elated by this discovery and the patient's reduced pain. These moments of emotion demonstrated a reciprocal relationship within an assemblage of emotion and mindlines: when mindlines worked, clinicians felt positive emotion and communicated that emotion to colleagues. These outward social displays reinforced the collective mindlines among the team. In this way, case reviews could be places to celebrate and thereby affirm positive practices:

GENERALIST NURSE 2: I... organised a home visit with the patient on Tuesday. Just before I went to see him, I rang to confirm. ... He just said, "Look darling ..."

SPECIALIST NURSE 1: (Laughs) Darling.

GENERALIST NURSE 2: "I'm enjoying my lunch. I'm doing really well, there's no pain, there's no constipation" (laughs).

SPECIALIST NURSE 1: (Laughs) It's like he knows [what you're going to ask him]...

GENERALIST NURSE 2: [He said], "I'm doing really well. There's no issue with me, I'm currently enjoying life with my family, and could I please have another visit on Wednesday?" So, I said, "Yeah, that's okay. As long as you're doing well". I don't want to disturb him if he's just enjoying time with family.

SPECIALIST NURSE 1: No. So, any treatment?

GENERALIST NURSE 2: Ah no, didn't mention about chemo or anything at this stage.

SPECIALIST NURSE 1: Pain's well controlled?

GENERALIST NURSE 2: Pain's well controlled.

SPECIALIST NURSE 1: Excellent. ... So, you're happy?

GENERALIST NURSE 2: Yep

SPECIALIST NURSE 1: I like it.

Within this case review excerpt, the senior nurse's demonstration of joy after learning of the generalist nurse's practice and humour around the patient's knowledge of the palliative-care script and about the familiarity between the patient and nurse were flash points of success. Recognising the patient was "doing really well" and "enjoying life" without "issue" was a victory for the nurses. These moments further demonstrate the reciprocity of mindlines and emotions: mindlines that worked fostered positive emotion, which in turn bolstered mindlines among the team:

> It's really nice to have that validation from [the specialist team] that I'm doing the right things. The fact that they support me so much means I'm doing the right thing and [will] keep doing that work.
>
> (*Generalist nurse 2*)

This reciprocal reinforcement was on display most often when nurses reflected on moments of holistic care. Nurses spoke with pride and humour about attending to unique aspects of care and the specialist team applauded these aspects of holistic practice. During one case review, a generalist nurse described a patient who experienced anxiety. Rather than discuss the immediate physical symptoms, she explained the patient was "scared of her mum". The nurse organised a visit from a social worker along with her own weekly visits to "calm [the patient] down". The specialist nurses took a moment to applaud the nurse's actions, addressing the physical symptoms and the "emotional issues in her life". These positive appraisals of holistic care motivated nurses and doctors to widen their scope of palliative care. These assemblages of mindlines and emotions directly impacted nurses' decision-making as they frequently engaged with patients' social, emotional, and spiritual well-being.

Case reviews were moments to review patient deaths to assess the nature of the deaths. These moments clarified the constituent arrangements of death and dying care mindline assemblages:

GENERALIST NURSE 5: [The patient] died peacefully at home. It was a good outcome because that's what he wanted.

SPECIALIST DOCTOR 1: He was not somebody who complains and that's how he went – at night, not bothering anybody.

GENERALIST NURSE 5: [The carer] said it was the first night she slept peacefully in ages. In the end, everyone rallied: the nephew, the sister. It was a really good outcome. I called over for a bereavement … visit but they stated they were, "Busy, busy, busy".

SPECIALIST NURSE 1: That's all you can do. It usually takes a little time once everyone has left after the funeral and everything when [the patient's death] is starting to sink in. That's usually the best time [for a bereavement visit].

The presentation of the patient's death as a "good outcome" was associated with peacefulness and patient choice, the family's involvement in patient care, and the carer's peacefulness. Also, the specialist medic's interjection reinforced the appropriate and individualised nature of the patient's death. These moments created a shared understanding around the goals of death, which feature patient choice and family involvement. Additionally, the notion of "peacefulness", the "rallying" of the carers, and the time taken to let it "sink in" indicated some of the emotions that clinicians privileged in this context: resilience and tranquillity during death and, in the time following death, grief. The moment enabled the specialist nurse to remind the generalist nurse about the timeframe for bereavement visits. Bereavement visits were home visits to carers after a patient died. They were a point of closure for carers and nurses, during which a nurse discussed how carers coped. During case review, palliative-care mindline assemblages were reformed with reference to emotion, connecting individuals to one another in purposeful relationships.

In our study, rationality and the relegation of emotions in clinician-to-clinician interactions aligned with physiological intervention or strictly clinical practices. When clinicians' emotions came to the fore during interactions, they often refocussed their attention towards matters they had not yet considered while discussing a patient together. In a 'holistic' specialty, where patient and carer issues could be innumerable, this tactic helped to prioritise colleagues' attention. Emotions during clinician-to-clinician interaction enabled formal and informal learning. Clinicians entwined emotions with 'professional' practices, validating their emotions by according them clinical significance.

Forming the limits of practice with emotion

Drawing from Deleuze and Guattari's notion of assemblage helped us to think about mindlines in terms of their conceptual and material limits – to ask what variations in ideas and practices a palliative-care mindline assemblage could accommodate. Formal and informal interactions were instructive opportunities to collectively form mindline assemblage limits in palliative care using emotion. These emotions were directed at a failure to address patients' symptoms, organisational barriers to effective care, a patient's non-compliance to clinical advice, or workload and fatigue, among other frustrating elements of practice. The clinicians supported many patients, many of whom experienced comorbidities. This workload exacerbated expressions of frustration and anger, stemming from hopelessness and powerlessness at a limited ability to act:

> I'm frustrated about [the patient's] pain management. She is on 50 milligrams of Fentanyl, which is really high and it's still not working. The carers are really inconsistent. She needs fulltime care. We're just watching her deteriorate. We asked [the specialist doctor] for advice, but she came out and just [arranged access to the government disability insurance scheme] and didn't really address the pain. [She] was more worried about the wound care and was wanting [the generalist nurses] to do the wound care everyday.
>
> (*Specialist nurse 1*)

> Every time you get on top of things, they just throw something else at you.
>
> (*Generalist nurse 4*)

"Something else" in this excerpt represented a patient's comorbidities and the structural barriers that limited effective care. Specialist nurse 1 was assigned to care for the patient. With specialist nurse 2, specialist nurse 1 decided to manage the patient's pain. They decided the patient could be admitted to a palliative-care unit with the resources to monitor the patient. Two inpatient units were in close proximity: the local public hospital and a specialist palliative-care unit. Despite bed availability at the local hospital, the patient was unwilling to be admitted. Specialist nurse 1 advised this might have been due to poor experiences with clinicians there in the past; this exacerbated her frustration:

SPECIALIST NURSE 2: I understand choice, but at the end of the day, we're not going backwards and forwards, backwards and forwards for another week. She makes a decision. Either she goes in or she doesn't. She's got a doctor who will accept her into [the local hospital] …

SPECIALIST NURSE 1: Everybody else that knows her for years goes "Aw, that's [the patient]". But I've gone out there [with] fresh eyes. Maybe I'm being conned by her, but she's popping 20 milligrams of Endone and it's not even touching [the pain] so, she must be in pain.

During specialist nurse 1's description of the situation, her voice began to break. She audibly and visibly fought back an overwhelming emotion. For specialist nurse 1, there were multiple pressing concerns in this case, including the patient's pain, her susceptibility to being "conned", and the patient's unwillingness to be admitted to the local hospital. These different concerns were important as the clinicians considered the patient's palliative-care status. Reflecting on the situation afterwards with specialist nurse 1, she was even more despairing than during the case review, rejecting the notion that the patient required palliative care:

> Someone should be taking care of these people and it shouldn't be us. I don't mean to be awful, but it shouldn't be us. We have become a dumping ground for these really chronic conditions and it's not fair. I don't have the time anymore to care for real palliative-care patients. … The government and the [government disability insurance scheme] have failed these chronic patients for so long.
>
> (*Specialist nurse 1*)

Specialist nurse 1's frustration and anger clarified some of the limits of compassion and humanistic care. Her self-assessment helped her to weaken her connection with the patient, suggesting she might have been "conned". However, specialist nurse 1 also used her palliative-care identity to legitimise her anger, citing disruption to her role and justifying her decision to stop providing palliative care to a patient who needed another kind of care. In this way, clinician emotions constructed collective boundaries of self-preservation to mitigate threats to their identity and work life. This contradicted the patient-centrism and humanism of palliative care. For specialist nurse 1, this was a limit of what could be done as a palliative-care clinician and, to preserve her palliative-care identity, she needed to identify this boundary. As a senior clinician, she established limits for herself and others during case reviews and informal conversations. Others shared specialist nurse 1's despair and frustration, noting the systemic failures, with one nurse calling it a "broken system". They also offered each other words of care and encouragement, potentially to approve or legitimise the boundaries:

> You're doing a great job. You are such an amazing nurse [Specialist nurse 1]. It's so inspirational for us junior nurses.
>
> (*Generalist nurse 4*)

Like other instances of expressed anger or frustration at the 'system', patients, carers, or other clinicians, this was a moment of bonding. Clinician hardships strengthened their connections. Moments of frustration were almost always followed by collective care and compassion. Ultimately though, these expressions of emotions created boundaries of practice, identity, and emotion, establishing the borders of mindline assemblages.

Emotionful learning in practice

The emotional timbre of formal and informal interactions between clinicians extended from the community health centre to patient homes. Clinicians were required to constantly rethink and re-feel palliative care in terms of the diverse challenges they faced, shifting the types of labour required while engaging with their patients. Patients, carers, and clinicians described diverse and constantly changing intensifications of feeling as a terminal illness progressed.

Delivering care in the community was an important part of the way nurses considered their identity, where humanistic care and rapport-building were enabled without the structures of established health-service practices. They proudly described their exploits when navigating unconventional situations – like the generalist nurse who was praised for delivering palliative care to a patient in a hotel:

> This guy was an alcoholic living in a hotel. I was so impressed with [Generalist nurse 13]; the way she handled that – just went in and made that connection with him despite the situation.
>
> (*Specialist nurse 3*)

Mindful of their role in the community, these stories evoked determination in the face of uncertainty and complexity as a learned conviction. This pride fostered a resilient capacity to navigate unusual situations, sometimes at their peril, as nurses would often confront risk. Some were caught in flood waters, entered homes with menacing pets, or delivered care in unsanitary conditions – yet each story demonstrated an ability to overcome adversity.

Although this nurse did not refer to it as professionalism, she also spoke of the need to avoid emotions to provide 'good palliative care':

> A good nurse can will those emotions aside. If you are walking into a patient's home who's dying, in tears, not coping, then it's going to be hard for the family because they may not trust what you are doing. You want to give confidence when facing that suffering or that despair.
>
> (*Specialist nurse 5*)

Clinicians who appeared to maintain positive relationships with patients and carers learned to embrace chaotic environments, adapting quickly to different emotional and physical contexts.

Palliative-care clinicians were connected with certain mindline assemblages that incorporated specific actions, values, and ethical positions. Contradictory embodied and emotional positions were often present, contingent on the context and moment, and the potential emotive capacities of individuals as professionals, clinicians, or just as people. Emotion as a productive force was only available when that productiveness could be embodied in actions – for instance, clinicians managing a patient's pain or trainees developing a carer's skills. This might explain the relegation of emotion during discussions of patient diagnoses, as diagnoses in palliative care were unchangeable; thus, becoming performatively emotional about them was fruitless. This is not to suggest that clinicians were uncaring, but rather they generally directed their emotions to elements of care that could be impacted through 'productive' mindline assemblages: those related to pain management, social support, rapport-building, death and dying care, and setting palliative-care limits.

Emotion and mindline assemblages in healthcare

As our research suggests, emotions were central to the ways palliative-care clinicians conceived and enacted care for dying patients. Within formal and informal interactions, mindlines were assembled with emotion as a productive mechanism to prioritise or limit certain kinds of care. A reference to a patient as "suffering" acquired a performative function, framing the patient as deserving of care. The performative function of the suffering patient was bound with the clinicians' embodied empathy, implicating a mindline that purposely addressed that suffering. Part of the 'realness' Wieringa and Greenhalgh (2015) described as being so important in mindlines is the emotion that is felt and attached to particular experiences and exchanges. This chapter demonstrates that the affective resonance of suffering is an immediate, present sensation that stabilises some of the humanism of palliative care, shaping clinicians' practice. Here, emotions are assembled with the pieces of information that were transformed into action.

Collier (2013) suggested that palliative-care clinicians need to meet the needs of dying patients, their families, and healthcare workers by "learning to be affected" (p. 204). Doing this requires an openness to learn from, and be in tune with patients' and carers' experiences of, for instance, pain.

Within other assemblages, other forms of evidence, such as experiential or emotional, took precedence for clinicians, fostering experimentation and joyful combinations of care. Becoming affectively attuned can raise awareness of the problems and remedies of suffering (Shusterman 2006). Being affectively attuned means having a capacity to be moved or activated by other bodies – however, this does not mean that clinical knowledge is relegated. Professionalism can be bound with emotionful caring. Clinicians should be encouraged to engage with the embedded emotionality within medical encounters (Wong, Broom, Kirby et al. 2020). Positive emotions in these contexts can generate knowledge and creative solutions to intractable problems (Hodgins and Dadich 2017).

By highlighting the performance and discursive production of emotions within mindline assemblages, this study extends Gabbay and le May's work. Learning – and mindlines – can be reshaped through collective affective emotional positioning through, for instance, moments of joy, fear, and sorrow. In our study, clinicians performed or foreshadowed patient sadness and suffering; they used joy to affirm specific values, and they showed frustration and anger to establish the limits of mindline assemblages. Emotion was central to negotiating care and establishing priorities, like prioritising the care of a disabled grandchild of a dying patient, and creating space for self-preservation. Gabbay and le May described collective identity as "a social process of continual mutual heedful interacting between those who share it" (2011, p. 163). In this sense, clinicians are 'heedful' of the internal limits of palliative-care mindline assemblages. During case reviews, these limits were pronounced when physiological ailments were melded with emotional detachment, establishing limits of what can be discussed, when, and how. Our study supports the notion that emotion inherently coexists within mindline assemblages along with clinicians' "skills, norms, attitudes, and infrastructural demands" (Gabbay and le May 2004 p. 193).

Considering mindlines in the context of Deleuze and Guattari's (1987) ideas provides an enlightening philosophical grounding for future clinical workplace learning. For participants in our research, good palliative care did not have a linear fixity, where healthy become sick, a cure is introduced, and sick become well. Instead, different assemblages of 'good' palliative care were remade as quickly as they were becoming unproductive. Contemporary literature speaks to the complex world of clinical practice, where patients and carers "live in the messy, idiosyncratic, and unpredictable world of a particular person in a particular family context or … in a context of social isolation and/or abandonment" (Greenhalgh, Snow, Ryan et al. 2015). This 'messy world' is realised in community-based palliative care, with patients in a fluctuating space of the home, contending with physical, mental, spiritual, and social threats to their personhood while living with a life-limiting illness. Within clinical interaction, multiple mindline assemblages were evoked in close proximity, sometimes as binaries, like professionalism and familiarity, as well as attention to the body and attention to the social. These differently segmented territories produced more or less clear delimitations on the clinician-self, resulting in ongoing variations in clinical practice and identity.

Health services must be attentive to how mindlines are assembled within different contexts by allowing for interpretative, flexible, and relative ideas of care within emotional contexts. We need to give clinicians the material and conceptual space to consider and engage with their emotions and share those emotions with their colleagues to enhance learning in all of its forms. We must work against the 'oppressive[ness]' of rigid policy (Scott 2010) and promote ways to create and examine joyful combination of bodies and ideas. Allowing clinicians to identify novel, exhilarating, and magic moments and practices that exceed expectation and increase agency is a useful starting point, evidenced by recent scholarship (Dadich, Fulop, Ditton et al. 2015; Dadich, Collier, Hodgins et al. 2020; Collier, Hodgins, Crawford et al. 2019; Fulop, Dadich, Ditton et al. 2013; Dadich, Collier, Hodgins et al. 2018). Clinicians should be allowed to learn to be affected in productive ways. Being affected can lead to important discoveries, some of which might provide opportunities for experimentation in developing mindlines and produce alternative ways to care.

Summary

- We present findings from a study on mindlines and emotion in community-based palliative care.
- We demonstrate how emotions were assembled with mindlines to direct the attention of peers, exemplify good practices, and establish the limits of care.
- When nurses or doctors became emotional during review of patients, it heightened conversation about the issue at hand, creating focal points for different mindlines to be involved or developed.
- Emotion during interactions between clinicians also established the limits of mindlines (i.e., delineating what was and was not palliative care), helping to establish a shared sense of identity for palliative-care clinicians.

- Our findings suggest that health services need to continue to be attentive to how mindlines are assembled within different contexts by allowing for interpretative, flexible, and relative ideas of care within emotional contexts.
- Rather than insisting on unemotional objectivity in discussions about patient care, there is a strong argument for creating the space and 'giving permission' for emotional dimensions of patient care to be included in clinical discussions. This has the potential to improve the pertinence of clinical mindlines in the many clinical situations that inevitably invoke emotional responses.

Acknowledgements

To the amazing patients, carers, nurses, doctors, administrative team, and managers who were involved either principally or peripherally in this project, we thank you from the bottom of our hearts.

Michael Hodgins' PhD was completed with the Western Sydney University School of Business, with the support of the Australian Government Research Training Program Scholarship.

Note

1 We use the term 'performance' to clarify our limited ability as ethnographic researchers to determine the "true" felt emotions of participants as we observe them. We can mostly only observe and document emotions as outward expressions for the benefit of other participants in social interactions. It also emphasises the considered way participants expressed emotions to underscore their mindlines.

References

Benozzo A Colley H. 2012. 'Emotion and learning in the workplace: Critical perspectives'. *Journal of Workplace Learning*, 24: 304–316.

Collier A. 2013. *Deleuzians of patient safety: A video reflexive ethnography of end-of-life care*. University of Technology Sydney.

Collier A, Hodgins M, Crawford G, Every A, Womsley K, Jeffs C, Houthuysen P, Kang S, Thomas E, Weller V, Van C, Farrow C, Dadich A. 2019. 'What does it take to deliver brilliant home-based palliative care? Using positive organisational scholarship and video reflexive ethnography to explore the complexities of palliative care at home'. *Palliative Medicine*, 33: 91–101.

Dadich A, Collier A, Hodgins M. 2020. 'Navigating and understanding organisational complexity in health services: The value of POSH-VRE'. *Journal of Management & Organization*, 26, 375–390.

Dadich A, Collier A, Hodgins M, Crawford G. 2018. 'Using positive organizational scholarship in healthcare and video reflexive ethnography to examine positive deviance to new public Management in Healthcare'. *Qualitative Health Research*, 28: 1203–1216.

Dadich A, Fulop L, Ditton M, Eljiz K, Fitzgerald A, Hayes K, Herington C, Isouard G, Karmi L, Smyth A. 2015. 'Finding brilliance using positive organizational scholarship in healthcare'. *Journal of Health, Organization and Management*, 29(6): 750–777.

Deleuze G, Guattari F. 1984. *Anti-Oedipus: capitalism and schizophrenia*. Translated by R Hurley, M Seem, HR Lane London: Athlone.

Deleuze G, Guattari F. 1987. *A thousand plateaus: capitalism and schizophrenia*. Minneapolis, University of Minnesota Press.

Fulop L, Dadich A, Ditton M, Campbell S, Curry J, Eljiz K, Fitzgerald A, Hayes K, Isouard G, Herington C, Karimi L, Smyth A. 2013. Working on the edge: positive organisational scholarship in healthcare (POSH) and looking for what's good in healthcare. *27th ANZAM (Australian and New Zealand Academy of Management) Conference*. Hobart, TAS.

Gabbay J, le May A. 2004. 'Evidence based guidelines or collectively constructed "mindlines?" Ethnographic study of knowledge management in primary care'. *British Medical Journal*, 329:1013–1016.

Gabbay J. le May A. 2011. *Practice-based evidence for healthcare: clinical mindlines*. London; New York: Routledge.

Greenhalgh T. 2013. 'Why do we always end up here? Evidence-based medicine's conceptual cul-de-sacs and some off-road alternative routes'. *International Journal of Prosthodontics*, 26: 11–15.

Greenhalgh T, Snow R, Ryan S, Rees S, Salisbury H. 2015. 'Six "biases" against patients and carers in evidence-based medicine'. *BMC Medicine*, 13: 200.

Hochschild A. 1983. 'Comment on Kemper's "social constructionist and positivist approaches to the sociology of emotions"'. *American Journal of Sociology*, 89: 432–434.

Hodgins M, Dadich A. 2017. 'Positive emotion in knowledge creation'. *Journal of Health Organization and Management*, 31: 162–174.

Hökkä P, Vähäsantanen K, Paloniemi S. 2020. 'Emotions in learning at work : a literature review'. Vocations and Learning, 13(1): 1–25. https://doi.org/10.1007/s12186-019-09226-z

Kemper TD. 1981. 'Social constructionist and positivist approaches to the sociology of emotions'. *American Journal of Sociology*, 87(2): 336–362.

Parkinson B. 1995. *Ideas and realities of emotion*. London: Routledge.

Pile S. 2010. 'Emotions and affect in recent human geography'. *Transactions of the Institute of British Geographers*, 35: 5–20.

Savage J. 2004. 'Researching emotion: the need for coherence between focus, theory and methodology'. *Nursing Inquiry*, 11: 25–34.

Scott T. 2010. Conclusion. *Organization philosophy: Gehlen, Foucault, Deleuze*. London: Palgrave Macmillan UK.

Shusterman R. 2006. 'Thinking through the body, educating for the humanities: a plea for somaesthetics'. *Journal of Aesthetic Education*, 40: 1–21.

Thrift N. 2004. 'Intensities of feeling: towards a spatial politics of affect'. *Geografiska Annaler: Series B, Human Geography*, 86: 57–78.

Wieringa S, Engebretsen E, Heggen K, Greenhalgh T. 2018. 'Rethinking bias and truth in evidence-based health care'. *Journal of Evaluation in Clinical Practice*, 24: 930–938.

Wieringa S, Greenhalgh T. 2015. '10 years of mindlines: a systematic review and commentary'. *Implementation Science*, 10: 45.

Wong WT, Broom A, Kirby E, Lwin ZJH. 2020. 'What lies beneath? Experiencing Emotions and Caring in Oncology'. Health, 24:4; 348–365.

Zembylas M. 2007. 'Theory and methodology in researching emotions in education'. *International Journal of Research & Method in Education*, 30: 57–72.

7

RETHINKING NURSES' MINDLINES ABOUT THE LIVERPOOL CARE PATHWAY

The knowledge behind the care

Marianne Brattgjerd

Introduction

In this chapter, I draw on findings from my PhD project, in which I explored nurses' thought processes when using the Liverpool Care Pathway (LCP) in Norwegian nursing homes. This came about initially because of the controversy surrounding the LCP and a desire to understand better how nurses think about their practice when caring for patients at the end of their lives. By using a philosophical research technique that seeks to understand the many causes that lie beneath the surface of what we observe, I was able to consider the place of clinical mindlines when nurses use evidence-based practice.

Using an integrated care pathway for dying patients

The LCP is an integrated care pathway designed to ensure high-quality end-of-life care during the last days and hours of life (Ellershaw and Wilkinson 2011). The pathway was initially developed in the United Kingdom (UK) in the late 1990s to transfer palliative-care principles derived from hospice care into general healthcare settings, such as hospitals, home-care services, and nursing homes. It is currently in use in at least 17 countries worldwide (Husebø, Flo and Engedal 2017). In Norway, it is implemented in 459 institutions, including 23 hospitals, 330 nursing homes, and 106 home care municipalities (KLB 2019).

The core of the LCP is structured guidance for organising and coordinating palliative care, including comfort measures, anticipatory prescribing of medication, discontinuation of inappropriate interventions, and psychological/spiritual and family care (Ellershaw and Wilkinson 2011). The care pathway consists of three parts: (1) initial assessment of the patient's condition, including a plan for further treatment and care; (2) ongoing assessment of the plan of care; and (3) assessment

DOI: 10.4324/9781003158721-7

after death (Ellershaw and Wilkinson 2011). In Norway, the pathway is based on the 11th version of the LCP, translated and adapted to the Norwegian context. We refer to it as *Livets siste dagar* ("The last days of life").

Despite its promise of high-quality care, the LCP has drawn substantial criticism in recent years, including suggestions that it has led to deteriorating standards of care and the concealment of staff incompetence (Neuberger, Aarnovitch, Bonser et al. 2013; Nilsen 2015; Husebø, Flo and Engedal 2017). Specifically, the LCP has been accused of promoting a tick-box approach to palliative care without genuine concern for the care of patients or their relatives (Craig 2008a; Craig 2008b; Millard, Cole, Hargreaves et al. 2009; Devlin 2009; Phillips 2012; Neuberger, Aarnovitch, Bonser et al. 2013). Concerns have also been raised about hastening patients' deaths by denying them fluids and food and using syringe drivers to give continuous terminal sedation, without regard for the possibility of a wrong diagnosis (Millard, Cole, Hargreaves et al. 2009; Neuberger, Aarnovitch, Bonser et al. 2013). One consequence of such box-ticking may be that it becomes a self-fulfilling prophecy, where death is the inevitable outcome of care (Devlin 2009; Phillips 2012; Neuberger, Aarnovitch, Bonser et al. 2013). Accordingly, the UK government withdrew the LCP from all healthcare settings in 2014, stipulating that it should be replaced with a personalised end-of-life care plan (Neuberger, Aarnovitch, Bonser et al. 2013). No other country using the LCP has made a similar decision.

My review of the scientific literature revealed no evidence of poor care in relation to using the LCP. On the contrary, it highlighted several studies indicating that LCP could improve general end-of-life care (Brattgjerd 2021) This finding confirmed a positive national evaluation of the care pathway in Norway (Melby, Das, Halvorsen et al. 2016). More specifically, healthcare professionals reported that the structure of the pathway enabled them to become more alert to the holistic needs of dying patients (Brattgjerd and Olsen 2016; Andersson, Lindqvist, Fürst et al. 2018b; Olsson, Kling, Grundel et al. 2019). The LCP also ensured that healthcare professionals regularly assessed the needs and condition of dying patients (Gambles, Stirzaker, Jack et al. 2006; Veerbeek, Van Zuylen, Swart et al. 2008; Clark, Marshall, Sheward et al. 2012a; Clark, Marshall, Sheward et al. 2012b; Mayland, Williams, Addington-Hall et al. 2013; Andersson, Lindqvist, Fürst et al. 2018b; Olsson, Kling, Grundel et al. 2019; Brattgjerd, Olsen and Danielsen 2020). It seemed particularly useful to nurses, providing a clear plan for palliative care and, hence, preventing anxiety about what to do next (Walker and Read 2010; Iversen and Haugen 2015; Brattgjerd and Olsen 2016). Family members also reported positive attitudes towards the LCP (Veerbeek, Van Zuylen, Swart et al. 2008; Watson, Hockley and Murray 2010; Mayland, Williams, Addington-Hall et al. 2013; Costantini, Pellegrini, Di Leo et al. 2014a; Costantini, Romoli, Leo et al. 2014b; Ekeström, Olsson, Runesdotter et al. 2014; Brännström, Fürst, Tishelman et al. 2016; Andersson, Lindqvist, Fürst et al. 2018a). Several studies showed that they experienced a reduction in the symptom burden of dying patients when healthcare professionals used it (Veerbeek, Van Zuylen, Swart et al. 2008; Watson, Hockley and Murray et al. 2010; Mayland, Williams, Addington-Hall et al. 2013; Costantini, Romoli, Leo et al. 2014b; Brännström et al. 2016), as well as improved overall palliative communication (Ekeström, Olsson, Runesdotter et al. 2014). Other studies noted that family members saw their dying relatives treated with respect, kindness, and dignity when healthcare professionals used the LCP (Costantini, Pellegrini, Di Leo et al. 2014a; Costantini, Romoli, Leo et al. 2014b).

Overall, therefore, the picture is contradictory. On the one hand, there are serious criticisms that the LCP leads to deteriorating standards of care. On the other hand, the scientific literature indicates that the LCP contributes to high-quality end-of-life care. However, LCP studies generally tend to be evaluations based upon surface-level empirical data, giving little in-depth understanding of the thought processes and causal mechanisms that underlie the actions of nurses using this standardised approach to end-of-life care. It was a desire for deeper insights into what underpinned the way that nurses apply the LCP that laid the foundation of my PhD within Nord University's doctoral programme in professional praxis.

Methods

The project consisted of four qualitative empirical studies, of which three have been published (Brattgjerd and Olsen 2016; Brattgjerd, Danielsen, Næss et al. 2019; Brattgjerd, Olsen and Danielsen 2020). The three empirical studies used individual and focus-group interviews to gain in-depth insight into the use of the LCP in Norwegian nursing homes (Brattgjerd and Olsen 2016; Brattgjerd, Danielsen, Næss et al. 2019; Brattgjerd, Olsen and Danielsen 2020), involving 34 nurses working in 18 nursing homes (long-term ward, short-term ward, and palliative ward). These were sampled randomly from a comprehensive list supplied by a competence centre in western Norway that is responsible for the implementation and use of the LCP. The interviews lasted approximately 45–90 minutes and were audio-recorded and transcribed verbatim. All studies were conducted following the Declaration of Helsinki (WMA 1964/2013) and approved by the Norwegian Centre for Research Data.

The fourth study, for which a manuscript is in preparation, was a scoping review to map the available evidence regarding the use of the LCP for dying patients across healthcare settings. A total of 489 articles were screened for eligibility, and 29 studies were included in the review.

Dispositionalism

My research used a method designed to arrive at a deep understanding of individual cases, based on Mumford and Anjum's (2018, 2011) theory of causal dispositionalism. Dispositionalists work on the assumption that particular events occur as a result of multiple contingent causes, or 'causal dispositions', that come together to make them happen. So, to understand the causes of any particular event, the individual involved, be that the practitioner or the patient, is a key source of evidence about that particular set of causes (Anjum, Copeland and Rocca et al. 2020). This means exploring in depth the individual case, its unique context, and the causal dispositions that led to it. To abstract the findings in order to do that, I used what Danermark and colleagues term 'retroduction', a form of intuitive thought-operation, where essential data are extracted from the overall findings (Danermark, Ekström, Karlsson et al. 2015). The goal is not to generalise data to a population level ('empirical generalisation') but to generalise the findings to a theoretical level ('analytic generalisation'). The overall intention of this method was to delve beneath superficial observations to explore underlying causes, their meaning, and their sources (Anjum, 2016).

In short, this method enabled me to use my qualitative data as a way to generate a deeper level of knowledge, explanation, and understanding. More specifically, I was using this approach to explore and understand the thinking that underpinned the practice of nurses using the LCP in end-of-life care.

Episteme, techne, phronesis

Within this methodological framework, it was also possible to introduce a philosophical tradition that goes back millennia, but which still has contemporary currency, especially in the Scandinavian literature. Thus, perhaps unexpectedly for many readers, I synthesised the findings using an Aristotelian framework to interpret the meaning of the observed data at a deeper and more abstract level.

Aristotle regarded the human being as a living substance that comprises matter and form (Martinsen 1991). A person's 'matter' is the physical body that has mass and takes up space, whereas their 'form' is their rational soul (Feser 2019), which in modern parlance is typically translated as 'consciousness' or 'mind'. In Aristotelian terms, this is what gives the person life (Martinsen 1991), and it entails three forms of knowledge: episteme, techne, and phronesis (Ando 1965). **Episteme** deals solely with the theoretical and the unchangeable; it seeks to understand, on a general level, universal or essential principles of specific substances both inert (e.g., stones and houses) and living (e.g., trees, animals, and people). For episteme, the knowledge itself is the ultimate goal in its own right. **Techne**, however, is about the practical and the changeable; it seeks to understand not only universal principles but also the unique, contingent properties – what Aristotelians would have called the 'accidental principles' – of those specific substances. Techne, being a more instrumental type of knowledge – akin to a craft – that is external to the act itself and allows a person to cause things to happen, to create or change something. **Phronesis** also belongs to the practical and changeable domain. However, its value is more innate; phronesis is the kind of knowledge that tells a person what is intrinsically right or wrong about an event or act (Ando 1965). Thus, moral and good acts are dependent on phronesis being brought to bear in the decision-making process.

In short, when one is trying to understand a situation and decide what to do, episteme can be described as theoretical knowledge of its universal aspects, techne as the practical, contingent, instrumental knowledge, and phronesis as an understanding of the inherent ethical dimensions that require practical/political wisdom.

Results and discussion

Combining the dispositionalist approach with the aforementioned Aristotelian framework proved a surprisingly useful way to think about clinical mindlines. As a means of decision-making, mindlines could be seen as a way of representing causal dispositions within the nurses' minds – helping them to immediately assess the causes and forces affecting any given situation or action. Moreover, it was possible to see how mindlines allowed the nurses to simultaneously understand the universal principles (episteme) and contingent factors (techne) of a situation, and if possible (using phronesis) to make changes for the best.

The 'rigid-rational approach' or acting independently of the LCP?

All four of my studies revealed that the nurses experienced the LCP as a valuable tool in end-of-life care. They spoke about practice changing towards more proper and dignified care for dying patients and their relatives. These changes were most apparent in the long- and short-term wards but were also present in the palliative wards.

> It's so good! I mean, there is a plan to follow! We are now agreeing that we are not checking blood pressure, saturation, taking blood tests, giving antibiotics, you know. … And the prescribing of the medications – it's so good! The doctor is also very fond of it! Everything is well planned.
>
> *(Heidi, registered nurse, short-term ward, 19 years of experience)*

> I find the plan very useful … it helps us speak the same language when caring for the dying. … Looking for the same things … having focus on covering the same basic needs of the patients. … Before the introduction of the LCP … I think it was more chaotic. … There was no consensus on what to do.
>
> *(Karen, registered nurse, palliative nurse, short-term ward, 14 years of experience)*

Where nurses use only such knowledge as in the LCP, without thinking about the individual circumstance of each patient, I term it the 'rigid-rational approach'. However, the nurses in my studies did not use the LCP rigidly – nor indeed explicitly – in their ongoing bedside care of the dying patients. When the nurses' stories were thoroughly explored, it became evident that they were all acting independently of the LCP in the care of dying patients. More specifically, the interviews showed that they used the LCP in a manner that allowed them to work autonomously within its general tenets.

> What's good about the LCP is that it gives us important knowledge about end-of-life care. … I think this is especially important for the newly graduated nurses, but it is also a good reminder for the more experienced nurses.
>
> *(Lise, registered nurse, long-term ward, 24 years of experience)*

> When I enter the patient room, I am not thinking of the LCP … I mean. … How can I explain it? … I believe the points and the content of the LCP are in our heads in a way.
>
> *(Sarah, registered nurse, long-term ward, 14 years of experience)*

> I don't have the LCP with me in the patient's room. … I know the content of the plan … what to look for. … It has become automated in a way.
>
> *(Hannah, registered nurse, palliative nurse, palliative ward, four years of experience)*

Whilst clearly redolent of mindlines, these findings can also be interpreted using the philosophical lenses described in the previous section. The nurses were using the theoretical knowledge within this standardised instrument to extract and internalise universal principles into their clinical mindlines about end-of-life care. We might therefore view the LCP as a means to increase nurses' competence in end-of-life care by virtue of expanding their episteme. Through the dispositional lens, however, the episteme is itself part of the cause of the nurses' actions: it disposes them to think and act in certain ways. They must integrate that disposition with their other knowledge about each individual case, which enables them to construct ways of dealing with them individually.

The "flexible-rational" approach

The nurses' independence from the LCP was often related to the fact that dying patients have multiple comorbidities that are unique and cannot be solved by rigidly following universal principles or criteria. In line with Rittel and Webber (1973), we can consider these as 'wicked problems', meaning that they comprise both universal dispositions, which are common to all end-of-life care, and contingent dispositions that are unique for individual patients, which requires the nurses to be highly cognisant of each distinct situation.

> I always observe the patient. … Is he lying in a bad position? … Does he have pain? … you know. … You always have to be vigilant to the patient's situation.
>
> *(Anette, registered nurse, intensive care nurse, short-term ward, 30 years of experience)*

> You have to customise the care. … I give different care because people are different … so you have to make a judgement based on the full situation because every patient is unique.
>
> *(Martha, registered nurse, long-term ward, 15 years of experience)*

Aristotle emphasised this in his well-known quote: "Knowledge of health in general is not enough to cure a sick Socrates" (Dunne 1993, p. 282). In his terms, this can be interpreted as using techne, the practical rationality that is crucial to handling wicked or complex problems. Such techne is built up over time, through praxis.

When combining the universal principles extracted from the LCP with contingent, contextual factors, nurses can make sound decisions in highly complex situations. I have labelled this a flexible-rational approach in contrast to the rigid-rational approach (Brattgjerd 2021). The evidence is synthesised within the nurses' own clinical mindlines, which enables nurses to make sound decisions based on the best available practice-based evidence.

> I remember especially one patient. ... I have never seen anything like this. ... She had this terrible mucus ... and Robinul (an anticholinergic medication) had no effect. ... We do not usually suction the airways when patients are terminally ill because it often does more harm than good. ... But within this situation, we just had to. ... It looked like her own mucus suffocated her ... it was horrible! ... and I am glad we did because it removed the worst mucus, and she got a peaceful death within the end, so I am glad we did it.
>
> *(Ella, registered nurse, oncology nurse, palliative ward, 33 years of experience)*

However, using the LCP in a flexible-rational manner depends on having sufficient competence and training to interpret the patient's situation professionally. Nurses must also have enough time to deliberate when assessing the unique situation of the patient. This highlights the importance of having both sufficient competence and staffing in the ward. Otherwise, nurses are in danger of becoming more inclined to the box-ticking of the rigid-rational approach, leading to prescriptive and less thoughtful care, as was found in the UK (Neuberger, Aarnovitch, Bonser et al. 2013).

> If you don't have competence, the LCP can be a dangerous tool. I think you are more prone to use it rigidly.
>
> *(Aline, registered nurse, short-term ward, 12 years of experience)*

> Last summer, I was in charge of 32 patients ... and there was this patient on the LCP. ... I remember it as chaotic. ... They (assistants) could not dispense medications, nor did they know the patients or the routines. ... So I had to be everywhere! ... I did not have the time I wanted for the dying patient, nor his relatives. ... When I entered the patient's room, I only did what was most necessary. ... Turn the pillow and moisten the mouth. ... I remember when I was checking off the boxes at the end of the shift, I had this guilty feeling that I had not been doing a sufficiently good job.
>
> *(Lilly, registered nurse, long-term ward, three years of experience)*

Although a flexible-rational approach allows an understanding of the unique and distinct dispositions of individual patients' circumstances, it will always be merely instrumental by nature. Nurses using that approach do things to change things, such as alleviating pain and nausea; they find the means that work to efficiently achieve the end. However, the Norwegian pedagogue and philosopher Hans Skjervheim (2002) argues that while the instrumental approach is essential to professional practice, it becomes an 'instrumental fallacy' if used without including the ethical aspects that are prerequisites for morally good actions.

The value-rational approach

Kari Martinsen, a Norwegian nursing researcher, expands on this concern by contrasting two different approaches: 'seeing with the recording eye' and 'seeing with the heart's eye' (Martinsen 2000). Seeing with the recording eye can be described as the flexible-rational approach, which seeks to understand all the objective principles appertaining to the patient, with the overall purpose of alleviating or curing their symptoms. However, this 'recording eye' can lead to treating patients as objects, with no guarantee that an action is undertaken with genuine care. She argues that such a strategy can easily result in an emotionless and cold relationship between human beings; it is dehumanising. Martinsen (2000) asserts that genuine care of the patient depends on nurses seeing with the heart's eye, which means that assessing and treating them should be done with the intention of doing what is morally right and good. One needs, in other words, what I have called a 'value-rational approach'.

This approach can be equated to Aristotle's phronesis, the knowledge of the intrinsic moral value of the act itself. However, Aristotle did not think that one must choose between techne (flexible-rational approach) and phronesis (value-rational approach) as Martinsen argues. He believed that both strategies were important, but stressed that phronesis always has a higher position within the human soul (Ando 1965). This aligns with Skjervheim's (2002) thinking; he would maintain that the ethical approach is vital to prevent people from being objectified.

Based on these theoretical perspectives, one could say that the poor care found in the UK might not always have been related to a lack of competence or time when using the LCP. Perhaps the poor care came about through the lack of the value-rational approach so that patients might have been objectified without ethical and moral consideration; my research did not set out to answer this point. However, in interpreting my own Norwegian data, it appears that having a nurse who is acting with good values is a prerequisite for a patient to feel they are not being treated as an object. As human beings, we need others to confirm that our lives are worthy; life becomes empty and meaningless if people see and treat each other as objects. Hence, the value-rational approach should be the underlying foundation of all interactions, not least in healthcare settings when patients are in a vulnerable, dependent situation and their lives are in the hands of others.

As Martinsen (2003) reminds us, nursing at its core assumes that all human life has intrinsic value that goes beyond our looks, career, or material acquisitions. For the nurses in my study – and perhaps for all nursing – the value-rational approach depends on them having this view of human life integrated within their thinking. However, to put into practice what is morally required, this approach also depends on having the requisite time and resource; thus, for example, there must be enough staffing to enable nurses to include the value-rational dimension in their nursing practice.

The need for all three approaches

Together these theoretically informed empirical findings led me to a new model of the kinds of thinking and knowledge behind the nursing practice that I observed in end-of-life care. In that model, universal principles (from standardised instruments, for example) are used in a flexible-rational manner, but patients are also treated with the genuine kindness and respect demanded by a value-rational approach.

The model portrays the value-rational approach (phronesis) as the foundation, or the 'heart of nursing', that all the other approaches rest on. However, although the value-rational approach may be necessary for good nursing practice, it is not sufficient. Having a solid repertoire of moral virtues does not necessarily mean that the nurse also has proper nursing skills.

Professional nursing assumes an understanding of the patient's condition, their illness, and how to treat them correctly. This requires the kind of knowledge of universal principles (episteme) that is learned from books and scientific articles, from standardised instruments and guidelines, from talking with colleagues, or from being and acting in praxis (by using the senses). In these ways, nurses develop their knowledge about the mechanisms behind the dying process (e.g., circulatory failure, organ failure due to lack of oxygen), the symptoms (e.g., coolness, confusion, sleeping, incontinence, change in breathing), and the treatment (e.g., alleviating pain and other discomforts, managing mental, emotional, and spiritual needs).

We have seen, however, that acting purely on universal principles does not ensure proper nursing care. On the contrary, acting in a rigid-rational manner might lead to improper care of patients; it ignores the unique, contingent dispositions of the patient and their contexts. To ensure individualised healthcare based upon the best available evidence, nurses need also to amalgamate the flexible-rational approach (techne), combining universal principles with the unique dispositions of the situation. For example, there is consensus that parenteral fluids can cause more harm than benefits in the last stages of life due to potential fluid retention and pulmonary oedema (Helsedirektoratet 2018). However, this should not be treated as a universal principle applicable to all dying patients. On the contrary, research shows that some patients might benefit from small amounts of subcutaneous fluids in the last stages of life (Bowen, Mansfield and King 2014). Therefore, giving hydration as an intervention must be considered, depending on the unique dispositions of the patient and the situation. The flexible-rational approach assumes that nurses have the competence and the time to deliberate. Only then are they capable of customising the care to the individual patient.

Clinical mindlines in nursing practice drive all three approaches

From my analysis of how nurses used the LCP, I have suggested that the ancient concepts of episteme, techne, and phronesis help us understand the types of knowledge that underpin the three approaches that they used – rigid-rational, flexible-rational, and value-rational. Alternatively, one could say that this represents three key domains within the nurse's mindlines, or perhaps three overarching spaces within which their mindlines were constructed. Mindlines that lead to high-quality practice require all three types of knowledge. For example, if a nurse were invoking only the episteme, the nursing practice will tend towards a rigid-rational approach. However, if both episteme and the techne are being put into practice, the nursing practice will tend towards a flexible-rational approach. And finally, it is only when phronesis is also being invoked, thus supporting the value-rational approach, that 'the heart of nursing' starts to beat.

These findings support the idea that nurses' mindlines contribute and coordinate knowledge from a wide range of sources in order to give proper and morally good patient care. Gabbay and le May's (2011) original idea of the concept of mindlines portrayed them as social constructs. I prefer to think of them as real forces that drive nursing practice through a combination of rigid-rational, flexible-rational, and value-rational approaches. However, this conclusion must be further explored and confirmed by new empirical studies that move beyond this study of just one branch of nursing.

Summary

- I have explored the thinking behind nursing practice when nurses are using a standardised instrument, the Liverpool Care Pathway.
- Using a standardised instrument rigidly might lead to improper patient care (rigid-rational approach).
- Using a standardised instrument flexibly might lead to individualised patient care (flexible-rational approach).
- The flexible-rational approach is, however, instrumental in nature and is no guarantee of treating the patient with dignity and kindness.
- Only when also using the value-rational approach does 'the heart of nursing' start to beat.
- To be effective in helping nurses deliver good care, therefore, their mindlines need to comprise all three of these approaches.

Acknowledgements

I would like to thank my supervisors, Rose Marie Olsen and Inger J. Danielsen, for their dedicated support and guidance throughout the work on the doctoral project.

The PhD project was funded by Nord University, Norway.

References

Andersson S, Lindqvist O, Fürst C-J, Brännström M. 2018a. 'Family members' experiences of care of the dying in residential care homes where the Liverpool Care Pathway was used'. *International Journal of Palliative Nursing*, 24: 194–202.

Andersson S, Lindqvist O, Fürst CJ, Brännström M. 2018b. 'Care professional's experiences about using Liverpool Care Pathway in end-of-life care in residential care homes'. *Scandinavian Journal of Caring Sciences*, 32: 299–308.

Ando T. 1965. *Aristotle's theory of practical cognition*. The Hague, Netherlands: Springer.

Anjum RL, Copeland S, Rocca E. (Ed.). 2020. *Rethinking causality, complexity and evidence for the unique patient: a causehealth resource for healthcare professionals and the clinical encounter.* Cham, Switerland: Springer.
Bowen P, Mansfield A, King H. 2014. 'Using subcutaneous fluids in end-of-life care'. *Nursing Times*, 110: 12–14.
Brattgjerd M. (2021). *Standardisering av sykepleie. Hvordan påvirkes profesjonsutøvelsen?* Doktorgradsavhandling. Nord Universitet (Standardization in nursing. How is the practice affected? Doctoral dissertation. Nord University) https://nordopen.nord.no/nord-xmlui/handle/11250/2770986
Brattgjerd M, Danielsen IJ, Næss G, Olsen RM. 2019. 'Dokumentasjonspraksis og bruk av elektronisk tiltaksplan for døende pasienter i sykehjem–en mysteriefokusert studie', in R. Hellesø, R. Olsen (Eds.) *Digitalisering i sykepleietjenestenen–en arbeidshverdag i endring*. Oslo: Cappelen Damm Akademisk/NOASP (Nordic Open Acess Scholarly Publishing).
Brattgjerd M, Olsen RM, Danielsen I. 2020. 'End-of-life care and the use of an integrated care pathway'. *The Qualitative Report*, 25: 216–237.
Brattgjerd M, Olsen RM. 2016. 'Care at the end of life – a qualitative study of nurses' experiences in using the Liverpool Care Pathway in nursing homes'. *Tidsskrift for Omsorgsforskning*, 2: 189–201.
Brännström M, Fürst CJ, Tishelman C, Petzold M, Lindqvist O. 2016. 'Effectiveness of the Liverpool care pathway for the dying in residential care homes: an exploratory, controlled before-and-after study'. *Palliative Medicine*, 30: 54–63.
Clark J, Marshall B, Sheward K, Allan SG. 2012a. 'Staff perceptions of the impact of the Liverpool Care Pathway in aged residential care in New Zealand'. *International Journal of Palliative Nursing*, 18: 171–177.
Clark J, Marshall B, Sheward K, Allan SG. 2012b. 'Staff perceptions of end-of-life care following implementation of the liverpool care pathway for the dying patient in the acute care setting: A New Zealand perspective'. *Journal of Palliative Medicine*, 15: 468–473.
Costantini M, Pellegrini F, Di Leo S, Beccaro M, Rossi C, Flego G, Romoli V, Giannotti M, Morone P, Ivaldi GP, Cavallo L, Fusco F, Higginson IJ. 2014a. 'The Liverpool Care Pathway for cancer patients dying in hospital medical wards: A before-after cluster phase II trial of outcomes reported by family members'. *Palliative Medicine*, 28: 10–17.
Costantini M, Romoli V, Leo SD, Beccaro M, Bono L, Pilastri P, Miccinesi G, Valenti D, Peruselli C, Bulli F, Franceschini C, Grubich S, Brunelli C, Martini C, Pellegrini F, Higginson IJ. 2014b. 'Liverpool Care Pathway for patients with cancer in hospital: a cluster randomised trial'. *The Lancet*, 383: 226–237.
Craig G. 2008a. 'Palliative care and sedation: The Liverpool Care Pathway'. *BMJ*, 336: 781.
Craig G. 2008b. 'Palliative care in overdrive: patients in danger'. *American Journal of Hospice & Palliative Medicine*, 25: 155–160.
Danermark B, Ekström M, Karlsson JC, Jacobsen L. 2015. *Explaining society: critical realism in social sciences*. London: Routledge.
Devlin K. 2009. 'Sentenced to death on the NHS'. *The Daily Telegraph*.
Dunne J. 1993. '*Back to the rough ground': 'phronesis' and 'techne' in modern philosophy and in Aristotle*. London, University of Notre Dame Press.
Ekeström ML, Olsson M, Runesdotter S, Fürst CJ. 2014. 'Family members' experiences of the impact of the LCP in a palliative care unit and a geriatric ward in Sweden'. *International Journal of Palliative Nursing*, 20: 381–386.
Ellershaw J, Wilkinson S. 2011. *Care of the dying: a pathway to excellence*. Oxford: Oxford University Press.

Feser E. 2019. *Aristotle's revenge: the metaphysical foundations of physical and biological science.* Germany: Editiones scholasticae.

Gabbay J, le May, A. 2011. *Practice-based evidence for healthcare - clinical mindlines.* Oxon: Routledge.

Gambles M, Stirzaker S, Jack BA, Ellershaw JE. 2006. 'The Liverpool Care Pathway in hospices: an exploratory study of doctor and nurse perceptions'. *International Journal of Palliative Nursing*, 12: 414–421.

Helsedirektoratet. 2018. *Nasjonale faglige råd for lindrende behandling i livets sluttfase (National guidelines for palliative care in end-of-life care).* Oslo: Helsedirektoratet. https://www.helsedirektoratet.no/faglige-rad/lindrende-behandling-i-livets-sluttfase

Husebø BS, Flo E, Engedal K. 2017. 'The Liverpool Care Pathway: discarded in cancer patients but good enough for dying nursing home patients? A systematic review'. *BMC Medical Ethics*, 18: 1–13.

Iversen GS, Haugen DF. 2015. 'Staff experiences with use of the Liverpool Care Pathway in two Norwegian hospitals'. *Sykepleien Forskning*, 10: 144–151.

KLB. 2019. *Registrerte brukersteder for Livets siste dagar* [Online]. Available: https://helse-bergen.no/seksjon/KLB/Documents/Livets%20siste%20dagar/Brukersteder_Livets%20siste%20dager.pdf

Martinsen V. 1991. *Filosofi: en innføring.* Oslo: Kontekst.

Martinsen K. 2000. *Øyet og kallet.* Bergen: Faagbokforlaget.

Martinsen K. 2003. *Fra Marx til Løgstrup. Om etikk og sanselighet i sykepleien. 2. utg.* Oslo: Universitetsforlaget.

Mayland C, Williams E, Addington-Hall J, Cox T, Ellershaw J. 2013. 'Does the "Liverpool Care Pathway" facilitate an improvement in quality of care for dying cancer patients'. *British Journal of Cancer*, 108: 1942–1948.

Melby L, Das A, Halvorsen T, Steinhaug S. 2016. Rapport. Evaluering av tjenestetilbudet til personer med behov for lindrende behandling og omsorg. Available: https://helsedirektoratet.no/Documents/Nyheter/A27799%20Rapport%20lindrende%20behandling_revidert%202017.pdf

Millard PH, Cole A, Hargreaves P, Hill D, Negus E, Salisbury DL. 2009. 'Dying patients'. *The Daily Telegraph.*

Mumford S, Anjum RL. 2011. *Getting causes from powers* Oxford: Oxford University Press.

Neuberger JB, Aarnovitch D, Bonser T, Charlesworth-Smith D, Cox D, Guthrie C, Hameed K, Pentregarth H, Jackson E, Waller S. 2013. More care, less pathway: A review of the Liverpool care pathway. Available: https://www.gov.uk/government/uploads/system/uploads/attachment_data/file/212450/Liverpool_Care_Pathway.pdf [Accessed 21-11-16].

Nilsen L. 2015. Mener bruk av tiltaksplan bør stoppes. 07.02.15. *Dagens Medisin*

Olsson C, Kling E, Grundel PK, Larsson M. 2019. 'Impact of the Liverpool Care Pathway on quality end-of-care in residential care homes and home care—Nurses' perceptions'. *Nursing Open*, 6: 1589–1599.

Phillips B. 2012. 'Care? No, this is a pathway to killing people that doctors deem worthless'. Available: www.dailymail.co.uk/debate/article-2217748/Care-No-pathway-killing-peopledoctors-deem-worthless.html

Rittel HWJ, Webber MM. 1973. 'Dilemmas in a general theory of planning'. *Policy Sciences*, 4: 155–169.

Skjervheim H. 2002. 'Det instrumentalistiske mistaket', in J Hellesnes, G. Skirbekk (Eds.) *Mennesket.* Oslo: Universitetsforlaget.

Veerbeek L, Van Zuylen L, Swart SJ, Van Der Maas PJ, De Vogel-Voogt E, Van Der Rijt CCD, Van Der Heide A. 2008. 'The effect of the Liverpool Care Pathway for the dying: a multi-centre study'. *Palliative Medicine*, 22: 145–151.

Walker R, Read S. 2010. 'The Liverpool Care Pathway in intensive care: an exploratory study of doctor and nurse perceptions'. *International Journal of Palliative Nursing*, 16: 267–273.

Watson J, Hockley J, Murray S. 2010. 'Evaluating effectiveness of the GSFCJ and LCP in care homes' *End of Life Care Journal*, 4: 42–49.

WMA. 1964/2013. *The declaration of Helsinki. Ethical principles for medical research involving human subjects.* [Online]. Available: https://www.wma.net/policies-post/wma-declaration-of-helsinki-ethical-principles-for-medical-research-involving-human-subjects/

8

HOW MINDLINES WERE SHEPHERDED ACROSS COMPLEX NETWORKS, ENABLING NEW LEARNING ABOUT SEPSIS TO FLOURISH

Tricia R Tooman

Introduction

Many years ago, when working in the Continuing Professional Development (CPD) field, I began to wonder how, and if, CPD really did affect clinical behaviours. Study after study provided limited support for the role of ongoing education in affecting how doctors and nurses practised, but nothing really seemed to get to the bottom of how CPD worked, and how we could make it work better (Davis, O'Brien, Freemantle et al. 1999; Forsetlund, Bjørndal, Rashidian et al. 2009). Intuitively, we believed educational interventions helped clinicians' practice, but it was unclear how (Olson & Tooman 2012). As a result, I expanded my focus to see what answers could be found in the field of knowledge mobilisation. Here I 'met' the concept of clinical mindlines, which helped to capture and conceptualise knowledge in far more nuanced ways, addressing the complexity of knowledge *and* knowing. Hitherto, our often over-simplified ways of conceiving knowledge had in turn led to overly simplistic ways of training, examining, maintaining, and licensing clinicians (e.g., based on one's ability to regurgitate information). Eventually, I began my doctoral studies where I considered how knowledge is developed and used by looking at a particular area of practice.

I undertook a case study of a sepsis-focused knowledge network made up of interconnected research, policy, and practice communities. My fieldwork entailed documentary, observational, and interview data collection and analysis. The in-depth observations and interviews were undertaken in Scotland where a national policy network including policymakers and clinicians (the Sepsis Collaborative) was based. These data were augmented and contextualised by 'following' the internationally based sepsis-research community (the Surviving Sepsis Campaign). I did this by scouring publications, organisational websites, and related documents to trace the creation of a sepsis definition and guidelines from their inception through

DOI: 10.4324/9781003158721-8

their evolution over several decades (for the definition of sepsis, this was 1992, 2003, 2016, and for the guidelines, in 1992, 2001, 2004, 2008, 2013, 2017). The practice community I explored was a high-performing hospital in Scotland (named here as Aurora), which was a forerunner, since the 1980s, in addressing sepsis in the country. At Aurora, I collected data from interviews, observations, and documents over a 13-month period. Melding these data sources enabled me to understand better:

1. the many structures that enable interactions between people that facilitate mindline development and/or enhancement,
2. how mindlines in this case study were 'shepherded' within and across the networks to bring about high-performing sepsis care, and
3. how individual and collective mindlines work in tandem and tension.

In this chapter, I will elaborate on each of these key points.

The 'emergence' of sepsis

But first, let me tell you why sepsis is important. Although sepsis has been around for a very long time, killing tens of thousands of people every year, until the 1990s, it remained a puzzle shrouded largely by confusion and uncertainty. Considering sepsis was named in ancient Greek literature, it seems strange that as recently as 1989 Bone and colleagues were compelled to publish a piece declaring that sepsis was indeed "a valid clinical entity" (Bone, Fisher, Clemmer et al. 1989, p. 389). This publication marked the beginning of a collaborative process that paved a way to constructing a clear definition of sepsis, ways to promote early identification, and, importantly, recommendations for treatment (Tooman 2019, p. 110). This effort brought together the research, policy, and practice communities and provided me the opportunity to study how they learned, shared, and put their knowledge into practice. Table 8.1 illustrates critical aspects of the recent history of sepsis and tells something of the key influencers[1] over the last three decades. (A full account is available in Tooman 2019, Chapter 5.) Box 8.1 summarises the sample I used to explore sepsis further.

Enabling structures: people, processes, and materials

CPD is facilitated through many kinds of structures, e.g., formal courses and less formal learning and teaching opportunities, print, and online materials as well as protected time for study. Such components can link with structures in the workplace to build a supportive and interactive learning milieu. I was interested to see if (and where) the sepsis communities had such enabling structures where learning was facilitated and mindlines could be developed or enhanced.

I uncovered an array of structures – some expected, others not. These structures can be placed into three categories: the configuration of *people*, the interactional

TABLE 8.1 Influential groups, individuals, and events; key terms, and acronyms (see Tooman 2019 for greater detail)

Influential groups	
European Society of Intensive Care Medicine	ESICM is a medical specialist society based in Europe with an associated journal, *Intensive Care Medicine*. The ESICM and SCCM (their North American counterpart) jointly preside over sepsis definitions and guidelines work, with individual actors from each society engaged in both initiatives.
Institute for Healthcare Improvement	IHI specialises in quality improvement and patient safety. They partnered with ESICM and SCCM in the Surviving Sepsis Campaign to aid the application of guidelines in clinical care. IHI advocates the standardisation of care through, among other quality improvement techniques, the development of care bundles.
Society for Critical Care Medicine	SCCM is a medical specialist society based in North America with an associated journal, *Critical Care Medicine (CCM)*. In partnership with the American College of Chest Physicians (ACCP) SCCM organised the first sepsis-focused consensus meeting. Thereafter, it has been a co-lead with ESICM for sepsis definition and guideline development.
Surviving Sepsis Campaign	SSC is an international quality improvement collaboration spearheaded by ESICM and SCCM and was joined early on by IHI.
Scottish Patient Safety Programme	SPSP is a Scotland-based, quality-improvement programme established in 2008 with a partnership between NHS Scotland and IHI. The Sepsis Collaborative was part of the SPSP effort.
Notable individuals	
Bone	Roger Bone first articulated the concept of 'sepsis syndrome', conducted foundation clinical trials, and chaired the 1991 ACCP/SCCM Consensus Conference that proposed the concepts of SIRS (Systemic Inflammatory Response Syndrome). He died in 1997 and was described in this way by Marshall in his moving tribute: "Roger Bone's ideas transformed clinical research in sepsis. He led a revolution in the way we see the disease."
Dellinger	R. Phillip Dellinger is a former president of SCCM and a lead in the SSC collaboration. He has partnered with many in consensus-focused sepsis publications (in addition to his own clinical and lab-based work numbering 30 books and hundreds of articles) since 2001 and continues to this day. He was lead author for the SSC Guideline publications in 2004, 2008, and 2013.
Knaus	William A. Knaus in the 1980s created the first scoring system (the APACHE score) that rapidly predicted the severity of illness. Knaus was one of seven Session Chairmen in the 1991 Consensus Conference. The 1992 publication advocated the use of quantified measures (i.e., a scoring system) to identify patients at risk of sepsis, at least potentially because Knaus brought his expertise and ideas to their collaboration.

Marshall	John C. Marshall is a leading sepsis researcher and practitioner. He attended Bone's Consensus Conference in 1991 and co-authored the first sepsis definition and guideline materials and has remained active over the last three decades. He is a co-author of the most recent SSC Guidelines. His 2010 publication gave a first-hand potted history of the SSC, which proved valuable in my research.
Vincent	Jean-Louis Vincent is a highly productive researcher, intensive-care practitioner, and past president of the ESICM. Along with Dellinger, he joined the collaborative efforts noted here in the 2001 publication and remains active. Notably, he was a vocal critic of using SIRS to define sepsis and developed an alternative score, the Sepsis-Related Organ Failure Assessment (SOFA), which is now used to assess risk of sepsis.
Key events	
1989	Sepsis defended as "a valid clinical entity" by Bone and co-authors in *CCM*.
1991	ACCP/SCCM Consensus Conference took place in Chicago. The meeting resulted in the first definition of sepsis and related treatment guidelines. Spearheaded by members from two North American medical specialist societies, the SCCM and the ACCP, chaired by Bone and attended by Knaus, Dellinger, and Marshall, among other experts.
1992	Publication of first the sepsis definition ("SIRS", later interchangeable with term "Sepsis-1") and guidelines from 1991 ACCP/SCCM Consensus Conference.
1997	Vincent published an editorial in *Intensive Care Medicine (ICM)*, "Dear SIRS, I'm Sorry to Say That I Don't Like You". This publication indicated the difference of opinion regarding SIRS that existed within the research community.
1998	Bone and Dellinger responded to Vincent with their own editorial published in *CCM*, "To SIRS with Love".
2001	Publication and expansion of second set of sepsis guidelines.
2002	SSC officially launched.
2003	Publication of second sepsis definition ("Sepsis-2") that modified a SIRS-based definition to include an expanded list of diagnostic criteria.
2004	SSC Guidelines publication. First of the ongoing SSC series of publications.
2008	Next iteration of SSC Guidelines publication.
2013	Further iteration of SSC Guidelines publication.
2016	Most recent definition of sepsis, "Sepsis-3". The Sepsis Definitions Task Force markedly shifted by removing all connections to SIRS criteria. As a result, sepsis was no longer linked with SIRS.
2017	Most recent publication of SSC Guidelines. Discarded SIRS-based scoring system for SOFA.

(*Continued*)

TABLE 8.1 (Continued)

Key sepsis-related terms and acronyms	
SIRS	Systemic Inflammatory Response Syndrome was the first definition of sepsis agreed upon by Bone and colleagues in 1991 (published in 1992).
Observation Charts	Bedside monitoring tool used to record patient data, such as blood pressure, temperature.
Early Warning Scores	Quantitative risk-calculation scores based on measurements routinely collected via patient observation charts. Also called 'track and trigger tools'.
SIRS Score	The first early warning score for sepsis.
NEWS	National Early Warning Score developed by the Royal College of Physicians for the NHS in 2012. The Sepsis Collaborative in Scotland supported the use of NEWS scores for identifying patients at risk for developing sepsis.
SOFA	Sepsis-Related Organ Failure Assessment score developed by the ESICM. Vincent was lead author in SOFA development publications.
Care Bundles	An IHI quality improvement technique, care bundles simplify clinical practice guidelines into a set of defined tasks.

BOX 8.1 THE THREE INTERCONNECTED NETWORKS – MY SAMPLE

Interconnected Networks

SSC – An international research-based network that develops and distributes materials for use in policy and practice. Chaired by two professional specialist societies: the Society for Critical Care Medicine and the ESICM. Documentary data included key definition and guideline publications, hundreds of further sepsis-related publications and reports, and sepsis organisations' website content.

NHS Scotland (NHSS) Sepsis Collaborative – A national policy-oriented network that includes policy leaders and clinicians from every regional health board in Scotland. Data sources included publicly available documents such as NHS Scotland reports, guidelines, SPSP materials, and publications, including evaluation of the Sepsis Collaborative. I conducted five interviews with collaborative leaders and participants, and attended and observed three day-long meetings.

Aurora General Hospital – A local Scottish practice-based network of people providing sepsis-related care. Data sources included performance and audit data, materials developed onsite (e.g., patient observation charts and a sepsis sticker for their patient records), 25 formal interviews with those leading and involved in sepsis care at the hospital, and 13 months of observation via regular site visits.

processes, and the *materials* they use to coordinate the flow of their knowledge between them (see Paul Engel's 1997 work). The *people* are individual and collective actors who are clustered in specific departments, teams, and organisational memberships based on their knowledge (and often their roles). For example, at Aurora, the people included the Intensive Care Unit (ICU) and the Critical Care Outreach teams. Elsewhere, individual influencers, opinion leaders and researchers organised into collective actors such as NHS Scotland's Sepsis Collaborative, the SSC, and the various specialist medical societies. *Processes* are the activities and ways actors connect to develop, share, and use their knowledge. They include team meetings, specialised working groups, educational activities such as obtaining and maintaining licensure, procedures such as critical incident systems, calculating and tracking early warning scores. Further examples include consensus-building activities like voting, as well as the activity of reading other actors' work. *Materials* are the physical objects created by actors that are explicit presentations of actors' knowledge. Some examples are guidelines, journal articles, policies, checklists, audit data, patient observation charts.

Clinicians naturally draw on many sources and forms of knowledge to 'know' how best to do their work – this is at the centre of the mindlines model. I also saw this in my research as it became evident that sepsis-focused mindlines were influenced and shaped through *many* differing kinds of structures, specifically, the ways different people engaged and learned from one another, their processes, and materials.

For example, at Aurora, a senior ICU doctor in the 1980s noted that patients were deteriorating and dying, in his view, unnecessarily due to sepsis. Too often, patients would be rushed from a general ward to the ICU because they had deteriorated unnoticed until one or more organs began to fail. He reasoned that having different charts (e.g., for medications, fluid intake and output, breathing, and bowel function) made it difficult to put the pieces together and 'see' if a patient was struggling. Along with his ICU medical and nursing colleagues, they trialled a new combined chart to address this fragmentation of information. However, the combined chart did not alter the last-minute transfer of very unwell patients as they had hoped. They added colour (red, amber, green) where these numbers were placed on the patient chart to visually 'trigger' areas of concern, based on reading about 'trigger tools' in a medical journal. But the ward staff still found it difficult to identify a patient at risk of sepsis. In the mid-1990s, the same ICU doctor came across Bone et al.'s SIRS definition and went about incorporating the material into their observation chart. Their expectations were high. However, the problem continued. To share their specialist knowledge with others in the hospital, the ICU staff began in-house/hospital training sessions on how to use the chart to identify a patient at risk and what to do in response. And yet, to their frustration, patients continued to suffer. Funding was then put in place that allowed the ICU to share their specialist knowledge regularly and in person via an outreach team. The Critical Care Outreach Team (CCOT) started with one senior ICU nurse who would be physically present to support the ward nurses. Only then, with the CCOT structure, alongside the SIRS-reliant charting materials and processes, did Aurora begin to notice a turnaround in their sepsis-related deaths. Success at Aurora was based on using a range of organising structures. Structures like the CCOT facilitated connections between people by crossing the physical and thereby relational boundaries between the ICU and the general wards. Such structures compiled their collective knowledge into their materials and then embedded these materials within their processes (e.g., calculating SIRS scores when taking patient observations) to bring the personnel and the materials together.

Critically, I observed that the interactions between people, either one-to-one (e.g., the CCOT nurses providing on-the-job mentoring to the ward staff) or in groups (such as consensus-building meetings) were a central component of these structures. Such interactions enabled mindlines to not only be shared but also 'caught', developed, and expanded so the now collective mindline could be formally condensed and codified into guidelines (or similar) for wider mobilisation. One example was the process of developing sepsis definitions and guidelines. The Consensus Conference that Bone chaired in 1991 was the first time two professional organisations had been assembled to coordinate a sepsis effort (Bone, Balk, Cerra et al. 1992a, 1992b; Marshall, Dellinger & Levy 2010). The meeting brought together not just distinct professional societies but actors from different locales, roles, and specialisations. Attendees were medical-school leaders, researchers, practising clinicians, and pharmacists. They specialised in medicine, infectious diseases, emergency medicine, pulmonary, respiratory, and critical care, as well as pharmaceuticals (industry). Prior to this meeting, they were largely separated in their specialised siloes. But for the first time, actors with a shared concern for sepsis were brought together.

Publications from their ongoing work have provided an account of regular communication between actors. They use words and phrases such as "considerable debate" (Levy, Fink & Marshall 2003) and "vigorous debate" (Angus 2016), "elusive consensus" (Jaeschke, Guyatt, Dellinger et al. 2008), "passionate disagreement" (Marshall, Dellinger and Levy 2010) and "intentional compromise" (Angus 2016). Marshall, Dellinger and Levy (2010) describe the SSC community this way:

> The story of its origins, successes, and failures bears a resemblance to a work of classic theatre – part comedy, part high drama, both set against a backdrop of tragedy – [namely] the continuing toll of deaths from one of the leading causes of preventable death around the globe.
>
> *(p. 276)*

Together they learned and changed how they made decisions. Because group interactions could be dominated "by individuals with powerful personalities and intimidating reputations" (Jaeschke, Guyatt, Dellinger et al. 2008, p. 327), they instituted a Delphi process to generate consensus that provided a way that allowed all members of the group to speak their views. In these writings, we see hints that they experienced the full gamut of human engagement.

These interactions could be seen within Aurora as well. The CCOT provided opportunities for expertise (expert mindlines) to circulate through contact with others in the hospital. These relationships enabled the team to influence and shape other's mindlines about sepsis – how to see it and how to act on what they saw. The CCOT was a structure that provided not only a practical and knowledge-based resource for developing mindlines in others, but it also provided a level of reassurance and comfort that may have ameliorated the psychological and emotional uncertainties associated with such high-risk care: this amalgam enabled practitioners to use sepsis knowledge-in-practice-in-context.

Other informal, relational structures emerged as important. The hallways and corridors and the break room and canteens also provided space for interactions where connections were made, and trust was built. These kinds of low-risk contact-built relationships are critical to sharing and shaping ideas and mindlines not only because of the ease with which they occurred since they required little or no organisation but also because they were seen as largely acceptable and safe encounters. Many of the discussions were of a normal workplace sort – a mix of personal and professional – about holidays and children, as well as the patients leaving them feeling uneasy in Ward 10 or trying to make sense of the shift from one technique to another, e.g., SIRS to NEWS.

Collegial contact and discussions over time provided the 'relational oil' that smoothed communications (i.e., mindline sharing) when, later, they came under pressure. For instance, a CCOT nurse was advocating elevating care for a patient 'up' to the ICU. But the ward-based doctor responsible for the patient did not agree that urgent action was required. The CCOT nurse and doctor knew one another and had formed a relationship through prior work, corridor conversations, or other interactions. When the nurse found out that the doctor had blocked the patient transfer, she sought him out. He listened and, while he made clear he continued to have reservations, agreed to move the patient to the higher level of care as the nurse knew the ICU had capacity (another form of knowledge, a local mindline), and the ICU medical staff would almost certainly agree with her (they did). Soon afterwards, the doctor apologised to the nurse for not trusting her judgement immediately.

Shepherding mindlines

Interactions and relationships are of great importance to the development of mindlines, knowledge mobilisation, and learning; we have already seen in this case study they were central to bringing about high-performing sepsis care. I use the term 'shepherding' to describe how these inter-relational practices were enabled and made visible.

Shepherding could be understood as an integral part of a leadership role. And while some leaders may well shepherd (I did see this in my data), there were others who shepherded but were not in leadership roles. Instead, shepherding, I suggest, is a collection of practices, rather than a role, that cultivate the development, sharing, and use of knowledge at the actor-to-actor level. Shepherding is the relational connections that facilitate mindlines. These practices include nurturing, challenging, influencing, negotiating, and shaping knowledge, as well as growing trust. They were evident in all three communities. Boundaries can be addressed through shepherding, and tensions can be managed either by building them up or smoothing them down and by reducing resistance (or not). Shepherding entails seeking out connections between actors and working with them. This work includes challenging existing views, providing opportunities to modify understanding, knowing when to push and when to hold or wait for a better time, facilitating the re-binding of different forms of knowledge, and, in some instances, enabling relationships to mend. These, often subtle, social processes bring together different forms of knowing (tending the knowledge) and relevant actors and communities (tending the knowers). Box 8.2 shows some examples of shepherding. Additionally, and importantly, shepherding encourages the creation of interconnected networks of actors for mobilising knowledge and implementation. While the documentary sources from the SSC could not provide direct observation of their interactions, such as was available in the other two networks, these data nevertheless provided hints that shepherding practices supported actor engagement. What began as an early collaboration between two North American professional medical societies,

BOX 8.2 EXAMPLES OF SHEPHERDING

As seen earlier with the CCOT nurse, shepherding is sometimes confronting. But most often for the CCOT, it involved coming alongside the ward staff, helping, listening, reassuring. For the policy and research communities, shepherding involved the effort of connecting disparate actors, listening, and responding to criticisms, at times defending their processes and materials, but at other times, adjusting to enable further collaboration.

now involves 36 organisations that represent groups from every inhabited continent on the globe. Nursing and microbiologist professional societies joined the medical groups in 2004, and a patient representative was added to the guidelines committee in 2016. Shepherding knowledge, shepherding mindlines, meant bringing people and their ways of thinking together.

The longevity of the SSC further attests to the importance of relational work in underpinning their ongoing and long-lasting efforts around knowledge mobilisation. Furthermore, the SSC story shows that 'evidence' in the form of guidelines was created, interpreted, and moulded into material outputs emerging from the ongoing social (and occasionally public – see the next paragraph) interactions between actors.

Connecting via regular meetings and other forms of contact was part of sustaining the relationships between actors. And the SSC, as individuals and organisations, connected frequently. A sampling of face-to-face meetings mentioned in publications includes Chicago (in 1991), Paris (1997), Brussels (2000), Barcelona (2002), Amsterdam (2003), London (2003), Berlin (2011), Puerto Rico (2013), Honolulu (2017). Smaller groups met together in subcommittee meetings. The SSC literature mentions "teleconferences", and by the 2004 guideline document, there were regular "electronic-based discussions" (Dellinger, Carlet, Masur et al. 2004a, 2004b, p. 858) that took place amongst small subsets, as well as the full committee.

Such ongoing contact developed long-standing partnerships and professional friendships. Dellinger (2015a, 2015b) acknowledged his gratitude for their shared work saying,

> I thank Mitchell Levy, MD, Sean Townsend, MD, and Christa Schorr, RN, MSN, for their input on this Foreword, but even more importantly for the incredible journey we have shared together, along with our European SSC leadership colleagues, over the last 11 years with the Surviving Sepsis Campaign.
>
> *(Dellinger 2015b, p. 1789)*

Similarly, Marshall, Dellinger and Levy (2010) credited the SSC's success to

> the remarkable dedication of a diverse international group of practitioners to engaging in such a process of change.
>
> *(Marshall, Dellinger and Levy 2010, p. 279)*

The consensus-building process brought together actors' formal, informal, tacit, and experiential ways of knowing (their individual mindlines) and in the course of connecting, shaped their collective mindlines.

Unfortunately, because it is intensely relational, shepherding is not self-maintaining. It relies on an array of sometimes delicate social settings and subtle understandings, as well as the availability of people themselves. All of these are transient and must be understood, affirmed, and protected to be sustained. In addition, there is a need to capture the output from such relational work to pass on to others.

Aurora was well aware that the hospital could not rest on the laurels of its past success with sepsis. In part, this was because the enabling structures were always in motion. Those within the organisation who are shepherding their sepsis processes and materials retire and new nurses and doctors regularly join the ranks, whether as newly qualified clinicians or new posts. Their knowledge of sepsis and how to address it comes with their own sets of mindlines, some at least being influenced by other sources. Senior managers, who gather some of the praise for the good outcomes on their watch, move on too, and new leaders bring a different set of experiences and views on sepsis. They, perhaps, will hold different priorities and respond differently to centralised policies, possibly based on their own professional relationships and aspirations. As the people change, so does the material they draw upon.

NHS Scotland shifted to using NEWS during the 2010s, which involved an enormous reworking of the patient observation charts to match the data needed for the new scoring system. Soon afterwards, the new Sepsis-3 definition was published, so the reworking had to continue with that in place. Based on that experience, Aurora will continue to face such challenges and necessarily re-shape its evolving collective mindline, especially as staff leave and join. Perhaps newcomers' individual mindlines will be affected as they hear what is done at Aurora and learn from the success of, among other things, existing structures, e.g., the CCOT. Or perhaps future financial pressures might mean that new leaders will question the added expense of a CCOT. To date, the CCOT has worked well for shepherding ICU-based mindlines outside the ICU walls in Aurora. But the ever-changing structures will require ongoing adaptation and careful tending. These sorts of adjustments and refinements are always likely to be critical facets of dynamic collective mindlines.

Individual and collective mindlines work in tandem and tension

Researchers, policymakers, and clinicians did not 'know alone'; rather, they developed and used their knowledge while interacting with others. This is most readily traced in guidelines. My work followed three decades of sepsis guidelines and considered the people/experts involved, the processes they used, and the materials they drew on. Tracking the sepsis research community's materials over time provided a clear example of how individual mindlines affected or were incorporated into collective mindline outputs, such as guidelines (see Tooman 2019). Largely, this was done through consensus-building processes bringing together actors' formal, informal, tacit, and experiential ways of knowing (their individual mindlines) in order to shape their collective mindlines.

Sepsis guideline development involved individual and collective actors – experts, groups, and organisations. They created, refined, and set their collective mindline into codified forms through interactions, collaborations, and compromise. I was able to see how individuals' mindlines informed some collective documents (i.e., what then became the collective mindline). The following three examples show this.

EXAMPLE 1 THE BEGINNING

The first scoring system that quickly indicated the severity of illness (the APACHE score) was created by W. A. Knaus in the 1980s. Knaus was part of the first gathering of sepsis experts in 1991 and one of the seven session chairmen at the meeting. The 1992 publication from this group advocated the use of quantified measures (i.e., a scoring system) to identify patients at risk of sepsis, maybe because Knaus was involved in the materials production.

EXAMPLE 2 LONG-TERM PRESENCE AND PERSISTENCE MATTER

The second gathering of international experts to consider the definition of sepsis was in late 2001. They observed that since the first meeting in 1991, the definition based on SIRS had been widely adopted around the world. And yet, some experts sought modifications to this using the openly available media of the time – a journal – to facilitate debate. Jean-Louis Vincent was one particularly vocal critic of SIRS. Dualling editorials had already demonstrated a stiff difference in expert opinion. Vincent (1997) penned "Dear SIRS, I'm Sorry to Say That I Don't Like You" in the ESICM's journal, *ICM*. Dellinger and Bone responded with an editorial piece of their own (in the SCCM's associated journal, *CCM*), headed "To SIRS with Love" (1998), supporting SIRS. In the end, the 2001 conference attendees decided to keep the SIRS-based definitions.

But a compromise was appended to address some of Vincent's concerns. The lack of major revision was considered important, given some actors' considerable dissatisfaction with SIRS-related definitions (Abraham, Matthay, Dinarello et al. 2000): "The fact that no new definitions for sepsis are introduced in this conference report is noteworthy" (Levy, Fink and Marshall 2003, p. 537).

However, Vincent, along with others, eventually succeeded in their drive to redefine sepsis separately from SIRS (Vincent & Moreno 2010; Vincent, Opal, Marshall et al. 2013; Balk 2014). By 2016 a further sepsis definitions task force had convened. Dellinger and Bone were not involved (Dellinger focused on guidelines work, and Bone had died nearly 20 years before). But Vincent was. This group markedly shifted sepsis definitions and removed all connections to SIRS criteria, saying that SIRS had outlived its usefulness. In their 2016 *JAMA* publication Singer et al. (2016) agreed to discard SIRS as the basic definition for sepsis and a new definition was provided. Relatedly, a new early warning score system replaced the SIRS criteria – the SOFA score. This was developed by the ESICM (Vincent, Moreno, Takala 1996; Vincent, de Mendonça, Cantraine et al. 1998). We can see that Vincent's presence and involvement in the research community over many years, as a critic of SIRS and developer of SOFA, had an influence that brought about a significant change in their collective mindline.

And yet, the record shows that not everyone agreed. Some societies declined to endorse the new Sepsis-3 definition, including the ACCP, an original organising member for the two prior definitions (Bone et al. 1992; Levy, Fink and Marshall 2003). Publication titles illuminate how this remains an unsettled topic within the research community: "New Sepsis Criteria. A Change We Should Not Make" (Simpson 2016), "To SIRS with Love—An Open Letter" (Sprung, Schein, Balk et al. 2017), and "New Definition of Sepsis and Septic Shock: What Does It Give Us?" (Rodriguez, Martin-Loeches and Yébenes 2017). But persistence and presence were central for negotiating and bringing about the evolution and development of both collective and individual mindlines.

EXAMPLE 3 EXPOSING THE TENSIONS BETWEEN COLLECTIVE AND INDIVIDUAL MINDLINES

A further dispute centred on the time allocation given for completion of a bundle (a distillation of a guideline into a small set of practices to be completed together (Tooman 2019, p. 148)), specifically regarding the timing of antibiotic administration. The sepsis bundles have been revised with each new set of guidelines. In 2016, the time to complete the bundle was reduced to one hour. This time frame, known as the "golden hour" in sepsis care, was introduced in a research publication by Kumar and colleagues in 2006 (p. 1594). Their work showed a stepwise decrease in survival by 7.6% for each hour an antibiotic was delayed (p. 1592). The golden hour, although part of prior guidelines, had not been incorporated into the bundles before 2016.

Subsequent attempts to replicate Kumar's work have not shown the same relationship between antibiotic administration time and survival (Puskarich, Trzeciak, Shapiro et al. 2011; Sterling, Miller, Pryor et al. 2015). Furthermore, the then chief of critical care medicine for the US National Institutes of Health and named author (Masur) on earlier SSC Guidelines, co-authored a position statement on behalf of the Infectious Diseases Society of America (2017) failing to support the one-hour rule and consequently the 2016 SSC Guidelines. However, despite these factors, the next update to the SSC bundle upheld the reduction in time at one hour (Levy, Evans and Rhodes 2018).

Guidelines are the product of a group's agreed knowledge at a given place and time, and like people, they will change and evolve to remain contemporary. The longitudinal study of the sepsis guidelines helps us to see this. Guidelines can be likened to a snapshot in time, a reflection, of a moment in the evolution of a collective mindline. And as we see from the aforementioned examples, even when largely the same group meets on another occasion to do the same work, their individual mindlines will have evolved – shifting their knowledge, their collaborative process, and their outcomes to reflect that new position.

Furthermore, in the practice setting such as Aurora Hospital, the multifaceted weave of many forms of knowledge enabled them, as individuals and collectives (e.g., the CCOT or the ward nurses) to use their sepsis-based knowledge to benefit patients. Indeed, they relied upon each other. Different actors provided differing views, which both informed and shaped their collective sepsis activities. Intuition, or 'gut feelings'; past experiences; contextual values and procedures; patient concerns; and the sepsis research evidence all worked together for interpreting the most beneficial way to apply their *knowledge*-in-this-*practice*-in-this-*context*-for-this-patient. These actors' mindlines worked in tandem and (useful) tension. In other words, the tensions between many sources of knowledge contributed to, rather than impeded, high-performing care.

The value and importance of the mindlines model

The mindlines model provides a useful (and I would argue now sturdy) explanation of how science-informed sources can work in tandem and in productive tension with other forms of knowledge such as experience, judgement, wisdom, local values, from both individuals and collectives/groups. Using this model allowed me to assemble a picture of knowledge evolution and contemporary knowing in practice in relation to sepsis care. I was able to reach beyond traditional evidence sources and types of knowledge and consider the context in which knowledge from research, guidelines, and practical experience was sculpted for practice – and shepherded into practice at the bedside. These findings have implications for both learning and education.

Implications for learning and education

Understanding knowledge acquisition and use as a *process* (growing, shifting, sorting, etc.) – and indeed a relational process – rather than an *object* to be obtained, enables educators to shift away from focusing only on traditional structures for learning. When knowledge is viewed as socially constructed, emergent, and having meaning drawn from a particular context, then learning is both an individual and a collective process of transformation. This view shifts the focus from (only) individual knowledge acquisition to how individuals and groups change, transform, and learn as a result of connecting and engaging over a shared task.

If we are to encourage this transformation, we need to engineer and capitalise on structures to facilitate interactions between people, which in turn will facilitate mindline development and enhancement. Shepherding knowledge is a critical facet of both CPD and, as we have seen from the case study, of care. We need to devise ways to engage with and nurture shepherding practices and social processes which bring together different forms of knowing *and* relevant actors and communities. These include prioritising places and spaces for people to meet together. In the name of efficiency, many workplace coffee times and break rooms have been phased out. But informal 'chat' can provide vital, valuable connections and build trust that enables mindlines to flourish. Meeting together at conferences and the like, while perhaps tiring and inconvenient, provides a time for building and extending professional relationships, having ideas challenged or validated. Both formal and informal engagement bear fruit. Supporting relational contact will enable mindlines to move fluidly across networks, ensuring knowledge mobilisation and opportunities for the critique of that knowledge.

Finally, does CPD affect clinical practice, and if so, how? The answer in this case study was, yes, it did. But not in a straightforward, causal manner. Instead, the most productive learning about sepsis in this case study – the learning that actually appeared to have an impact on reducing deaths from sepsis – was part of a complex milieu at the intersection of individual and collective mindlines across several inter-related systems. The learning seemed to be less scientific than ecological. Such learning is dynamic and needs to be nurtured. The ground can be prepared, fertilised, and tended, allowing for growth and collective development rather than being simply a set of rules that, when an individual follows them precisely, can be replicated. Continued efforts are needed to deepen our understanding of the kinds of systems and structures that can be put in place to facilitate, nurture, and shepherd the many forms of learning and knowledge transformation that are needed for mindlines to develop. Understanding these better and using this understanding to underpin learning about and in practice may enable more effective construction and targeting of CPD in the future.

Summary

- To understand more about the connections between continuous professional development, clinical practice and mindlines, I undertook a case study of a sepsis-focused knowledge network made up of interconnected research, policy, and practice communities.
- The three study communities were the Surviving Sepsis Campaign, NHS Scotland (NHSS) Sepsis Collaborative, and a leading general hospital. I used documents, observations, and interviews to collect data.
- I uncovered three sets of structures important to mindlines development and enhancement: the configuration of *people*, the interactional *processes*, and the *materials* they use to coordinate the flow of their knowledge between them.
- I found that:
  - interaction facilitates mindline development and enhancement,
  - 'shepherding' mindlines within and across the networks brought about high-performing sepsis care, and
  - mindlines work in tandem *and* in tension by providing a form of checks and balances.

Acknowledgements

Acknowledgements and heartfelt gratitude to my thesis advisors, Professors Huw Davies and Sandra Nutley for their expert mindlines and kindness, to all my research participants who worked incredibly hard to prevent unnecessary deaths from sepsis, and the Darwin Mindlines Group for their partnership and fun.

Note

1 It should be noted that some of the controversy they generated still lingers, as can be seen in Box 13.1 in Chapter 13.

References

Abraham E, Matthay MA, Dinarello CA, Vincent J-L, Cohen J, Opal SM, Glauser M, Parsons P, Fisher Jr CJ, Repine JE. 2000. 'Consensus conference definitions for sepsis septic shock, acute lung injury, and acute respiratory distress syndrome: time for a reevaluation'. *Critical Care Medicine*, 28 (1): 232–235.

Angus DC. 2016. 'Defining sepsis: a case of bounded rationality and fuzzy thinking?' *American Journal of Respiratory and Critical Care Medicine*, 194 (1): 14–15.

Balk RA. 2014. 'Systemic inflammatory response syndrome (SIRS): where did it come from and is it still relevant today?' *Virulence*, 5: 20–26.

Bone RC, Balk RA, Cerra FB, Dellinger RP, Fein AM, Knaus WA, Schein RMH, Sibbald WJ. 1992a. 'American College of Chest Physicians/Society of Critical Care Medicine consensus conference: definitions for sepsis and organ failure and guidelines for the use of innovative therapies in sepsis'. *Critical Care Medicine*, 20: 864–874.

Bone RC, Balk RA, Cerra FB, Dellinger RP, Fein AM, Knaus WA, Schein RMH, Sibbald WJ. 1992b. 'Definitions for sepsis and organ failure and guidelines for the use of innovative therapies in sepsis. The ACCP/SCCM Consensus Conference Committee. American College of Chest Physicians/Society of Critical Care Medicine'. *Chest*, 101: 1644–55.

Bone RC, Fisher Jr CJ, Clemmer TP, Slotman GJ, Metz CA, Balk RA. 1989. 'Sepsis syndrome: a valid clinical entity'. *Critical Care Medicine*, 17: 389–393.

Davis D, O'Brien MA, Freemantle N, Wolf FM, Mazmanian P, Taylor-Vaisey A. 1999. 'Impact of formal continuing medical education: do conferences, workshops, rounds, and other traditional continuing education activities change physician behavior or health care outcomes?' *Journal of the American Medical Association*, 282: 867–874.

Dellinger RP. 2015a. 'The Surviving Sepsis Campaign: where have we been and where are we going?' *Cleveland Clinic Journal of Medicine*, 82 (4): 237–244. doi:10.3949/ccjm.82gr.15001.

Dellinger RP. 2015b. 'The future of sepsis performance improvement'. *Critical Care Medicine*, 43 (9): 1787–1789. doi:10.1097/CCM.0000000000001231.

Dellinger RP, Bone RC. 1998. 'To SIRS with love'. *Critical Care Medicine*, 26 (1): 178–179.

Dellinger RP, Carlet JM, Masur H, Gerlach H, Calandra T, Cohen J, Gea-Banacloche J, Keh D, Marshall JC, Parker MM, Ramsay G, Zimmerman JL, Vincent J-L, Levy MM. 2004a. 'Surviving Sepsis Campaign guidelines for management of severe sepsis and septic shock'. *Critical Care Medicine*, 32 (3): 858–873. doi:10.1097/01.CCM.0000117317.18092.E4.

Dellinger RP, Carlet JM, Masur H, Gerlach H, Calandra T, Cohen J, Gea-Banacloche J, Keh D, Marshall JC, Parker MM, Ramsay G, Zimmerman JL, Vincent J-L, Levy MM. 2004b. 'Surviving Sepsis Campaign guidelines for management of severe sepsis and septic shock'. *Intensive Care Medicine*, 30: 536–555.

Dellinger RP, Levy MM, Carlet JM, Bion J, Parker MM, Jaeschke R, Reinhart K, Angus DC, Brun-Buisson C, Beale R, Calandra T, Dhainaut J-F, Gerlach H, Harvey M, Marini JJ, Marshall JC, Ranieri M, Ramsay G, Sevransky J, Thompson BT, Townsend S, Vender JS, Zimmerman JL, Vincent J-L. 2008a. 'Surviving Sepsis Campaign: international guidelines for management of severe sepsis and septic shock: 2008'. *Critical Care Medicine*, 36 (1): 296–327, doi:10.1097/01.CCM.0000298158.12101.41.

Dellinger RP, Levy MM, Carlet JM, Bion J, Parker MM, Jaeschke R, Reinhart K, Angus DC, Brun-Buisson C, Beale R, Calandra T, Dhainaut J-F, Gerlach H, Harvey M, Marini JJ, Marshall JC, Ranieri M, Ramsay G, Sevransky J, Thompson BT, Townsend S, Vender JS, Zimmerman JL, Vincent J-L. 2008b. 'Surviving Sepsis Campaign: international guidelines for management of severe sepsis and septic shock: 2008'. *Intensive Care Medicine*, 34: 17–60, doi:10.1007/s00134-007-0934-2.

Dellinger RP, Levy MM, Rhodes A, Annane D, Gerlach H, Opal SM, Sevransky JE, Sprung CL, Douglas IS, Jaeschke R, Osborn TM, Nunnally ME, Townsend SR, Reinhart K, Kleinpell RM, Angus DC, Deutschman CS, Machado FR, Rubenfeld GD, Webb S, Beale RJ, Vincent J-L, Moreno R. 2012. 'Surviving Sepsis Campaign Guidelines Committee including the Pediatric Subgroup. Surviving Sepsis Campaign: international guidelines for management of severe sepsis and septic shock, 2012'. *Intensive Care Medicine*, 39: 165–228. doi:10.1007/s00134-012-2769-8.

Dellinger RP, Levy MM, Rhodes A, Annane D, Gerlach H, Opal SM, Sevransky JE, Sprung CL, Douglas IS, Jaeschke R, Osborn TM, Nunnally ME, Townsend SR, Reinhart K, Kleinpell RM, Angus DC, Deutschman CS, Machado FR, Rubenfeld GD, Webb S, Beale RJ, Vincent J-L, Moreno R. 2013. 'Surviving Sepsis Campaign Guidelines Committee including the Pediatric Subgroup. Surviving sepsis campaign: international guidelines for management of severe sepsis and septic shock: 2012'. *Critical Care Medicine*, 41: 580–637.

Engel PGH. 1997. *The social organization of innovation: a focus on stakeholder interaction*. Amsterdam: Royal Tropical Institute.

Forsetlund L, Bjørndal A, Rashidian A, Jamtvedt G, O'Brien MA, Wolf F, Davis D, Odgaard-Jensen J, Oxman AD. 2009. 'Continuing education meetings and workshops: effects on professional practice and health care outcomes'. *Cochrane Database of Systematic Reviews*, 2: CD003030.

Infectious Diseases Society of America (IDSA) Sepsis Task Force. 2017. 'IDSA position statement: why IDSA did not endorse the Surviving Sepsis Campaign guidelines'. *Clinical Infectious Diseases*, 66 (10): 1631–1635. doi:10.1093/cid/cix997.

Jaeschke R, Guyatt GH, Dellinger P, Schünemann H, Levy MM, Kunz R, Norris S, Bion J. 2008, 'Use of GRADE grid to reach decisions on clinical practice guidelines when consensus is elusive'. *British Medical Journal*, 337: 327–330.

Kumar A, Roberts D, Wood K, Light B, Parrillo JE, Sharma S, Suppes R, Feinstein D, Zanotti S, Taiberg L, Gurka D, Kumar A, Cheang M. 2006. 'Duration of hypotension before initiation of effective antimicrobial therapy is the critical determinant of survival in septic shock'. *Critical Care Medicine*, 34 (6): 1589–1596. doi:10.1097/01.CCM.0000217961.75225.E9.

Levy MM, Evans LE, Rhodes A. 2018. 'The Surviving Sepsis Campaign bundle: 2018 update'. *Intensive Care Medicine*, 44 (6): 925–928. doi:10.1007/s00134-018-5085-0.

Levy MM, Fink MP, Marshall JC. 2003. '2001 SCCM/ESICM/ACCP/ATS/SIS International sepsis definitions conference'. *Critical Care Medicine*, 31: 1250–1256.

Marshall JC, 1997. 'In memoriam: Roger C. Bone'. MD. *Sepsis*, 1: 7–10.

Marshall JC, Dellinger RP, Levy M. 2010. 'The Surviving Sepsis Campaign: a history and a perspective'. *Surgical Infections*, 11 (3): 275–281.

Olson CA, Tooman TR. 2012. 'Didactic CME and practice change: don't throw that baby out quite yet'. *Advances in Health Sciences Education*, 17 (3): 441–451.

Puskarich MA, Trzeciak S, Shapiro NI, Arnold RC, Horton JM, Studnek JR, Kline JA, Jones AE. 2011. 'Association between timing of antibiotic administration and mortality from septic shock in patients treated with a quantitative resuscitation protocol'. *Critical Care Medicine*, 39 (9): 2066–2071, doi:10.1097/CCM.0b013e31821e87ab.

Rodriguez A, Martin-Loeches I, Yébenes JC. 2017. 'New definition of sepsis & septic shock: what does it give us?' *Medicina Intensiva*, 41 (1): 38–40.

Royal College of Physicians. 2012. *National Early Warning Score (NEWS): standardising the assessment of acute illness severity in the NHS. Report of a working party*. London: Royal College of Physicians.

Simpson SQ. 2016. 'New sepsis criteria. A change we should not make'. *Chest*, 149: 1117–1118.

Singer M, Deutschman CS, Seymour CW, Shankar-Hari M, Annane D, Bauer M, Bellomo R, Bernard GR, Chiche J-D, Coopersmith CM, Hotchkiss RS, Levy MM, Marshall JC, Martin GS, Opal SM, Rubenfeld GD, van der Poll T, Vincent J-L, Angus DC. 2016. 'The third international consensus definitions for sepsis and septic shock'. *Journal of the American Medical Association*, 315 (8): 801–810. doi:10.1001/jama.2016.0287.

Sprung CL, Schein RMH, Balk RA. 2017. 'To SIRS with love—an open letter'. *Critical Care Medicine*, 45 (4): 736–738.

Sterling SA, Miller WR, Pryor J, Puskarich MA, Jones AE. 2015. 'The impact of timing of antibiotics on outcomes in severe sepsis and septic shock: A systematic review and meta-analysis'. *Critical Care Medicine*, 43 (9): 1907–1915. doi:10.1097/CCM.0000000000001142.

Tooman TR. 2019. Shepherding knowledge: a case study of social interactions that support knowledge mobilisation for sepsis care in Scotland. [Doctoral thesis, University of St Andrews] St Andrews Research Repository. doi:10.17630/10023-19246.

Vincent J-L. 1997. 'Dear SIRS, I'm sorry to say that I don't like you'. *Critical Care Medicine*, 25: 372–374.

Vincent J-L, de Mendonça A, Cantraine F, Moreno R, Takala J, Suter PM, Sprung CL, Colardyn F, Blecher S. 1998. 'Use of the SOFA score to assess the incidence of organ dysfunction/failure in intensive care units: results of a multicenter, prospective study. Working group on "sepsis related problems" of the European Society of Intensive Care Medicine'. *Critical Care Medicine*, 26: 1793–1800.

Vincent J-L, Moreno R, Takala J, Willatts S, de Mendonça A, Bruining H, Reinhart CK, Suter PM, Thijs LG. 1996. 'The SOFA (Sepsis-Related Organ Failure Assessment) score to describe organ dysfunction/failure'. *Intensive Care Medicine*, 22: 707–710.

Vincent J-L, Moreno R. 2010. 'Clinical review: Scoring systems in the critically ill'. *Critical Care Medicine*, 14: 207.

Vincent J-L, Opal SM, Marshall JC, Tracey KJ. 2013. 'Sepsis definitions: Time for change'. *Lancet*, 381: 774–775.

9

ON BECOMING A (PHYSIO)THERAPIST

Mindlines changing education

Joost van Wijchen and Maria Nordheim Alme

Introduction

A physiotherapy training programme is the first step to being socialised into the physiotherapeutic community, building the necessary competence and experience to provide good healthcare. Within such programmes, scheduled pre-designed pathways for development of physiotherapeutic knowledge, skills, and competences are usually considered a safeguard for ensuring that all students become competent physiotherapists. The mandate and role of the physiotherapy profession are the key basis for this training. However, like all healthcare professionals, physiotherapists need to work within changing and uncertain contexts and to take responsibility in unfamiliar situations, and we have found that many newly educated physiotherapists do not feel competent although they have the diploma in their hands. The gap between their education and clinical practice becomes too big. Our contention is that this gap exists because they do not yet have the individual and collaborative mindlines that would allow them to think and practise in the face of uncertainty, and that appropriate mindline creation should therefore be an explicit part of the professional socialisation in the training programme.

At HAN University of Applied Sciences in the Netherlands, we wanted to improve our support for students in understanding what it means to be a capable physiotherapist, so in 2015, we started an alternative learning landscape, the Delta-stream, for BSc physiotherapy education. The Delta-stream focuses on the process of becoming a physiotherapist who can practise with confidence and take responsibility in known and unknown situations. Students are seen as upcoming physiotherapists and future colleagues, and they share a joint responsibility for their own learning paths. There is an analogy between the mindlines construction within early education and in later professional practice, and by working within this analogy, we help bridge the gap between education and practice. In this chapter, we

DOI: 10.4324/9781003158721-9

will discuss how the programme is designed and how it supports our students in developing their mindlines while becoming capable physiotherapists. We start by discussing the ideas and experiences that led us to question our predominant educational structure and allowed us to change it.

From reflections to change

First reflections

During informal meetings with students, we found that the subject of confidence often arose. Students were telling us that although they had passed their exams, they did not feel competent in their physiotherapeutic tasks, especially in unfamiliar contexts. This happened despite well-planned courses, training sessions, and practice periods within the physiotherapy programme. We started to discuss how we could improve our support for upcoming physiotherapists, and we started to discuss how we saw the process of *becoming* a physiotherapist, what this means, and how we could better support this. To understand what it means to become a professional, we can turn to Gloria Dall'Alba: "we are continually in a process of becoming; more specifically we are already (oriented to) what we are not yet" (Dall'Alba 2009, p. 36). "Becoming" can in this way be understood as moving beyond the simple acquisition of knowledge and skills; it is about being able to act in dynamic contexts and accept the ambiguities involved. This involves a development within the student, a process leading to a broader understanding of what it means to be a physiotherapist.

A change within the Dutch healthcare system had a large influence on us during this time. The Dutch healthcare system, policy, and education of healthcare professionals were in a transition (Kaljouw and Vliet 2015) fuelled by a different way of seeing health. A description of health by Huber played a central role. She described health as "the ability to adapt and to self-manage in the face of social, physical, and emotional challenges" (Huber, Knottnerus, Green et al. 2011). Huber provided a key for us by mentioning "the ability to adapt and self-manage". Physiotherapists play a role in supporting people to do this, and to manage this, they also need to be able to adapt and self-manage themselves. This is fundamental to the process of becoming, and facilitating it was an educational challenge. We needed a concept to express our thoughts, and we found this in the concept of mindlines (Gabbay and le May 2011). Gabbay and le May express the importance of ongoing collaboration during the developmental process, and that socialisation is an inherent aspect of mindlines development (2011, p. 78). As such, becoming a physiotherapist involves the construction of one's mindlines alongside others' as part of the process of socialisation. This way of thinking led to a change in our understanding of teaching and learning and for our roles as educators. We started to reflect around our own mindlines concerning teaching, and the various roles we could play to support the process of becoming. We discussed the power balance between students and teachers, and we saw an analogy between the patient-physiotherapist and the student-teacher relationship. We see the socialisation within education as directly relevant for the interaction physiotherapists build with their clients in clinical practice. This is important because it directly points to a responsibility for us, as teachers, beyond the transfer of knowledge and physiotherapeutic methods. We should therefore support our students to construct their mindlines based upon the principle of creating an equitable relationship and use the strengths and experiences they have in the process of becoming.

A new way of thinking

To understand how students can build their mindlines, we conceptualised what it means to be a physiotherapist by taking a step back and looking at our educational programme with the eyes of a stranger. By doing that, we were free to ask critical questions, to evaluate the meaning of what we saw, and to re-examine our own roles (Curzon-Hobson 2017). By managing to leave behind our expectations, we found it became easier to reflect open-mindedly on our practices, and we could move onwards to, for us, uncharted areas. In this way, we avoided the new way of thinking just becoming something troublesome, as often is the case when one explores new ways of thinking. Still, we got confronted with our own selves as we challenged our beliefs and convictions about teaching. At some point, we felt that we lost part of our identity as teachers because so much of our identity was linked to the specific knowledge we have. We were teachers in rehabilitation, in neurology, in physiology and anatomy, in communication, and now we realised that these subjects were not the key factors within the education; they were more assets in the process of becoming a physiotherapist. We, therefore, experienced some resistance in ourselves when realising that our specific knowledge took second place. Of course, we are not saying that just anyone could teach the physiotherapy programme; our competence and experience were certainly needed, but we had to reduce the focus on these. On the other hand, we were free to ask questions about the meaning of the content, tasks, assignments, and evaluations within our own education, and we were free to look a bit more broadly at our identity. It became inspiring and safe to ask questions and to go into discussions that we may have feared previously, especially around the role of content and our role as teachers. We found that seeing through this lens promoted real discussions about why we were doing what we did, and we experienced ourselves becoming a team with a common responsibility of creating a space for socialisation into the physiotherapy profession.

Person-centred education

In our physiotherapeutic practice, we know that each patient is unique. Although the intended outcomes for the patients can be similar, for example in rehabilitation, the methods, and the strategies to reach the desired outcome will vary depending on the individual and the context. Despite this, within our physiotherapy programme, we had been focusing on standardisation and control as a way of ensuring that all students would have the necessary competencies when going into practice. So students lacked the responsiveness to practise in unfamiliar settings, and they told us that the structured certainty from their education could feel like a 'hoax' when they met variation, complexity, and uncertainty in their encounters with patients. Gloria Dall'Alba expresses it like this: "[W]e have to promote learning by all and not only those who learn despite our teaching" (Dall'Alba 2007). We realised that doing the best for our students demanded incorporation of contextual variation and unfamiliarity in such a way that the students would feel comfortable in uncertainty and happy to engage with complexity later in their clinical practice. We realised that we needed learning pathways that could embrace variations from the start, not just when the students ended their education. This is not in conflict with established learning outcomes or descriptions of the physiotherapy profession; we rather believe it better covers the range of the therapeutic competence needed to meet the variations within our societies. We became more observant of the landscape of the outcomes we aimed for, and that several methods and paths would be beneficial for reaching more of the outcomes in this landscape. We neither searched for, nor wanted, an educational path where all students would become similar. This also better appreciated the variations between upcoming physiotherapists that we knew existed, and it reminded us to build on this difference as a resource. In addition, it allowed us to think differently about the support students needed in their process of becoming – some more intensively than others and some more often.

The paths to learning to self-manage are different within the group of learners. It is often considered unfair if some students get more supervision than others, but we argue that it is a necessary personalisation of education. Of course, we need to ensure that all get the support that is needed, some might not ask for the support they should have, but we hope this does not stop a more individualised understanding of education and learning to become. It is an interesting question whether students who have experienced this kind of personalised education also will be better in providing personalised health support later in their practice.

We designed a study to investigate how undergraduate students of physiotherapy perceive their development of self-efficacy in physiotherapeutic competences. We found a shift in perception and motivation around becoming a physiotherapist during the education. This became visible during internships in the third year. In this process, a transition from being a student of physiotherapy into a becoming physiotherapist became clear. In seeing themselves as students of physiotherapy, they had their focus on assessments, and learning was described as an external obligation they had to consume. In contrast, when they looked at themselves as a becoming physiotherapist, they showed an internal engagement, with an eagerness to keep learning and develop, to offer service for future clients. Their focus shifted from obligations and assessments to eagerness and professional responsibility (van Wijchen 2013). We realised that motivation and effort are to a large extent based on a sense of ownership of the process of becoming, a freedom to choose how to reach the necessary competence levels. The connection between choice, ownership, and togetherness provides important process elements of becoming (Biesta 2015).

We, therefore, focused on these key points in the design of a new educational landscape. Here the students would have roles as becoming physiotherapists right from the beginning. In the process, we saw the need for looking beyond competences and towards capabilities. Competences are often connected to high levels of agreement and certainty, leading to descriptions of outcomes in an explicit way where contextual variations are lost, or not even considered. Capabilities are connected to lower levels of agreement and certainty around contextual variations, being concerned with acting in familiar and unfamiliar, complex, and uncertain situations (Fraser and Greenhalgh 2001). Developing an educational landscape mainly connected to certainty and agreement would fit poorly with the purpose of building capability to work within a field (physiotherapy) that is so dependent on the context. To acknowledge the contextual and dynamic nature of reality, we needed a different perception of the curriculum. We, therefore, moved from a convergent curriculum, with a focus on an endpoint, towards a divergent curriculum with an open view. During this process, we were in close dialogue with the formal structures of the physiotherapy programme management and administration at HAN University to stay in line with the regulations (EHEA 2005; ENPHE 2012; KNGF and SROF 2017; NVAO 2018; HAN University of Applied Sciences 2019).

The Delta-stream

When large rivers meet the ocean, they lose speed, and the sediments they have carried with them end up fashioning new land formations and a plethora of new smaller river branches at the transition between land and ocean. The Ganges-Brahmaputra delta is the world's largest delta, formed by the two rivers Ganges and Brahmaputra in the Bengal region of South Asia. The sediments and rich access to fresh water, have turned this region into the most fertile soil in the world and therefore the region also goes under the name 'the green delta'. This was an important inspiration when we sat down to design the new physiotherapy stream at HAN. As Nijmegen is situated in the lowlands (Netherlands) right between the rivers Maas and Waal, the area of fertile grounds is dependent on yearly flooding, a process that – for people who are not from the area – might seem more damaging than useful. Through the past centuries, the rivers and streams have meandered, changed, and connected in multiple ways. This has continued up to the time the Dutch built dikes to control the rivers, limiting flooding and space for the river. In the last decades, policy has changed from controlling the river to giving the river space. This transition in ecological thinking strengthened our idea of a Delta-stream, in which we stepped back from control and gave space to learning and variation. The goal was to create a rich learning landscape where it could be possible to become a physiotherapist along different routes, where all participants in the education are active parts, rather like sediments in a river delta. In addition, the various elements that build capability within each learner can be seen as a sediment in their individual physiotherapeutic landscape, or in their physiotherapeutic mindlines. We wanted to use the resources within each of the students and teachers and the contextual elements we encounter, and to use these in the process of becoming in a divergent way. The Delta-stream was born.

Physiotherapy students at HAN University can choose to sign up for the Delta-stream or the Alpha-stream (regular education programme) (Box 9.1). The Alpha-stream is structured around transfer of formal knowledge and skills, and training in specific physiotherapeutic methods. The process of learning and becoming is secondary, and to a large degree left to the individual student. The Delta-stream has its prime focus on the process of becoming a physiotherapist, where mobilisation of knowledge and skills have a supportive role. In the Delta-stream, there are no classes, no schedules, and no topics being taught at fixed times. There are no standardised assignments, but there is room for a multitude of challenges and learning questions. The education is designed by the students in consultation with the teachers. Students learn by doing what is needed to demonstrate and achieve the intended learning outcomes. Depending on the situation, the teachers take on roles as challenger, scout, coach, and expert, thus serving the learning process of the students. Students can also take these roles, which is a useful preparation for their later role as physiotherapists. An important element for constructing mindlines is the formation of individual and collective intellectual resources that enable practitioners to be contextually adroit. Each experience, interaction, and engagement creates contextual and situational references that may provide security and self-efficacy to bring into practice.

BOX 9.1 *HAN NUMBERS*

In the Netherlands, entry-level physiotherapy education is provided at universities of applied sciences. It is an undergraduate programme of four years (240 European Credits Transfer System) and leads to a BSc physiotherapy degree. The undergraduate physiotherapy programme at HAN University of Applied Sciences in Nijmegen has around 800 students. The programme has a 'numerus fixus', meaning that each year 240 new students are selected from an average of 700 prospective students to start their education. Currently within the programme, 140 students follow the Delta-stream programme and 680 students the regular Alpha-stream. The resources used per student are the same in the two programmes. Entry to practice has the same threshold for all students.

(KNGF and SROF 2017)

Evaluation and testing are often seen as stable and controlled entities. They can, however, be more open and considered as formative learning processes where the goal is further development (Van Der Vleuten, Schuwirth, Driessen et al. 2012). During the first years, the Delta-stream students had the same standardised exams as the Alpha-stream students. In 2018, the results between the two streams were compared and showed no difference (Van Lankveld Maas, van Wijchen et al. 2019). However, we experienced that this way of evaluating the students was not in line with the capabilities they were trained for, and we wanted to design an evaluation protocol that also had its focus on the process of learning and development of the students. We implemented programmatic assessment in the Delta-stream in 2019 and, based on this experience, in the Alpha-stream in 2020. In programmatic assessments, portfolios and feedback are influential for learning and evaluation (Heeneman, Oudkerk Pool, Schuwirth et al. 2015). During the first year, we assess students' portfolios quarterly, and thereafter twice a year. In between the portfolio assessments, the students evaluate their own capabilities, and they gather feedback from their peers, teachers, external experts, and their own reflections, which helps them get a broad picture of their capabilities. The portfolios differ between the two streams. The Alpha-stream students have their focus more on the products. In the Delta-stream the focus is on the learning process and how it relates to the intended learning outcomes.

The portfolios differ between students, as they provide a connection between the learner and their individual intended learning outcomes. As such, the portfolios do not have prescribed content, but we rather ask the learners to provide multiple sources of evidence of their capabilities and professional development. During the assessments, we ask the students what they are proud of and what they experience as difficult, and we use this as a route to discussing the boundaries of their capabilities. The latter is an important safety threshold for professional practice, knowing one's present limits of autonomy and one's needs for support or guidance. These portfolio conversations bring up discussions about what it means to be capable, which is an important step for the learning process because it gives the student a direction linked not to a grade but to future practice.

Constructing mindlines

The Delta-stream was designed as a learning landscape for constructing physiotherapeutic mindlines, and the developmental processes within each learner can be seen as sediments building the landscape. We have been focusing on the students' construction of therapeutic mindlines, but as the reader probably already has realised, this process was equally important for the teachers. The building of therapeutic and educational mindlines share the same sediments: socialisation through togetherness, freedom to choose, coping with uncertainty, and the ability to adapt.

Socialisation through togetherness

Essential for mindlines development within a profession is togetherness, a socialisation process where one builds on the strengths of each other (Gabbay and le May

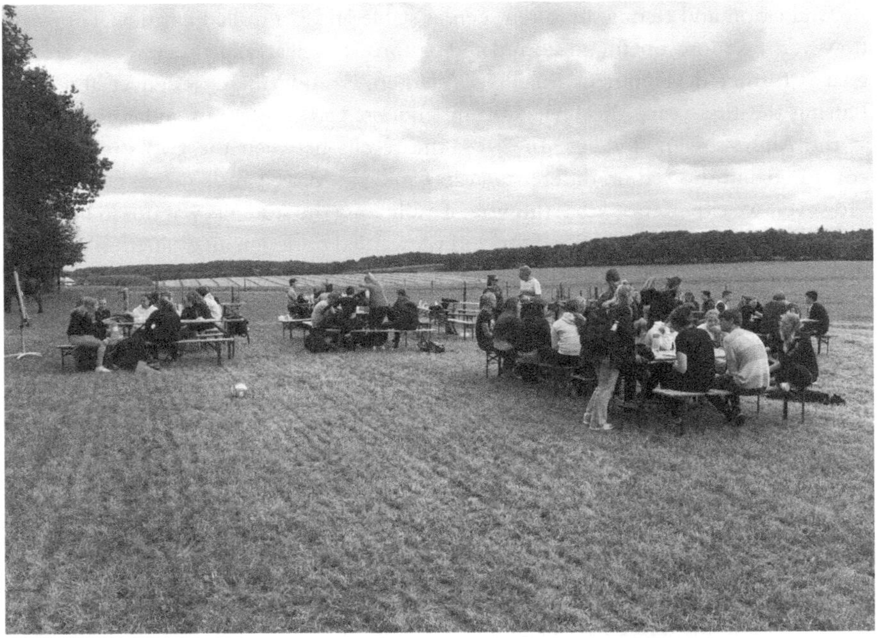

FIGURE 9.1 Delta-stream education on a grassland, education without walls.

Source: Joost van Wijchen.

2011). During the first week, we take the Delta-stream students to a farm where we spend the days together on a grassland — education without walls (Figure 9.1). The main goal is to create a social and cultural milieu of learning where the new students are invited into the existing communities of practice within the programme. When we come to this farmland, we start by sharing expectations and needs, and we want the students to immediately understand their own important role in creating the learning environment. For some, this can be a bit frustrating, but with the support from the more senior students, trust and a sense of togetherness – a community — is built.

As each student is unique, their process of learning unfolds in different ways during the four years of their study. One key point is to see these differences, to use them actively, and to support the students to see how they can use both their own and others' experiences to continue their development. We have students with an academic master's degree or bachelor's degree, students with previous vocational education, and students coming immediately from secondary education. And of course, everyone comes with a range of non-educational experiences. From one of the students, who has a background as a professional dancer, we learned new ways of expressing exclusion, fear, uncertainty, and human needs. Another student, a sportswoman at the international level, brought the skills of discipline for deadlines and internal motivation. Her need for pre-planned activities in relation to her training also provided insight in personal planning for others. The experiences the students bring have a natural place within their education, and we try to use these experiences actively in the learning environment.

How the group of students collaborate with each other also differs. Some prefer a stable group of collaborators, while others move more between groups. This structure encourages caring, togetherness, critical thinking, and promotes collaborative modes of practice. In this structure, individuals and groups discover that they are part of a community. They discover their own and others' paths of becoming capable, and they experience the variety in learning paths in their group of peers. They get experience in asking questions arising from internal interests, societal dilemmas, and the interactions they are exposed to. We focus on building connections, much the same as we do as clinicians when we build a therapeutic alliance, a network of trusted colleagues or a community of practice. As the students are connected to a professional domain and share passion about practice, they learn to practise better through regular interaction (Wenger 1998). They become part of a community in which collaborative modes of practice evolve in collective mindlines. These trusted networks and the interactions within, are a crucial part in collective mindlines development (Gabbay and le May 2011). Within this community, each student will be able to *become* in terms of qualification, socialisation, and subjectification (Biesta 2020). This entails not only becoming qualified but also being a member of the community that further develops collective mindlines. As influential others, teachers are observing, waiting, and critically judging when and how to engage (van Wijchen and Oerlemans 2010). The teachers can provide examples of how to support community building and interactions. Here we see the analogy between the roles of the teacher and physiotherapist in being an influential other. Within the learning context, teachers help the students to become aware of the possibilities within the situations they face, just as physiotherapists do for their patients.

Freedom to choose

Making decisions could be easy if we acted and lived within a certain and singular context. However, life does not bring us such kinds of contexts, and in clinical practice, one must make decisions in contexts that are highly complex and multifaceted. The uncertainty this brings can be challenging, especially for novices. Therefore, the educational programmes need to create opportunities where learners experience decision-making in complex and uncertain situations. We realised that instead of streamlining education into smooth paths that become more challenging over time, we needed to embrace constraints and ambiguities in our learning opportunities from day one. Therefore, we are purposefully not solving contradictions and ambiguities in advance. We perceive the conflicts that arise as important catalysts for constructing malleable mindlines. By means of these experiences, students get trained in seeing what they need to work on to be capable, which includes seeing where they are currently not competent. They discover their own questions, interests, and necessities. Being currently incompetent is unpleasant though its realisation can also be a step to become capable. Our goal is that students start developing their mindlines at an early point within their education.

Having multiple educational streams provides the students with a choice, and we immediately make it clear that there are several ways of becoming a physiotherapist. The first challenge new students face is therefore which stream to choose. Students have told us that this is a difficult choice as they get confronted with a lot of uncertainty, especially concerning the consequences and implications of their choice. We, therefore, provide support from teachers and peers, and students can opt to change their stream during education (preferably within the first year). The choices provided create a sense of freedom and responsibility, in which students are invited to reflect upon where they stand and how they would like to become a physiotherapist.

Coping with uncertainty

The Delta-stream has a home base which can be used during university opening hours. This consists of a former classroom (around 70 m^2) and a common vicinity open for all. The home base is the home for all the Delta-stream students (140 in total) and is therefore too small for all to use at the same time. This is an example of a constraint that does not necessarily fit the expectations of the students. The limited physical space helps to segment people's presence during the day and to encourage the use of available common space within and outside the university buildings. The students are encouraged to find and create space in the vicinity by using the space constraint as an incentive for creating solutions.

> When I entered the classroom the very first day, I first thought I had come too late. I tried to understand who the teacher was, but I couldn't really tell. There were so many people, all doing different things, some chatting, others were sitting behind their computers. In a corner, people were doing a physiotherapeutic consultation, while in another corner a group was busy with anatomy. I thought I was in the wrong place when a senior student invited me to join their group.
>
> *(Student starting the Delta-stream)*

We have heard several variations of this story throughout the years, and the one who invites the newcomer in probably remembers very well the unease of not completely understanding the situation, and the relief of being included. For some, this apparent lack of structure is scary; for others, it is inviting, and it inspires. A need for structure is a recurring theme. Based on extensive discussions throughout the years, we have understood that the expressed need for structure often is a need for security and comfort in uncertain situations. Students, like many professionals, prefer to avoid uncertainty. This often leads to a conceptualisation of knowledge as unidimensional, missing the contextual variations that are present in professional practice. By purposefully creating uncertainty about the practice students engage in, their needs and assumptions are challenged. When the students become aware of this, they find acceptance for their needs, and it becomes easier to have critical conversations about needs, expectations, and coping strategies. In this way, students realise that they need flexible and malleable structures to engage in practice. This forms an important step towards the embodiment of mindlines as knowledge-in-practice-in-context.

Ability to adapt

An important part of the capabilities of healthcare professionals is to be able to act upon societal challenges and changes, and to provide the best possible healthcare to all, even when context changes. This demands a high ability to adapt. To do that, it is important that students experience variations and ambiguities during their education. During the first months in the Delta-stream, the students are confronted with several situations where they already get the chance to construct mindlines through deliberately varied experiences. This could be variations in communication strategies, diseases, symptoms, physiotherapeutic thinking, and practice. When we have patients, we try to show variation and complexity within the clinical caseloads. For example, they can choose a case of a 35-year-old woman experiencing functional limitations related to shoulder pain after a sports accident and another of a 52-year-old man suffering from long-lasting idiopathic shoulder pains. Such variations are well known for a trained physiotherapist, but for a fresh student, it can be an important eye-opener at the very beginning of their studies. They immediately experience how patient cases involve more than symptoms and causes, and that rehabilitation strategies need to be personalised and contextualised. By having these experiences right from the beginning of one's developmental path, professional practice will be construed as varied in nature.

When students ask questions and discuss matters with a group of teachers or peers, seeking the 'best' or 'correct' answer to their question, they often get different answers. We experience this as important for mindlines construction. As each situation and each patient brings their own context, a tolerance for variation will help students to learn to adapt their practice to the situation at hand. To support this, the group of teachers is also varied, and we support the different ways of teaching and the different perspectives that are found within the group. We do not try to become similar, or 'speak with the same voice'. This might be interpreted as a lack of a common view or a lack of structure, and in some students, this can create tension. We meet such tensions with open discussions to support the students to increase their tolerance and adaptabilities to variations. After some time, most students discover that "best" relates to the context and practice at hand. They also become more reflective about their frustrations of not understanding, and we see that experiencing variation in this way is an effective catalyst in the process of becoming. We think this is one of several reasons why the Delta-stream students converse a lot and that they dare to try out their meanings and experiences openly within the group of peers.

The importance of adaptability became clear to both students and staff during the COVID-19 outbreak in March 2020. The COVID-19 situation forced societies across the world to take protective actions and rapidly shut down. For most educational courses all practice training stopped. From the first day of lockdown, the Delta-stream students felt the obligation to serve the global community to the best of their abilities. Within three days, they created a global support network for people in quarantine to support mental and physical health (QuaranTrain 2020; van Wijchen, Kerry and Nordheim Alme 2020). Alongside this, they got in contact with the university hospital in Nijmegen, where they heard that there was a critical need for help. Students in the Delta-stream asked for training in patient care at the intensive care unit and supported the staff on the floor in three consecutive periods during the two years of COVID-19 pandemic. Both these activities were added to the portfolio for the students who took part.

Future courses and conclusion

We believe the journey we have undertaken with the Delta-stream fits the Dutch culture of progressive education. The dynamic nature of the Delta-stream demands a continuous development of the programme, and the Alpha-stream is developing in relation to the Delta-stream. Based on our experience, we transformed the HAN BSc in Physiotherapy into six vertical communities of practice in 2021–2022, where the Delta-stream is one. The Delta-stream has gained interest, but also had its fair share of scepticism, leading to critical and developing conversations. The Maastricht University Bachelor of Medicine degree programme is being redesigned, building on the underlying principles of the Delta-stream, and we have created a collaborative partnership in which we share experiences. A partnership also emerged with the BSc Physiotherapy degree at Western Norway University of Applied Sciences (HVL) in Bergen, Norway, starting with one of the authors (MNA) becoming a critical friend. Currently, we are exploring how principles of mindlines can enrich the learning landscape at the physiotherapy programme at HVL. Through sharing experiences, we challenge and construct collaborative mindlines across educational programmes and across national borders.

Our intention to start the Delta-stream was to start bridging the gap between education and clinical practice. Based upon the journey we have undertaken so far, we conclude that for students: (a) it encourages robust mindline development, and it works; (b) it improves their emerging confidence, competence, and resilience as practitioners; and (c) it enhances their sense of responsibility for the needs of persons and populations, and active engagement towards an equitable and sustainable society. Besides the impact on students, the journey also had an impact on us, the educators. The principles of mindlines have been shown to be fundamental to a rich learning landscape within the context of physiotherapy at HAN. We teachers started to enhance our competences concerning educational practice to be more flexible, malleable, and contextual, as such altering our own educational mindlines. Our educational mindlines keep us open and curious to explore how we can further enrich the learning landscape by means of mindlines principles. Changing the prime focus of education towards the process of becoming has proven to be a means to support students to become capable physiotherapists who can practise with confidence and take responsibility in known and unknown situations.

Summary

- Physiotherapists and other healthcare professionals are responsible for providing good healthcare for all populations within our societies, often in changing and uncertain contexts.
- The creation of individual and collaborative mindlines is an important part of any professional socialisation, as they represent the ways professionals think and practise. This helps to bridge the gap between education and practice.
- The Delta-stream within the undergraduate physiotherapy education at HAN University of Applied Sciences in the Netherlands is designed to provide a learning environment where students start developing their physiotherapeutic mindlines from day one.
- The Delta-stream focuses on four key points within mindlines development: socialisation through togetherness, freedom to choose, coping with uncertainty, and the ability to adapt.
- The demonstrably successful experiences and ideas from the Delta-stream are now being explored in other healthcare educational programmes, providing educationalists with a model for flexible education in a changing society.

Acknowledgements

This work was not possible without the collaboration of the Delta-stream team of present and future colleagues, especially Wim Oerlemans, Aukje van Pelt, Volcmar Visser, Hans Joosten, Steven van Moorsel, Lieke Dekkers, Anke van Erp, Wiebke Oswald, Joost Andriessen, Marjo Maas, Samantha Meijer, Hanneke van de Haar, Meike Geurtsen, Mees van Wijchen, Sterre Stoffels, Hannah Hanekamp, Jesse Weenk, Huub Stout, Simone de Groot, Ruud Sanders, Max Hendrickx, Marre de Vries, Robin Klaassen, and Siem van Wijchen. We thank Herman Berndt and Menno Pistorius for their managerial support in this journey. In the process, the ideas and inspiration from late Harrie Hendriks were a huge motivation. Finally, we thank David Nicholls, Michael Rowe, Paul Beenen, Patricia Almeida, Ann Gates, Jack Chew, Joletta Belton, Roger Kerry, Michel Landry, Filip Maric, Djenana Jalovcic and Matthew Low for all their critical support.

References

Biesta G. 2020. 'Risking ourselves in education: qualification, socialization, and subjectification revisited'. *Educational Theory*, 70(1): 89–104. https://doi.org/10.1111/edth.12411.

Biesta GJJ. 2015. *Beautiful risk of education*. New York: Routledge.

Curzon-Hobson A. 2017. 'The experience of strangeness in education: Camus, Jean-Baptiste Clamence and the little ease.' *Educational Philosophy and Theory*, 49(3): 264–272. Doi:10.1080/00131857.2016.1215897.

Dall'Alba G. 2007, November 21. Teachers' duty is to enable learning. *The Australian*, 27: 27. https://espace.library.uq.edu.au/view/UQ:170322

Dall'Alba G. 2009. 'Learning professional ways of being: Ambiguities of becoming.' *Educational Philosophy and Theory*, 41(1): 34–45. doi:10.1111/j.1469-5812.2008.00475.x.

EHEA. 2005. *The framework of qualifications for the European Higher Education Area*. EU

ENPHE. 2012. 'The Enphe : European qualification framework for life long learning in physiotherapy final report towards a qualification framework culture', (October). Available at: https://www.enphe.org/uploads/media/final-report-eq-fg_def_16012013.pdf

Fraser SW, Greenhalgh T. 2001. 'Coping with complexity: educating for capability.' *BMJ (Clinical research ed.)*, 323(7316): 799–803. Available at: http://www.ncbi.nlm.nih.gov/pubmed/11588088 (Accessed: 8 April 2019).

Gabbay J, le May A. 2011. *Practice-based evidence for healthcare: clinical mindlines*. Routledge.

HAN University of Applied Sciences. 2019. *Degree statute and education and examination regulations of the bachelors degree physiotherapy (DUTCH) 2019–2020*. Netherlands.

Heeneman S, Oudkerk Pool A, Schuwirth LWT, van der Vleuten CPM, Driessen EW. 2015. 'The impact of programmatic assessment on student learning: theory versus practice.' *Medical education*, 49(5): 487–498. doi: 10.1111/MEDU.12645.

Huber M, Knottnerus JA, Green L, Knottnerus JA, Horst HVD, Jadad AR, Kromhout D, Leonard B, Lorig K, Loureiro MI, Meer JWMVD, Schnabel P, Smith R, Weel CV, Smid H. 2011. 'How should we define health?' *BMJ*, 343. doi: 10.1136/bmj.d4163.

Kaljouw M. Vliet van K. 2015. 'Naar nieuwe zorg en zorgberoepen: de contouren.' *Minsterie van Volksgezondheid, Welzijn en Sport*, 74. Available at: http://www.rijksoverheid.nl/documenten-en-publicaties/rapporten/2015/04/10/naar-nieuwe-zorg-en-zorgberoepen-de-contouren.html

KNGF and SROF. 2017. *Dutch national diploma supplement national transcript physiotherapy*. Amersfoort: KNGF.

NVAO. 2018. *Assessment framework for the higher education accreditation system of the Netherlands*. The Hague: NVAO.

QuaranTrain. 2020. *QuaranTrain–home support program*. Available at: https://quarantrain.org/ (Accessed: 22 March 2020).

van Lankveld W, Maas M, van Wijchen J, Visser V, Staal BJ. 2019. 'Self-regulated learning in physical therapy education: A non-randomized experimental study comparing self-directed and instruction-based learning'. *BMC Medical Education*, 19(1). doi: 10.1186/s12909-019-1484-3

van der Vleuten CPM, Schuwirth LWT, Driessen EW, Dijkstra J, Tigelaar D, Baartman LKJ, van Tartwijk J. 2012. 'A model for programmatic assessment fit for purpose'. *Medical Teacher*, 34(3): 205–214. doi: 10.3109/0142159X.2012.652239.

van Wijchen J. 2013. *Students' development of self-efficacy in physiotherapeutic competencies*. University of Brighton https://www.dropbox.com/s/ojlsb0664az9qnh/Students'%20development%20of%20self-efficacy%20in%20physiotherapeutic%20competencies%20.pdf?dl=0 van Wijchen J, Kerry R, Nordheim Alme M. 2020. 'QuaranTrain: an international community of practice for learning'. *OpenPhysio Journal*. doi: 10.14426/ART/1552.

van Wijchen J, Oerlemans, W. 2010. Physiotherapy students performance coaching, project report. HAN University of applied science Physiotherapy. https://www.dropbox.com/s/grbu5jd2y9nzwbr/Physiotherapy%20Students%20Performance%20Coaching%20van%20Wijchen%20Oerlemans%202010.pdf?dl=0

Wenger E. 1998. 'Communities of practice: learning as a social system'. Ewenger. Available at: http://www.ewenger.com/pub/pub_systems_thinker_wrd.doc

10

IMPURE GUIDANCE? HOW MINDLINES INFORM GUIDELINES

Sietse Wieringa

Introduction

Having worked as a general practitioner (GP) and researcher in varied roles in the Netherlands, the UK, Curacao, and the USA, I became very aware that medical facts and recommendations vary greatly, even when based on the same international research evidence and clinical guidance. I noticed that most of my clinical decisions could not avoid the use of other kinds of knowledge and began to wonder how I and fellow clinicians could be sure that any of the knowledge that we use is true. For example, in Curacao, three medical traditions collide: northern American, southern American, and European (mainly Dutch). It was clear that each tradition had developed its own set of truisms with honest and ardent believers based on good research. As a result, implementation and change proved difficult and slower than expected.

I became more and more interested in concepts of knowledge creation in medicine as practised and preached by the dominant Evidence-Based Medicine (EBM) movement and embarked on a PhD to find, understand, and critique what lies beyond. Early on, I encountered the concept of mindlines, which turned out to be a very useful way to view what is meant by the 'medical knowledge' on which we base our clinical decisions. I decided to use mindlines to research the fundamentals of EBM by watching guideline developers in action. In this chapter, I revisit and use this material to explain the philosophical necessity for – and place of – mindlines in the production of guidelines.

Another essential concept for me was what Tonelli and Upshur have called "epistemic uncertainty", which they define as "[t] he challenge of applying clinical research results to individual patients; dealing with multiple sources of (at times conflicting) information, guidelines, and principles; and determining what level of

DOI: 10.4324/9781003158721-10

confidence to have and convey in a medical conclusion" (Tonelli & Upshur 2019). Whereas literature on epistemic uncertainty usually addresses the clinical encounter (Eddy 1984; Djulbegovic, Hozo & Greenland 2011; Engebretsen, Heggen, Wieringa et al. 2016), I applied an analytic lens to study efforts to reduce epistemic uncertainty in the guideline development process. I looked at the ways that panellists framed and gave meaning to knowledge, how they reasoned, and what criteria they used to evaluate the trueness of their recommendations (Wieringa, Engebretsen, Heggen et al. 2021). For this chapter, I explore mindlines as an intermediary for explicit and tacit knowing shared among social groups of practitioners, which reinforce norms of good practice in a fluid, dynamic, and constantly evolving way, especially where there is epistemic uncertainty. That, it turned out, was indeed true not just for practitioners but for guidelines-development panels.

Methods – a study of guideline development

This research was a conventional ethnography using participatory as well as observational methods to study panels involved in developing guidelines and related documents. Our research questions included the following:

1. How do guideline development panels combine (or why do they find that they are unable to combine) different kinds of evidence such as non-randomised controlled trial (RCT) research designs, routinely collected data, patient-experience data, and clinical experience and wisdom?
2. How is the work of guideline development panels influenced by different perspectives on epistemic hierarchies and approaches to uncertainty?

We used purposive sampling (Palinkas, Horwitz, Green et al. 2015) to select highly-regarded guideline development organisations that used rigorous and high standards of EBM methods and panels working on a variety of topics ranging from diverticulitis to hip fractures and from cardiovascular risk management to malnutrition screening. We also wanted to include several countries since processes for guideline development and the recommendations they produce on the same clinical entity vary considerably internationally, influenced by cultural factors including habits, patient expectations, and the healthcare system (Burgers, Grol, Klazinga et al. 2003; Christiaens, de Backer, Burgers et al. 2004; Qaseem, Forland, Macbeth et al. 2012).

Through our international networks and connections with members of the Guideline International Network, we gained approval to study panels at the National Institute for Health and Care Excellence (NICE) in the UK, the Dutch College of General Practitioners (NHG) in Netherlands, and the Norwegian Directorate of Health. NICE produces and publishes national clinical guidelines as well as guidance on the use of health technologies, social care, and public health. The Norwegian Directorate of Health produces guidance on public health. NHG produces all primary-care guidelines in the Netherlands and provides significant input on most guidance in secondary care and public health. At NICE, we were able to conduct participatory as well as observational research, as I was already a member of a guideline panel. At NHG and the Norwegian Directorate of Health, we conducted observational ethnography only.

Ethical approval

Having obtained formal ethical approval in each country, we asked guideline panel members at the outset to discuss whether this study would be acceptable to perform in collaboration with the institute's management. Before attending the panel, we explained in writing or in person to the organiser or the chair the design and purpose of the study and its value for research, and we asked the group as a whole, as well as individual members for consent. We answered further questions and gave feedback beforehand, during, and after meetings. We discussed our findings with a guideline-development coordinator at each institution to get feedback on results, analysis, and conclusions as well as to make sure our publications upheld participant anonymity as required by each of the organisations. To maintain the anonymity of all participants and interviewees, procedures were followed to mask conditions, interventions, and outcomes related to the guideline topic whenever possible. We asked all panel members to fill out a consent form. Consent was also explicitly obtained from online members whose verbatim quotes we intended to use in publications. Additional official consent procedures at the guideline-developing organisations were also followed. We discussed with the senior managers whether publishing our findings could have any unintended risks for the individual, the panels, and the organisation now or in the future.

Data collection and analysis

Between September 2016 and February 2019, we collected data from 19 panel meetings, along with documents and interviews with their members, covering a broad range of topics relevant to primary and secondary care, public health, and social care. I collected data both as a participant in my existing panel role on a NICE Clinical-Guidelines Update Team and as an observer of other guideline panels in the UK and the Netherlands. Two senior researchers helped to collect further observational data from two meetings in the UK and three in Norway. Together we observed 19 panel meetings (13 in observer role and 6 in participant-observer role). We also undertook semi-structured interviews (remotely or face-to-face) with a maximum-variety sample of ten participants recruited iteratively as the study unfolded, and we collected relevant documents. We used purposive sampling to organise the semi-structured interviews (via Skype, telephone, or in-person) with members from the guideline panels, technical committees, and managers from the organisations. Their recruitment occurred throughout the study via informal contact or formal nomination of the appropriate person by the guideline-developing organisation.

To disturb the process as little as possible, panel meetings were not audio-recorded, but we made detailed contemporaneous field notes that recorded the main discussions (including selected near-verbatim quotes), narratives, impressions, explanations, and alternative interpretations. The analysis of documents focused on publicly and non-publicly available documents produced by the organisation, committees, and group members. At NICE, this included the 'Leading Evidence to Recommendations' (LETR) tables designed to record the considerations of the guideline panels when they make a recommendation.

The panels that we observed varied greatly in setup and size. NICE panels (UK) were large (up to 25 people) and multidisciplinary (consisting of NICE staff, experts from several disciplines including health, economics, and lay members). In contrast, NHG panels (Netherlands) were usually smaller (5–15 members) and consisted of only GPs, although there was also one larger multidisciplinary panel. In Norway, the meetings were multidisciplinary (but without lay members) and had up to 15 members. The sample size did not allow comparison between countries. Findings discussed in the next section mainly draw on the NICE data, as it was larger but also because it included data from a special pilot panel aimed at following EBM principles more strictly.

Findings

Panels are expected to focus on RCTs/frequency data

Unsurprisingly, research evidence was the main type of knowledge discussed, usually randomised trials and data from other research papers. At NICE, these would most often be selected via review protocols. These generally limited the permissible study types to RCTs (and, occasionally, observational cohort studies) – a measure that was supported by panellists, who quickly learnt not to introduce non-RCT evidence.

> We only talk about research evidence, not other forms of evidence. That is the function of these groups.
>
> (*NICE panel member*)

The chair often reminded members not to bring in other knowledge (from experience or research not meeting the inclusion criteria, such as observational studies) in order to adhere to the analysis as defined in the research protocol. In practice, this proved to be quite a challenge. For instance, a panel struggled with insufficient evidence on outcomes for operating on people with cognitive impairment. As they were not allowed to make recommendations based on consensus, they looked at tendencies in the available studies instead:

PANEL MEMBER 1: Do we have enough evidence to keep cognitive impairment as a factor?

PANEL MEMBER 2: They weren't in the [X] study.

CHAIR: We're not allowed to make consensus statements, but the studies showed more positive results for operations in the cognitive impaired. (*Discussion at a NICE guideline panel)*

Of all the observed panels, the NICE Clinical Guidelines Update Panel most closely espoused the goal (in the words of a senior member) "to eliminate mindlines from that translation". It has to be stressed again that these panels were a pilot project within NICE and significantly different from standard panels at NICE. These Clinical Guidelines Update Panels consisted of a NICE technical team, topic experts, lay people, and non-expert standing committee members, working to make rapid updates of parts of existing guidelines. The standing committee members (consisting of clinicians, methodologists, lay people, and commissioners) without topic expertise were there to counterbalance the potential dominance of the contributions of the topic experts over the NICE team (who were viewed as less biased). A NICE staff member said, "Mixing specialists with neutrals, reduces evangelistic, religious belief. It can lead to standoff but that's better than using evidence [selectively] to support beliefs."

Panels have workarounds to use other sources of knowledge

However, in all countries we observed that panels still found and used other ways to include other literature, research, and expertise. Members could be assigned to ask external experts for literature on a specific topic, do some snowballing based on literature already discussed, look up other literature online during meetings, or even bring in personal work.

Much like Gabbay and le May's observations of clinicians (2004, 2011, 2016), guideline panel members did not usually read the actual research papers. At NICE, they would work with extracted data from research papers provided via email in advance of the meetings or in handouts during the meetings in the form of overviews, GRADE tables, forest plots, and other graphs produced by staff members. But extracted data could also be provided by a dedicated panel member who would be assigned to research a sub-question, or by external experts brought in to provide information on a specific topic, or by non-panel members from other organisations. At NICE, the latter included, for instance, systematic reviews produced by the Cochrane Collaboration. At NHG, as there was no budget to give every guideline panel a dedicated staff member to do this, GRADE tables could be produced by a separate team within the organisation, or as we once observed, by GP trainees who produced a "critically appraised topic".

Guideline panels would discuss papers that were excluded, especially when only a few studies made the cut, or when major studies could not be included according to the criteria in the organisation's research protocol. This could happen for instance because the follow-up duration of the study did not cohere with the research protocol, which would have been established without prior knowledge of the evidence. In these situations, panel members would put pressure on to revise the review protocol to include those studies. This was sometimes successful.

Panellists bring their mindlines into guideline production

Gabbay and le May (2011) found that mindlines would be formed by amalgamating all kinds of knowledge such as guidelines, personal memories, and experience, what experts had told them, and a lot of practical and tacit knowledge (that is, knowledge that is hard to write up, i.e., not 'explicit'), and other diffuse sources. In every one of the panels in all three countries, we observed this same phenomenon.

Such amalgamation of evidence usually happened in the context of discussing and challenging the findings from the systematic reviews or single studies. There were only a few instances where personal or individual cases were raised and discussed in detail, apart from the laypersons' experiences at NICE panels. More often panel members would share their professional experience to explain what is currently done, what could work in practice, or how they would deal with the problem.

> If I do not succeed, I will [try to place the device] a second time, and then I will do it with [specific drug] and then I usually succeed.
>
> *(NHG panel member)*

In this quote, NHG panellists discussed how they would place a device, a topic not covered in the evidence they were asked to use. This quote also serves as an example of how panellists would often simply mention what they would do in a certain situation without providing a reference to specific evidence to support their claims.

The final guideline would contain less information on the panel's discussions than the original minutes. But on several occasions, some significant knowledge discussed at the panel meetings was deliberately not included in the minutes, nor the tables that linked evidence to recommendations, nor the draft update or the final guideline. Particularly sensitive issues, such as suspected financial (instead of clinical) motives to do certain operations and procedures, appeared to be omitted. However, although the focus of most guideline panels was on handling and judging explicit (i.e., written, explainable) knowledge while observing clear rules and transparency, we found that many more kinds of knowledge were required to make recommendations. For instance, in this example, clinical panel members discussed how to advise on whether to operate on a patient:

Panel member 1: It's about transparency of that decision-making; it's inherent judgement, implicit. We should put something about that in the guideline.
Panel member 2: Can I challenge you on that? It's a bed-end decision.
Panel member 1: Is that implicit, is that transparent?
Panel member 2: I would have some idea if someone smells of alcohol.

Panel member 3: There is no clear evidence about what is driving that.
Chair: But we can make that statement, that we're concerned.

(*NICE guideline panel discussion*)

Here, the first speaker wanted recognition for the role of implicit knowledge in clinical decision-making even in the light of evidence. The second panel member tried to explicate this implicit judgement through contextual knowledge, such as the smell of the patient. This kind of knowledge is typically not included or considered in RCTs. The chair then suggested putting a statement in the documentation of the guideline apparently trying to leave room in the guidance for tacit knowledge and get around the problem of including knowledge that was not presented in the research evidence.

Our observations of nuanced actions by guideline panel members also suggested awareness of the influence of social group processes on knowledge creation. For example, a chair would adjust where members sat in order to support certain members to speak up and bring knowledge in or to oppose a dominant member. It was interesting to note that dominant members would not necessarily be topic experts. Furthermore, throughout the succession of the clinical update panel meetings, members appeared to become socialised into what was expected of them. They seemed increasingly more experienced in the processes of guideline making and acted more in ways that were expected from them by the guideline-developing institution, such as not bringing in alternative research data after the research protocol had been established. Panellists would ask more questions that would be of benefit later in the process (such as explicating the terms of the PICO – an EBM model to standardise clinical questions: People, Intervention, Comparison, Outcome – before looking at the data to prevent bias). They also grew into routines for arriving at shared recommendations more efficiently. (See also Judith Hughes' findings in Chapter 11.)

Guideline developers dealing with the influence of mindlines on guidelines

Although formally having a mostly 'fact-based' approach, there was subtle recognition at NICE that other forms of evidence had value and that excluding other kinds of knowledge was impossible, or even unwanted. For instance, a NICE Commissioning Guidelines manager discussed the recent 'controversial' asthma guidelines, which were not well received by all clinical groups:

> We draw upon robust evidence in the meetings, but what physicians [externally] don't realise is that at the meetings, we do draw on a wider range of knowledge. They just see the research evidence we draw upon. But actually, we are confident that our recommendations are sound by drawing on clinical as well as research knowledge.
>
> (*NICE Commissioning Guidelines manager in panel meeting*)

Reflecting on the contrasting views on kinds of knowledge, reasoning, and truths at play in the guideline process, a guideline maker observed lots of internal debate on the many different guideline committees' approaches all being practised in the same institution depending on the topic at hand:

> First there were the easier questions, there were the RCTs, that's where everybody started. They're easier to understand, because of things like CONSORT. They're easier to make decisions, because you've got rules. Before GRADE you had statistics, that we all understood, we all thought we understood p-value, we understood what effectiveness was. But all the time guidelines have tackled harder questions, they moved into public and social care. I think the pendulum swung in order to answer those harder questions; you have to use different types of study design. Now the reproducibility of RCTs is more of a hot item and it swings back [to a purer epistemology].
>
> *(NICE guideline developer)*

It is not just the types of knowledge but the ways of processing/handling the knowledge that often went against the transparent methods EBM aspires to. Guideline making is supposed to be a very different (rational, explicit, predominantly technical) process from the development of mindlines (subjective, emergent, predominantly deliberative) (Gabbay & le May 2004). However, a multitude of nuanced, ambiguous remarks by individual panel members appeared to significantly shape the discussions to understand the findings from the systematic reviews. These voices, however, generally did not end up as such in the final recommendations or LETR sections. LETR sections would instead present summarised deliberations on how to interpret the findings as concise arguments from a seemingly united panel. This was the case in the sense that panel members were given the opportunity after the meetings to amend the sections that portrayed the group discussions and needed to confirm their agreement with the final guideline as a whole, including those reflections. A NICE lay member however explained that due to the large size of the update reports, with a lot of medical jargon and given only a limited time frame, at least for lay members, it was uncertain if they had completely understood what was agreed upon in the guideline. Similarly, our field notes of the discussions appeared at times different from the content of the LETR.

Furthermore, deliberations were unstructured and could not be clearly separated from group interactions outside panel meetings. For instance, panel members would make use of the informal time before the meeting to discuss relevant cases that they had experienced themselves. During the meeting, they drew on such personal experiences to challenge the data presented and make alternative recommendations. Issues and context emerged in organic and unstructured ways. This was despite attempts that were made to capture deliberations and decision-making in a structured way. For instance, when RCTs or observational studies were not available, one Norwegian panel turned to the Delphi method, another to the DECIDE tool. These tools involve a kind of prioritising, valuing certain outcomes over others on pre-specified domains such as acceptability, feasibility, and resource use (Treweek, Oxman, Alderson et al. 2013). Panel members would receive training for these tools, but we did not see them successfully applied in our sample. Rather, the discussions to develop recommendations remained organic and unstructured much like the way mindlines are usually shaped.

Implications

The finding that other kinds of knowledge are embedded during guideline production is supported by other studies. Social scientists who have analysed the practices of guideline development (Atkins, Briss, Eccles et al. 2005; Moreira 2005; Nairn & Timmons 2010; Knaapen 2013) have repeatedly shown how knowledge other than systematic reviews, controlled trials, and other designs in the evidence hierarchy is unavoidably incorporated into guidelines. These other types of knowledge are used not just to challenge the evidence (e.g., using biological mechanisms and personal experience) but also to act as justifications (e.g., ethical principles and practice standards) for recommendations.

Researchers have also observed that panellists often perceive the evidence that they are expected to evaluate to be deficient. Indeed, based on one such ethnographic study of guideline development panels in Canada and the Netherlands conducted between 2007 and 2011, Knaapen identified four kinds of evidence that might be (though which were not necessarily) accepted by panellists as eligible for incorporating into the guideline: clinical trial findings, biological and pathophysiological principles, ethical issues relating to the research process (e.g., whether informed consent was obtained from trial participants), and "knowledge of the clinic" (i.e., current standards of practice and care pathways) (Knaapen 2013).

Contrary to what is generally assumed, therefore, the guideline production process is not – and indeed cannot be – restricted to purely frequentist data and objective judgements (see also Chapter 11). Our findings not only confirmed that but also suggest something further. They indicate that much more implicit knowledge beyond Knaapen's types of evidence was required to make recommendations, including an awareness of the subjective nature of decision-making and the importance of contextual knowledge. Panel members also brought to bear their accumulated caseload of personal clinical experience and their intuitive or emotionally driven hunches, collective deliberation, knowledge of pathophysiology, and so on. In short, panellists embedded their mindlines in guidelines, just as guidelines are embedded into their clinical mindlines.

To the extent that this is true (and that may vary considerably depending on the topic), the question arises of how to produce guidance that supports clinical decision-making in a meaningful way. Guideline producers could attempt to make their processes more transparent than they already do (to obtain "regulatory objectivity"). But whilst caution is needed against any attempt to 'over-script' this complex and emergent process, guideline production could be subjected to more radical solutions, including (1) rethinking what form guidance should take, (2) making better use of virtual networks of clinicians, (3) starting a dialogue on purification and uncertainty, and (4) rethinking the nature of knowledge translation. The latter might also stimulate reflexive practices that highlight the need for a critical awareness of fundamental philosophical assumptions about the nature of clinical reality. I discuss each suggested solution here in more detail.

New forms of guidance: from guidelines to a new genre of tools

If we acknowledge an unavoidable interaction between guidelines and mindlines, we need to consider the shape and form of guidelines too. Some re-tooling has already taken place within the EBM paradigm, as knowledge tools to facilitate this have been developed. The "just in time" and "just enough" tools such as medication-choice cards and option-grid decision aids (Wyatt, Branda, Anderson et al. 2014; Elwyn, Wieringa and Greenhalgh 2016a; Elwyn, Wieringa and Greenhalgh 2016b) and NHG guidelines are characterised by being short, flexible and accessible; they address the reason for the clinical encounter (not a textbook condition), and they compare alternative options (Elwyn, Wieringa & Greenhalgh 2016b). However, for new forms of guidelines to interact in a meaningful way with clinicians' mindlines, several further challenges would need to be dealt with to support evidence-based decision-making in the clinical encounter. In a previous paper, I argued, with others, that not only should guidelines include other kinds of knowledge and reasoning, but they also have to work with imperfect knowledge, be able to deal with unique single-case scenarios, and deal with multiple options as well as multiple actions (Elwyn, Wieringa & Greenhalgh 2016b). If, and exactly how this can be achieved remains a topic for further research, but it may mean that recommendations will give more leeway and provide contingent arguments that support going against them when appropriate.

Virtual social networks linking guidelines to mindlines

To allow this new genre of tools to be produced fast and frugally and in collaborations with patients and clinicians, many creative software formats have been developed, which contrast with guideline panels that typically take years to arrive at definitive recommendations (Elwyn, Wieringa & Greenhalgh 2016b). However, their processes may not necessarily link them to the mindlines of communities of clinicians or patients. The far less structured interactions on the virtual social networks of clinicians or patients may be of use for guideline development as they represent a broad understanding of knowledge and perhaps the mindlines of groups. Research shows that not all networks will provide deep, rich knowledge, but the idea of analysing selected virtual social networks as part of guideline update processes could help to better frame and synchronise recommendations with the mindlines of clinicians and patients (Wieringa, Engebretsen, Heggen et al. 2018). It would raise basic and fundamental questions: How would we define a virtual social network? What does a good network look like? How should we study these networks?

Some principles of internet research could help to develop an appropriate methodology to do this. As Christine Hine wrote, "Internet research has arguably been a valuable reflexive opportunity for the traditional disciplines that have fed its development" (Hine 2005 p. 239). Guideline developers could consider experimenting and set up collaborations with these networks. Further research would be required to examine whether using virtual social networks in this way in guideline production processes is feasible and produces meaningful guidance.

Towards a dialogue on purification and epistemological uncertainty

At the same time, new knowledge tools and virtual networks remain purifications of reality, unable to fully substitute for the judgement, experience, sensitivity, and humanity (Elwyn, Wieringa & Greenhalgh 2016b) of the mindlines in a real face-to-face encounter in clinical practice. Purification is a term Bruno Latour (2013) used to indicate that we as 'modernists' tend to divide reality in nature (which has always been) and human culture (which is man-made) while also trying to bring them together again (which he calls translation) (Wieringa, Engebretsen, Heggen et al. 2017). Ultimately, we never succeed in fully doing either, as the findings from the guideline panels show too. While attempting to objectify – that is purify – conditions such as a hip fracture or diverticulitis using the PICO as much as possible throughout the process, they had to see any condition not only as obeying the rules of physics but of societal maxims too. Latour would say that each is in reality a "quasi-object" that we artificially pull apart in nature and human culture. A dialogue within the EBM movement is needed about the role, the paradox, benefits, and harms of the modernist practice of purification. Rather than a sequence of research-driven abstract decisions, guideline makers should conceptualise clinical decision-making based on mindlines as a situated practice, always starting from the real problems of individual real patients (and real organisations and systems) in their real contexts.

This dialogue should start with undergraduate students, teaching them about epistemological uncertainty (the problem of making predictions) which lies at the heart of what it is to practice excellent medicine (Tonelli & Upshur 2019). Much of the training we offer students in EBM, however, can be thought of as a systematic approach to reducing the patient's presenting problem to a series of PICO questions. Critics argue that this training encourages them to over-value knowledge that can be made explicit and quantified, ready for frequentist reasoning – much as guidelines panels set out to do.

Instead of a limited practice of 'evidence-basing', evidence-based clinical decision-making could concern itself with 'inference in healthcare' as the many ways to explicate and mitigate epistemic uncertainty (Tonelli & Upshur 2019). In the process of building capability to cope with clinical complexity ("the ability to adapt to change, generate new knowledge, and continuously improve performance" (Fraser & Greenhalgh 2001 p. 799)), students should at least be able to debate and consider some of the broader philosophical assumptions underpinning clinical decision-making in healthcare, including knowledge as conceptualised in mindlines.

From knowledge translation to exploring the fundamentals of prediction and reality

Knowledge translation typically views knowledge as detached packages, held by no one individual, but there for anyone to use (Greenhalgh & Wieringa 2011). Think for instance of guidelines, papers, or medical webpages that exist out there for general use. The findings from the panels urge us to dismiss this narrow conceptualisation; medical knowledge is much broader than that. Mindlines can be conceived as a pragmatic container of knowledge, sufficiently flexible to dynamically hold many theories of knowledge. Instead of being defined in terms of an entity (fact-out-there) or as a property of an object (a single brain or computer), knowledge as in mindlines could be seen as a property of an interaction (like force and energy in physics): not directly observable but guiding and manifesting itself in real-world decision-making. Previous research had already shown that it is difficult to see EBM taking place directly in clinical consultations (Zwolsman, van Dijk & de Waard 2013). This suggests a move away from the current conception of decision-making in EBM, and indeed from the materialist and atomistic philosophy of science derived from classical physics that theories within the social sciences, including decision theory, still float upon. In classical physics, the world is perceived as consisting of many singular objects (molecules, apples, planets) that obey the laws of Newton. This extends to an idea that human brains are nothing more than molecules (the hardware) that determine knowledge (the software). As molecules have clear and separate states, decision-making in this view (simply put) is nothing more than choosing from clear predetermined singular preferences. Mindlines would fit modern, quantum physics, which sees particles as merely excitations in fields, like a large wave in a sea. Just as waves don't have clear delineations and are always connected to other waves, this would also apply to clusters of particles, like brains (hardware) and knowledge (software). Patients and clinicians would have implicit and unspecified preferences that only become actual and clear in the process of making the decision, like the big wave that results from interaction between many other waves from many directions. The underlying assumption is that it is not objects or thoughts themselves that are real; only their probabilities are real. What comes to be (that which we wish to infer) exists only as part of a set of interactions, not as a stand-alone entity. This conceptualisation challenges the use of decision aids and classic probability theory, which in contrast require distinct and independent, objectified options (Wendt 2015; Aerts, Beltran, Geriente et al. 2018).

As mindlines permit knowledge to be individually held and collectively shared at the same time, and are able to be played out differently in different contexts, the concept also allows us to question whether guideline makers and researchers can ever be independent and avoid conflict of interest and maintaining a 'scientific disinterest'. Perhaps it should be accepted that different panels will make different recommendations based on the same evidence, even in similar contexts (Reynen, Robson, Ivory et al. 2018) not only because of interaction but also because of the probabilistic nature of reality itself. This is complex but not chaotic – some recommendations and predictions of outcomes are more likely than others. Further research could develop new models and examine decision- and prediction-making in light of alternative concepts of reality and of the tensions between guidelines and mindlines during the clinical encounter.

Summary

- I present findings from an ethnographic study on guideline panels, and how they were using mindlines in their deliberations.
- The panels struggled with a fundamental problem – namely, that the rules expected them to eliminate mindlines from knowledge translation and use only explicit knowledge, but due to limited available research evidence, and clinicians inevitably working with their own mindlines, they could not actually come up with sensible guidelines if they adhered to that rule.
- Depending on their organisational context and their own personal predilections, they all solved the inability of only using explicit knowledge in different ways and produced guidelines that – had they been done by other panels – would almost certainly have been different.
- As mindlines of clinicians were inevitably part of guideline production, the final guideline recommendations depended partly on mindlines, just as clinical mindlines depend partly on guidelines.
- I have put forward some implications of these conclusions, including new forms of guidelines, the use of virtual social networks of clinicians and patients, to consider purification and uncertainty as well as to rethink fundamental assumptions about knowledge, reality, and, the relationship between the two, to gain more reflexivity in guideline production.

Acknowledgements

Many thanks to senior researchers David Wright and Gina Fraas Henrichsen for their contributions toward data collection. I also thank Toni Tan and Nichole Taske at NICE, Margriet Bouma at NHG, and Frode Forland, specialist director infectious diseases and global health, Norwegian Institute of Public Health in Oslo, for making this research possible. Research for this chapter was funded by European Union Seventh Framework Programme (FP7-PEOPLE- 2013- COFUND), Grant/Award Number: 609020 and the National Institute for Health Research Biomedical Research Centre, Oxford, UK (grant NIHR- BRC-1215-20008).

References

Aerts D, Beltran L, Geriente S, Bianch MS, Sozzo S, van Sprundel R. 2018. 'Quantum theory methods as a possible alternative for the double-blind gold standard of evidence-based medicine: outlining a new research program'. *Foundations of Science*. Springer Netherlands, 24(2): 217–225. doi: 10.1007/s10699-018-9572-0.

Atkins D, Briss PA, Eccles M, FLotttorp, S, Guyatt GH, Harbour RT, Hill S, Jaesche R, Liberati A, Magrini N, MAson J, O'Connel D, Oxman AD, Phillips B, Schünemann H, Edejer TTT, Vist GE, Williams JW, Cobley UT, the GRADE working group. 2005. 'Systems for grading the quality of evidence and the strength of recommendations II: pilot study of a new system'. *BMC Health Services Research*, 5(1): 25. doi: 10.1186/1472-6963-5-25.

Burgers JS, Grol R, Klazinga NS, Mäkelä M, Zaat J, AGREE Collaboration. 2003. 'Towards evidence-based clinical practice: an international survey of 18 clinical guideline programs'. *International Journal for Quality in Health Care*, 1:31–45. doi: 10.1093/intqhc/15.1.31. PMID: 12630799.

Christiaens T, de Backer D, Burgers JS, Baerheim A. 2004. 'Guidelines, evidence, and cultural factors'. *Scandinavian Journal of Primary Health Care*, 22(3): 141–145. doi: 10.1080/02813430410006521.

Djulbegovic B, Hozo I, Greenland S. 2011. *Uncertainty in clinical medicine, philosophy of medicine*. Elsevier B.V. doi: 10.1016/B978-0-444-51787-6.50011-8.

Eddy DM. 1984. 'Variations in physician practice the role of uncertainty'. *Health Affairs*, 3(2): 74–89. doi: 10.4103/0970-0218.112447.

Elwyn G, Pickles T, Edwards A, Kinsey K, Brain K, Newcombe RG, Firth J, Marrin K, Nye A, Wood F. 2016a. 'Supporting shared decision making using an Option Grid for osteoarthritis of the knee in an interface musculoskeletal clinic: a stepped wedge trial'. *Patient Education and Counseling*. Elsevier Ireland Ltd, 99(4): 571–577. doi: 10.1016/j.pec.2015.10.011.

Elwyn G, Wieringa S, Greenhalgh T. 2016b. 'Clinical encounters in the post-guidelines era'. *BMJ*, 3200(June): i3200. doi: 10.1136/bmj.i3200.

Engebretsen E, Heggen K, Wieringa S, Greenhalgh T. 2016 Uncertainty and objectivity in clinical decision making: a clinical case in emergency medicine. *Med Health Care Philos*. 4:595–603. doi: 10.1007/s11019-016-9714-5. PMID: 27260370; PMCID: PMC5088215.

Fraser SW, Greenhalgh T. 2001. 'Coping with complexity: educating for capability'. *BMJ (Clinical research ed.)*, 323(7316): 799–803. Available at: http://www.pubmedcentral.nih.gov/articlerender.fcgi?artid=1121342&tool=pmcentrez&rendertype=abstract.

Gabbay J, le May A. 2004. 'Evidence based guidelines or collectively constructed "mindlines?" Ethnographic study of knowledge management in primary care'. *British Medical Journal*, 329(7473): 1013. doi: 10.1136/bmj.329.7473.1013.

Gabbay J, le May A. 2011. *Practice-based evidence for healthcare: clinical mindlines*. Abingdon: Routledge.

Gabbay J, le May A. 2016. 'Mindlines: making sense of evidence in practice'. *British Journal of General Practice*, 66(649): 402–403. doi: 10.3399/bjgp16X686221.

Greenhalgh T, Wieringa S. 2011. 'Is it time to drop the "knowledge translation" metaphor? A critical literature review'. *Journal of the Royal Society of Medicine*, 104(12): 501–509. doi: 10.1258/jrsm.2011.110285.

Hine C. 2005. 'Internet research and the sociology of cyber-social-scientific knowledge'. *The Information Society*, 21(4): 239–248. doi: 10.1080/01972240591007553.

Knaapen L. 2013. 'Being "evidence-based" in the absence of evidence: the management of non-evidence in guideline development'. *Social Studies of Science*, 43(5): 681–706. doi: 10.1177/0306312713483679.

Latour B. 2013. *We have never been modern*. Cambridge: Harvard University Press

Moreira T. 2005. 'Diversity in clinical guidelines: the role of repertoires of evaluation'. *Social Science and Medicine*, 60(9): 1975–1985. doi: 10.1016/j.socscimed.2004.08.062.

Nairn S, Timmons, S. 2010. 'Scientific uncertainty and the creation of resuscitation guidelines'. *Social Theory and Health*, 8(4): 289–308. doi: 10.1057/sth.2009.4.

Palinkas LA, Horwitz SM, Green CA, Wisdom JP, Duan N, Hoagwood K. 2015. 'Purposeful sampling for qualitative data collection and analysis in mixed method implementation research'. *Administration and Policy in Mental Health*, *42*(5), 533–544. https://doi.org/10.1007/s10488-013-0528-y

Qaseem A, Forland F, Macbeth F, Ollenschläger G, Phillips S, van der Wees P, Board of Trustees of the Guidelines International Network. 2012. 'Guidelines International Network: toward international standards for clinical practice guidelines'. *Annals of Internal Medicine*. Apr 3;156(7):525–531. doi: 10.7326/0003-4819-156-7-201204030-00009. PMID: 22473437.

Reynen E, Robson R, Ivory J, Hwee J, Straus SE, Pham B', Tricco AC. 2018. 'A retrospective comparison of systematic reviews with same-topic rapid reviews'. *Journal of Clinical Epidemiology*, doi: 10.1016/j.jclinepi.2017.12.001.

Tonelli MR, Upshur REG. 2019. 'A philosophical approach to addressing uncertainty in medical education'. *Academic Medicine*, 94(4): 1. doi: 10.1097/acm.0000000000002512.

Treweek S, Oxman AD, Alderson P, Bossuyt PM, Brandt L, Brożek J, Davoli M, Flottrop S, Harbour R, Hill S, Liberati A, Liira H, Schünemann HJ, Rosenbaum S, Thornton J, Vandvik PE, Alonso-Coello P, Cobley UT, DECIDE Consortium. 2013. 'Developing and evaluating communication strategies to support informed decisions and practice based on evidence (decide): protocol and preliminary results'. *Implementation Science : IS*, 8(6): 1–12. doi: 10.1186/1748-5908-8-6.

Wendt A. 2015. '*Quantum mind and social science'*. *Unifying Phisical and Social Ontology*. doi: 10.1017/CBO9781316005163.

Wieringa S, Engebretsen E, Heggen K, Greenhalgh T. 2017. 'Has evidence-based medicine ever been modern? A Latour-inspired understanding of a changing EBM'. *Journal of Evaluation in Clinical Practice*. 23(5):964–970. doi: 10.1111/jep.12752. Epub 2017 May 16. PMID: 28508440; PMCID: PMC5655926.

Wieringa S, Engebretsen E, Heggen K, Greenhalgh T. 2018. 'How knowledge is constructed and exchanged in virtual communities of physicians: qualitative study of mindlines online'. *Journal of Medical Internet Research*; 20(2):e34 doi: 10.2196/jmir.8325

Wieringa S, Engebretsen E, Heggen K, Greenhalgh T. 2021. 'Clinical guidelines and the pursuit of reducing epistemic uncertainty. An ethnographic study of guideline development panels in three countries'. *Social Science & Medicine*. Elsevier Ltd, 272(January): 113702. doi: 10.1016/j.socscimed.2021.113702.

Wyatt KD, Branda ME, Anderson RT, Pencille LJ, Montori, VM, Hess EP, Ting HH, Le Blanc A. 2014. 'Peering into the black box: a meta-analysis of how clinicians use decision aids during clinical encounters'. *Implementation Science*, 9(1): 1–10. doi: 10.1186/1748-5908-9-26.

Zwolsman SE, van Dijk N, de Waard MW. 2013. 'Observations of evidence-based medicine in general practice'. *Perspectives on Medical Education*, 2(4). doi: 10.1007/s40037-013-0078-8.

11

THE GUIDELINE DEVELOPMENT PROCESS

Building a lexicon of mindlines

Judith Hughes

Introduction

Guideline development depends upon heterogenous groups of health and allied health professionals, patient and carer representatives, and guideline process experts. While the guideline development scenario is very different from the clinical context in which the mindline concept was conceived, it is inevitable that the participants will bring to the table their prior knowledge, experience, and assumptions about specific diseases in specific contexts. They will, in short, have the implicit resource of the clinical mindlines that guide their own practices. This has the potential to influence the final guideline, as Sietse Wieringa has shown in the previous chapter. Moreover, whilst considering the evidence that underpins the guidelines, the participants will also have different – sometimes conflicting, sometimes converging – roles to play, which could be an important contextual factor not only in the final product but also in the revision and negotiation of their own clinical mindlines. How might that impact on the agreed guideline that emerges from the group?

Around the time that Wieringa was doing his fieldwork, I was also embarking on PhD research that involved non-participant observation of a series of NICE Guideline Committee meetings within my own specialty of ophthalmology. My thesis revealed new insights into the social processes of guideline development. It provided:

> a detailed account of how the guideline group – working within an environment that includes influential external stakeholders – interpreted evidence, interacted and functioned as a group, and made consensus decisions on guideline recommendations. The study revealed that the ready availability (and acceptability) of evidence shapes the extent of reliance on expert opinion. In circumstances of low evidence availability, expert opinion is relied upon and

DOI: 10.4324/9781003158721-11

> factors such as group composition and dynamics, resource availability and external network challenges appear to be particularly important in the guideline development process and in shaping the guideline recommendations.
>
> (*Hughes 2018, abstract*)

During the fieldwork, I came across Gabbay and le May's accounts of mindlines (2004, 2011), and its relevance to what I was observing struck me immediately. I discussed this with them at the time and began analysing and interpreting the emerging data through the mindlines lens. As is often the way, however, my PhD research took a different direction, so the observations that I made were never analysed or written up within the theoretical framework of mindlines. When offered the opportunity to do so by revisiting the data as a contribution to this book, I agreed, and am grateful for the help they gave me in developing this chapter.

Methods

The committee I observed was developing a guideline for the diagnosis and management of a common ophthalmic disease. The committee followed the NICE generic structure for a guideline development group and consisted of a range of expert clinicians, primary-care physicians, allied health professionals, health economists, and laypersons. Also included as subjects for my research were the NICE personnel associated with the committee. This aimed at providing a more rounded view of the guideline development process. Ethical approval of this research was granted by the University of St Andrews.

My fieldwork took a real-time, case-study approach. This had the advantages of less emphasis on any particular outcomes, greater ability to use emerging themes to bring out the nuances of the data, and less reliance on interviewees' memories. The methods of data generation combined direct observation of the committee at work, semi-structured interviews of group members to validate observations, and review of documents pertinent to the guideline's development. I observed multiple committee meetings over 17 months, comprising 120 hours of observation. I held 22 formal interviews (average 40 minutes) and 25 ad hoc interviews (each 5–10 minutes). Documentary review covered over 1,500 pages of various documents. I used manual thematic analysis, following Braun and Clarke (2006, 2014), as the optimal way to maintain close contact with the data.

In the account that follows there is no verbatim group-discussion material included, as I was not permitted to use this. All verbatim quotes are from subject interviews or my research notes. Where there are interview quotes, I have included some indication of the committee member being quoted, but to preserve anonymity, I have omitted details of their professional and/or committee roles.

Mindlines, being so often inarticulable, present researchers with the problem of recognition and explication. In trying to make the mindline process in guideline development more transparent, I attempted to use the techniques of critical incident narrative (CIN) (Flanagan, 1954). This can explore significant differences, or turning points, in a situation, and I hoped it might provide a useful method to examine the reshaping of individual mindlines. Whilst observing certain topics of discussion at the committee meetings, I noted critical points of difference in practice plus a collective agreement on a *new* course of action, behaviour, or practice. In the subsequent interviews, I explored with the respondents an actual, or intended, change of behaviour suggesting acceptance of a new clinical practice. This, then, could possibly be considered to be a negotiation and refinement of an individual's clinical mindline for a specific topic, arising from the NICE committee process. It didn't work particularly well (CIN tends to be used to theoretically underpin extreme crisis situations), but it did help me recognise examples of the renegotiation of individual clinical mindlines.

Different types of mindlines

When I revisited my data to write this chapter, I was able to see a confluence of different kinds of mindlines intersecting and interacting while the guideline evidence was being appraised, assimilated, and transformed into guideline recommendations. These might include not only the clinical mindlines both of practitioner and patient committee members – but what I will call '*process mindlines*', which include '*chairing mindlines'*, and '*participant mindlines*', all of which had an unseen influence on the guidelines that eventually emerged.

Clinical mindlines

> [T]here's going to be a guideline written and it's got to be based on the knowledge of people around the table and any sort of evidence that's out there to inform that.
>
> *(Layperson)*

> Obviously, the recommendations are very contextual and it involves a lot more areas of expertise than just the evidence.
>
> (*Allied health professional*)

My data confirmed that committee members were clearly drawing on their own clinical mindlines in their discussions. For example, during one meeting, a clinician commented that he and one other clinician on the committee had very different rules for starting and stopping treatment. Both sets of rules were debated, as were – on another occasion – the different tests they did, and at which point in diagnosis and management. In both these examples, there was a paucity of data for the committee to discuss; hence, many were saying what they would do or what their local hospital did. One intriguing, and related, new insight was that interview comments from committee members suggested the possibility of geographical differences influencing the final consensus about any given guideline:

> Also, I've noticed a number of times, what has come up is the differences in practice around the country and, therefore, if you have people from the Northwest or the Northeast or a heavy preponderance of those people, perhaps you'll get one certain view. I don't know whether that's considered when NICE are putting together the group or not. I've been quite amazed by the difference, the variation in practice around the country.
>
> (*Layperson*)

> There is a lot of variation between how patients are treated, how they are managed and diagnosed. It's huge.
>
> (*Clinician*)

Committee members seemed to take for granted that their own experience and views were relevant. As one interviewee put it,

> So, because it's quite interesting, you know, a conundrum, isn't it? I guess if you're part of a group that's making consensus decisions, either you fight tooth and nail during the meeting and you turn it to the way that you feel or you go with the consensus which might mean that you have to change your own practice and the question is whether one does that or one doesn't do that.
>
> (*Clinician*)

Discussions did have an impact on the members' individual mindlines and perhaps hence their own practice. Box 11.1, which includes material from observation notes as well as interview data, is an account of the discussion about the recommendation of the guideline committee to revise existing disease classification systems to one simpler classification. It illustrates how individual clinical mindlines were being negotiated as part of the guideline-development process and revised by social interaction. The committee members appear to have agreed on a collective mindline that reshaped some individuals' mindlines, at least as demonstrated by the intent of individual committee members to change their own practice to what the group had newly agreed.

Whilst it is impossible to say whether that interviewee followed through and used the new classification in practice, the intent was present; their mindline had altered. Another example, however, suggested an actual change in practice after group discussions. Here, the group had discussed the diagnosis and symptoms of the disease and how patients could self-monitor and had agreed that self-monitoring was to become part of one of the guideline recommendations. During that discussion, one of the clinician members had suggested what patients could look out for e.g. a distorted image. At a subsequent meeting, another clinician member – an allied health professional – told how s/he had absorbed this into their clinical practice, saying,

> I tell all of my patients this now; it's great, thanks
>
> (*Observation notes*)

BOX 11.1 DID THE NICE COMMITTEE ON DISEASE CLASSIFICATION ALTER THE PARTICIPANTS' OWN CLINICAL MINDLINES?

There are various classification systems in use for the pathology of the disease and for chronological stages of the disease. The use of so many systems adds confusion to an already complex disease and the experience of the 12 co-opted experts on the committee suggested that different classifications are used by different parties in different circumstances. For example, when discussing the disease with patients, the ophthalmology nurse used one classification, but the clinical experts used a different classification when discussing the disease with colleagues. One lay member, whose charity produces information about the disease for patients and carers, used yet another classification.

The discussion at the committee meeting was around the unacceptability of using all the different classifications to support a guideline recommendation for disease classification. There was a proposal from NICE team members that creating a *new* classification would be a reasonable approach. Long discussions ensued about what that new classification would be and how it was intended that it would be used, and by whom, and in what circumstances. The group reached a consensus, and they discussed how all would sing from the same hymn sheet. A laminated copy of the new classification was produced and distributed to the committee members at their next meeting. Individual clinicians and other eye-care professionals said they fully intended to use the new classification system straightaway in their own practice. This was confirmed during follow-up interviews:

Interviewer: "Do you think this particular guideline will change your own practice?"

Interviewee (clinician): "My own clinical practice as an individual clinician?"

Interviewer: "Yes. You mentioned earlier about having a crib sheet for the new classification system. Would that change your practice?"

Interviewee: Yes! Definitely.

An example of how the formation of collective mindlines in the committee reshaped individual mindlines came during the discussions about barriers and facilitators to patient treatment. The discussion was about patients' experience of coming into hospital. Research data capturing this was qualitative in nature and given a low acceptability/quality score by NICE. There was little interest or input in the discussions from the clinicians but much animation from non-clinicians (including patients) to relate their own experiences. Some discussion was around accessibility of transport to hospital, especially for those who were blind or partially sighted. After some quite heated discussion, everyone on the committee (including the clinicians) recognised that this was something that they had not considered previously to be a barrier to treatment. This resulted in consensus wording in the guideline that individuals' accessibility to services, such as transportation, should be taken into account when treatment is planned or monitored. However, this is another example of intent; I was not in a position to check actual practice.

In a similar vein and for the same barriers-and-facilitators-to-treatment section of the guideline, there was discussion around whether the eye-injection treatments caused pain. Those having experienced pain themselves or others, like ophthalmic-nurses or eye-clinic liaison officers to whom patients had spoken about it – as opposed to the patients (not) talking to the clinicians giving the eye injections – very clearly said there was pain associated with these injections. This was dismissed initially by clinicians in the discussions held but gradually there was acceptance of the pain of injection being a possible barrier to treatment.

> [M]y interpretation of the [qualitative] study was that intolerance to treatment was because of pain on injection and, as I have experienced that too, I wanted to give support to future patients and add something to the rec[ommendation].
>
> (*Patient interview*)

The collective mindline that emerged in the discussions resulted in the guideline incorporating a recommendation for promotion of peer support for new patients having injections. Again, whether this resulted in a change in clinical practice is hard to say.

Such data suggested that individual experience of the sort that strongly influences clinical mindlines not only played a part in the guideline negotiations but was also influenced by the collective discussion. The distinction between the guideline, ostensibly based on high-quality research data, and the collective and individual clinical mindlines was a blurred one, and the influence between them was bidirectional.

But the question I then asked myself was whether it was possible that mindlines other than *clinical* mindlines might also be playing a part. So, for example, might mindlines be identified that relate to the guideline-committee process and functioning, such as the NICE process of evidence sifting, review and recommendation crafting, or the chairing process, or individuals' internalised guidance about how to participate effectively in the group?

Process mindlines

One key inductive theme extracted from the data was 'process'. It referred to the way the NICE technical process was presented, embedded, discussed, accepted, and used, beginning with how the disease-topic technical evidence was presented and received and ending with crafting the wording of guideline recommendations.

Individual expert members came to guideline development with their own ideas of what would be involved. Changes to those beliefs and values around the process resulted from the garnering of knowledge by formal learning, such as from the NICE manual, and by social interaction with the NICE team associated with the guideline and with other experts on the committee. The collective way of 'doing' the guideline-development process became embedded and endorsed. Numerous examples of this were found in the interview data:

> You just have a certain way to write certain things.
>
> (*NICE team member*)

> They [NICE] are incredibly process-driven, that's nice in a way. They're so process-driven and if you understand the process, you understand exactly where they are coming from.
>
> (*Allied health professional*)

> We have to stick to NICE-approved terminology, 'NICE-speak'
>
> (*Lay member*)

> So, they're bringing, presumably, a structure that they've used with other guidelines but are prepared to have it tweaked to be relevant for this particular condition. So, they're steering us in terms of providing a framework but are open to that framework being stretched or challenged.
>
> (*Allied health professional*).

> I take them at their word that they've looked through the appropriate stuff in the first place and weeded it out to the stage that they're then prepared to share with us. So, I don't have any qualms with that part of the process.
>
> (*Lay member*)

> But we do rely very much on that sifting process because, you know, out of those three thousand, two hundred studies, we end up with seventeen studies, for example. Who's to know that one of the good studies hasn't been picked out in the sifting, so we have to take the word of our NICE internal team to trust that they've done a good sift and they've not thrown out some of the good studies that we really needed to have seen?
>
> (*Clinician*)

Observations of that process in my research notes hinted strongly that a notion of 'how we do things here' was being collectively and individually internalised. A clear example was apparent when draft recommendations were being produced during the meetings. A NICE team member would enter the wording of the recommendation electronically and project it onto a screen so all the committee could contribute to its revision. The group would revise words and phrases until they reached a consensus that the wording reflected both the supporting evidence and what they wished to convey as guidance. An Editing Team would then ensure that the language used in the draft recommendation aligned with NICE standards for writing style and had the necessary clarity for the different audiences who access guidelines.

> It starts with so many ways/thoughts of how to write the draft recommendation and what should be the content. The committee are brought around to the NICE way of writing them, e.g., using active verbs at the start of a sentence, and clearly words matter, e.g., "routinely", as they mean something particular to NICE.
>
> (*Observation notes*)

As the group matured and got used to this procedure, they were learning how to handle the process in a similar way to how Gabbay and le May have described the formation of clinical mindlines.

> The group became faster at developing recommendations with less discussion (is this apathy, acceptance of the process, or knowledge that editors will change it later anyway?).
>
> (*Observation notes*)

The committee members often described the crafting of the wording of the recommendations as "problematic". Many of them had many negative views of the process, although they all subscribed eventually to the NICE way of doing it (although that may have been because they were not sure they had that much leverage to change it):

> I think that's when it gets quite tricky because then no one is coming up with a sentence. I find phrasing things very difficult. I think we all seem to be very good at talking through the evidence and then, there's that moment when you have to say what you are actually going to recommend. That's when it seems to be very difficult and everyone goes a bit quiet.
>
> (*Clinician*)

> So, there is an awful lot of constraining of what we're allowed to say and not allowed to say.
>
> (*Allied health professional*)

> I think it makes it difficult because the phrases that you're not allowed to use, because they're not NICE-speak, seem to be the ones that we would all naturally choose to use. So that makes it difficult. … I think it's fine then when someone tells you what it should be but I think it just seems a bit alien. They never seem to be the phrases you would naturally choose.
>
> (*Allied health professional*)

> Recommendations. It feels like a complete free-for-all at times, you know. Everybody just pitches in with what they would like to say and then somehow it is edited down. The re-editing moments of those recommendations are really interesting in that they come back to us after going through NICE. The people at NICE criticise whether the language is good enough. It comes back and we approve it but, of course, that's two or three meetings afterwards and you no longer have the evidence in front of you, so those subtleties of wording then actually make a massive difference.
>
> (*Allied health professional*)

The group seemed to move from individualistic ways of approaching the drafting of recommendations to a faster process within a collectively negotiated and accepted set of parameters. Thus, I began to think that maybe the way that recommendations were written was possibly an example of process mindlines in action. Although it is perhaps debatable whether this may be labelled as a mindline, it shows characteristics of how individual knowledge is influenced by others, in context, in practice. It also shares two other key characteristics of clinical mindlines. First was the way the committee moved beyond meticulous thinking and painstaking argument towards forging rapid and flexible solutions. Second was how this so often arose from what appeared to be a tacitly negotiated way forward when – both for the group as a whole and the individuals within it – there were conflicting demands that could not be met by simply following protocol or formal NICE procedures. A recurring feature of the process was the need to resolve tensions between what the individual members felt would be the most appropriate process, and what they were being required ideally to do. The interview quotes in Box 11.2 reveal, for example, tensions over:

- the acceptability of different types of evidence,
- the lack of availability of high-quality evidence,
- how to handle areas of practice that lack good evidence,
- the degree of deference to experts within the committee,
- meeting the varied needs of the guidelines' intended audiences,
- knowing whose judgement to trust and why,
- handling relations with stakeholders outside the committee,
- accommodating the pharmaceutical industry's perspectives,
- managing political and economic constraints,

- working within strict time constraints, and
- agreeing on the final recommendation.

BOX 11.2 TENSIONS IN THE GUIDELINES DEVELOPMENT PROCESS

1. *It is difficult and that's always the danger between being too prescriptive and saying this is what you have to do, versus, recognising that there is variation in practice.*
2. *I don't know whether they do or it is an impossible circle to square: writing for a patient but really it's a clinician [as the intended recipient]. They ... want to be wholly evidence-based, as well as use expert opinion, but still not upset regulatory frameworks. It's a very difficult balance to strike, isn't it? It's a very narrow tightrope to walk. Do NICE understand that there's a difference between the audiences? I think that they probably do but I don't think they're ever going to solve it. I don't think they can.*
3. *... the quantitative data's not that robust. You do things to three decimal places and all that kind of thing and [it's] how people then interpret those differences and understand them.*
4. *... in terms of the presentation of evidence that we've had, there doesn't seem to be anything that's particularly strong evidence ... you know, it's all sort of, moderate to low quality.*
5. *I think, depending again on the particular bit of evidence that we've been looking at, it's shocking in some respects that there isn't more that is of a better quality.*
6. *There's always a bit of a worry for me around quantitative data that appears to, sort of, overly infer a sense of accuracy which doesn't exist.*
7. *I think it's [qualitative data] an important source of information and it can often highlight and shine a light on things that you can't get from purely quantitative analysis.*
8. *... obviously they are deferred to a lot, aren't they, the clinical experts? So, it is a problem when there's only one there, I think.*
9. *I don't know if many more would have been better in terms of clinical experts because there'd be a real tendency for that group to completely dominate the committee.*
10. *... we haven't particularly drilled down on that in terms of, you know, what treatment regimes are being used in the* ***real*** *world. How many people in the real world actually are treated to plan. ... You should include it [Medisoft data] because it does mirror what happens, I think, a lot in the real world.*
11. *What I think is difficult is that a lot of this is tied because it has to be about [name of disease]. So, there are lots of studies out there that might show that doing certain things is helpful. The studies have looked at whole populations of*

people with poor vision or what support you have in poor vision needs but they aren't going to be included in this because they're not purely [name of disease].

12. *I'd find it obviously colossally difficult to provide guidance on any number of the other questions we've looked at in this guideline which have no robust evidence base at all. We're entirely reliant on the expertise of the people who deal with it day by day.*
13. *The impact on the guideline comes back to the limitations of which clinician you have round the table and how many ophthalmologists you have. That to me is a massive limitation. If it's left to expert opinion, that's what you're left with and the experts in the room then really, really matter.*
14. *I've heard it said by NICE team members that you round the table are there to give your expert opinion, but then ... we don't want it.*
15. *... we need that expert opinion when it comes to evidence-free zones or even evidence-poor zones. When it comes to the stuff that is well-evidenced, yeah, actually adding expert opinion on top of that tends to be more of an irritant.*
16. *I think, possibly, the ability to interpret the evidence is an issue and I feel that for myself. I'm reliant on other people accepting that the evidence [is] saying that it means what it says it means. I don't have the ability to do that. I'm not a statistician so, I find that difficult to challenge. I guess that's why there are lots of us but it does mean that I am ceding judgement to other people in lots of cases.*
17. *I think there's some who are overshadowed by a lot of professionals because they work in the field, they have more knowledge and expertise.*
18. *I think, getting stuff done in time is a big pressure. The influence on this is from line management. How we deal with that pressure comes from the line management. So, one approach [presenting all evidence] is safe but possibly means more work than necessary. One approach [extract the most useful evidence and present less to the group] is more risky but would mean less work. If any of those risks blew up in your face then you're set back ... it's difficult, so, your line manager guides you through that.*
19. *I think the challenge is the amount of work we have to do in the time space.*
20. *... all the trials point to monthly treatment being the most effective so I was quite concerned about the recommendation of three-monthly [name of drug] [which would be cheaper] and that, I guess, that came from the analysts rather than the committee. I felt at that point, well, it was left unresolved and, in some ways, the opinions of the committee were being superseded by the approach by NICE.*
21. *I mean NICE does not exist in isolation, they're part of a society and NICE is paid for by the taxpayer ... so there is a political drive, there is an economic drive, there is a capitalistic influence.*
22. *I try not to really consider cost or, you know, resource in terms of space or people because what we're wanting to do is to develop the best guidelines we can. But, obviously, we are constrained by resources.*

23. ... *there were two ophthalmologists recruited initially and one person had to resign and they have struggled, they've interviewed several but conflict of interest is a major problem in the field.*

These tensions, expressed by different members of the panel, were ever present, and just as Gabbay and le May suggest that clinical mindlines were a way to resolve "the often incompatible roles and goals that inform clinical decision making" (2011, p. 44), so – I would argue – process mindlines enabled the committee members to reduce the conflict between their personal knowledge-in-practice-in-context and the strict procedures and constraints that the NICE process required. Was the committee developing what might be described as collective process mindlines that could help them become adept at resolving such tensions to find an acceptable way of working? My research was not focused on this question, but the examples in Box 11.2 do suggest that it may be worth pursuing that notion, and also investigating the diversity and interactions between the mindlines of, say, clinical experts, experts by experience, or the NICE personnel/secretariat, which could greatly impact upon the eventual guidance.

Chairing mindlines

The role of the chair was sufficiently noteworthy in the guideline development to merit being singled out here as a specific sub-category of the process mindlines. In the committee I attended, the person appointed was a clinician who had vast experience in chairing all sorts of committees, political as well as clinical and, also, commissioning groups. The chairing role was clearly key to managing social group interactions and moderating discussions. Committee members thought likewise:

> I suspect that, in some cases, it might be difficult finding people who are appropriately skilled as expert in the subject and appropriately skilled as a chair but I think that role is so vital.
>
> (*Clinician*)

> I often come down on the side of having a good chair rather than having a clinician; somebody who keeps order and understands process and that's really what you want a chair to be there for, to keep everything going and keep everything together.
>
> (*Allied health professional*)

In this committee, my observations suggested that the chair's control of the process was limited. Not only did they feel it inappropriate to be directive (which is not always the case in such committees!), but the control lay with the NICE process and therefore the NICE personnel to whom the chair in this group would frequently defer. The chair was very good at getting the group to work collaboratively, making sure all were heard, giving extra time for discussion when needed and so on:

> My role as chair is really to try and get everyone's views heard, as you do in a magistrate's court, and then facilitate everyone, the whole committee coming to a right answer. I try very hard not to be directive myself, although I can be, but one of the things that you've probably noticed me doing is letting people talk because I want people to be heard. ... [...]... What I do is I scan, I'm constantly scanning the table, constantly looking around to make sure everyone's having their say and anyone who wants to, you know, if I get any inkling from a facial expression or their hand movement that someone wants to say something, I will look in their direction and pick up the cue. If I do, then I will bring them in so that they get their views heard. It's really important to, for me, to maintain that. So initially, I didn't know what to expect in terms of how controllable the group would be, as it were.

Interviewer: Had you been given any training by NICE?
Interviewee: No, no, I haven't but I think my role in the [non-NHS organisation] actually helped me a lot.

The chair here had definite views on how the role should be played based on their previous experience (what I am calling their chairing mindlines). However, it would be difficult to assess whether their individual chairing mindlines were (re) shaped as a consequence of learning what being a NICE chair meant and as a result of the social interactions in their role.

Others on the committee would, of course, have had their own chairing mindlines based on their own experiences of chairing meetings. They also had views on how this particular chair undertook the role:

> [They've] done good work in jollying things along and keeping the group together.
>
> (*NICE team member*)

> [They don't] have that thing that some chairs do: they have to be in charge all the time, sit there and stamp over stuff ... [they do] let conversations just flow and [they] will interject and ask questions just to keep it and everything going.
>
> (*Clinician*)

> Their attitude is not wanting to get in there and say: "no you're wrong", which I think is a good thing. It has allowed us to be more collegiate, but the chair seems a bit too mild-mannered.
>
> (*Allied health professional*)

It is possible to argue that any chair would have process mindlines guiding their practice of chairing. As with clinical mindlines, they would be a rapid, efficient, and flexible way of dealing with complex, fluid, and sensitive matters. They would include assumptions about the competencies required, previous experience of being a chair in the guideline development scenario, or in different organisations and circumstances, as well as formal knowledge gained through reading or undertaking training. Just as clinical mindlines are revised, chairing mindlines might be influenced by interactions with those managing and overseeing the process, such as the specific guideline project manager or others participating in the process; they would also be affected by the experience of chairing as the guideline process proceeds. The experience of chairing that particular guideline would then play back into that person's individual chairing mindlines and might change the way they chair subsequent meetings. Furthermore, the chairing mindlines of all those participating in the process would have been open to influence and revision as they interacted with the chair during the development period. It was difficult to ascertain if committee members' process mindlines changed as a result of learning/observing/experiencing the way a NICE committee was chaired.

Conclusions

The opportunity to use a mindlines lens when revisiting the data gathered from my ethnography of a NICE Guideline Committee has been both revealing and tantalising. This revisiting of the data certainly corroborates what others have described, including not only that clinical mindlines play a significant part in the construction of guidelines (see also Chapter 10) but also in sometimes revising the committee members' own collective and individual clinical mindlines. It has also tantalisingly suggested that the members of the committee, and especially the chair, may have been developing their own collectively agreed modus operandi and that this was rooted in an emerging set of mindlines about the process – one that whilst unique to that particular group of people, was also constrained by NICE's overall ethos and process guidance. One could argue that what I have described is not so much process mindlines as a local modus operandi, but there may be much in common with the way clinical mindlines are developed and used. Not only did the collectively evolving process help participants deal more quickly, efficiently, and frictionlessly with complex problems, just as clinical mindlines do, but it enabled individual participants to develop their own process mindlines, whether as chair or participant. And, like clinical mindlines, the result was a collectively negotiated set of accepted parameters about the process that all participants came to accept (even if reluctantly), and which allowed them to handle conflicts between what the system required and what they felt was needed.

This conclusion is necessarily tentative, as the case study had not been designed to examine that phenomenon. Nevertheless, there is enough evidence to suggest that the question is worth pursuing. In the development of mindlines theory, a challenging overall question is how, in our understanding of guidelines, it might be possible to represent the interactions of all such different mindlines – not just the clinical mindlines, but the process mindlines (see Chapter 4). More specifically, it would also be worthwhile to consider the differences between the individual process mindlines of, say, the members and the secretariat, or to explore possible external influences from beyond the committee itself, such as how the process mindlines were related to those that committee members were using in the healthcare organisations, commissioning groups, charities, or other organisations they belonged to. My findings suggested they were; however my observations were not focused on such questions, nor on how the participants learned to carry out those roles, how they moderated or developed them whilst in those roles, or what induced a change in the practice of those roles.

One thing, however, is already clear: the relationships between guidelines and mindlines – not just clinical mindlines but maybe many kinds of process mindlines – is complex, and the distinction between them is much more blurred than we had imagined. To the extent that process guidelines turn out to be a significant influence on the actual guidelines that emerge, my conclusions may have important practical implications for the future constitution and running of guideline committees. Although guidelines authorities may understandably strive for standard systems and methods, the way their procedures are interpreted and operationalised may inevitably vary depending on a committee's make-up, personalities, and individual mindlines – something that needs to be systematically taken into account by those who produce, promote, use, and monitor guidelines.

Summary

- In this chapter, I use a mindlines lens to revisit the data I gathered for my PhD, where I observed a guidelines-development NICE committee, revealing the social processes that led over time to their consensus decisions about the guidance.
- I highlight the confluence of different kinds of mindlines intersecting and interacting while the guideline evidence was being appraised, assimilated, and transformed into guideline recommendations.
- These included clinical mindlines (even though this was discouraged). The committee appear to have agreed on a collective mindline that reshaped some individuals' mindlines.
- There were also 'process mindlines' that strongly influenced how committee members took account of the evidence presented to them – a collective way of 'doing' the guideline-development process.
- Over time, the committee members developed their process mindlines, which became embedded and endorsed. Some committee members had misgivings about the process for arriving at the recommendations but eventually subscribed to it.
- The 'chairing mindline' was particularly influential on the eventual output in terms of the recommendations made – or not – by the committee.

- In the application of the mindlines model to the work of guidelines development, a challenging overall question is how to represent the interactions of the clinical mindlines and the process mindlines.

Acknowledgements

I thank the research participants, NICE, and the Specific Committee of Study, University of St Andrews. The study was not directly funded, except for a fee scholarship from the University of St Andrews for PhD research.

References

Braun V, Clarke V. 2006. 'Using thematic analysis in psychology'. *Qualitative Research in Psychology*, 3:7–101.

Braun V, Clarke V. 2014. 'What can "thematic analysis" offer health and well-being researchers?'. *International Journal of Qualitative Studies on Health and Well-Being*, 9:26152.

Flanagan JC. 1954. The critical incident technique. *Psychological Bulletin*, 51(4): 327.

Gabbay J, le May A. 2004. 'Evidence based guidelines or collectively constructed "mindlines? Ethnographic study of knowledge management in primary care"'. *BMJ*, 329:1013.

Gabbay J, le May A. 2011. *Practice-based evidence for healthcare: clinical mindlines*. Abingdon: Routledge.

Hughes JD. 2018. '*Exploring the clinical guideline process: influences and interactions*'. PhD Thesis. University of St Andrews.

12

REGRESSIVE LOGIC, COMMON SENSE, AND EVIDENTNESS

Thoughts of a guideline-writing epidemiologist

Elizabeth Matovinovic

Introduction

In my work producing guidelines using the methods of Evidence-Based Medicine (EBM), I often thought something was missing. Although, while working in the US, I enjoyed the international demographics of the working groups, it felt strange how interchangeable we all were; none of us seemed to have a particular 'identity' since each of us could contribute equally well to the process regardless of our clinical and cultural backgrounds. It was as though our individual experiences outside the world of guidelines weren't relevant, so any one of us had an equal chance of getting the 'right answer' for how to proceed within this particular development framework. This, of course, was because the guidelines development system was designed to try and strip out any personal expertise and admit only objective, scientific knowledge.

Not only were guidelines developers expected to stick as far as possible to research-based evidence, but the process itself was rigorously structured to ensure transparent objectivity. Throughout the process I seldom had any 'aha' moments of understanding how these guidelines might be applied to a clinical setting. I also noticed that instead of being guided by a natural flow of thoughts to lead me to the right answer, I relied more on memorising 'framework' rules and sentence structures, using mnemonics to help make things stick. I thought perhaps as an epidemiologist who merely worked with clinicians that I lacked the actual clinical experience to solidly know the answers to all the questions asked during the process or to know how our outputs would be applied in the real world. But then over time, it became clear that many clinicians also felt similarly when applying our guidelines to their practice. The connections between guidelines and their implementation in practice seemed fragile, as did the theory behind their construction.

DOI: 10.4324/9781003158721-12

My apprehensions about a mismatch between what goes on in the guidelines' construction arena and the real world of application were heightened when I realised that others were also seeking to restore these connections between the theory and practice of guidelines.

Underlying this was a distinction that I wish to explore here – namely, the contrast between formal, scientifically supported evidence and other forms of evidence that can be loosely grouped under the term 'common sense'. For reasons that will become clear, I include here not only the naturalistic, intuitive understanding that we all have of the everyday world but also, for example, the collective professional view of appropriate clinical practice. Under the rubric of EBM, guidelines developers had fingered such common-sense and unsystematic clinical experience as a main source of error in practice. It was to remedy that propensity for errors that the more purist proponents of EBM determined to exclude personal experience and common sense as evidence sources and focus instead on formulating guidelines based on scientific evidence from published studies that were systematically assessed to determine their rigour using pre-determined scales and tools. Good guidance, however, must be not only robust but also relevant and useful, which can't be determined just by the rigour of its creation process. And that means it needs to include much more pluralistic evidence than some purists demanded.

So, was the elimination of personal knowledge even desirable, let alone feasible? Clinicians, like other humans, rely on common sense to gauge situations; they use all sorts of evidence, including those derived from the senses, as well as personal and collective experiences to make decisions. By excluding common sense, the guidelines movement risked throwing aside the knowledge gleaned from practice and (often systematically) diminishing its relevance – which is why the notion of mindlines became so widely discussed. There isn't a dichotomous relationship between guidelines and mindlines, but somehow things had evolved in that direction and caused confusion. Some purists wanted to push clinical practice and indeed organisational policymaking towards extreme reliance on guidelines and de-emphasised the pluralistic, sometimes tacit, evidence sources and processes inherent in mindlines to the extent that in some circles it was regarded as almost blasphemous even to publicly mention them. Others in the guidelines world, however, were wondering like me whether it was appropriate for practice to be based only on research evidence. After all, the originators of EBM had been very clear that clinical judgement was always a necessary part of the application of research evidence. One solution to the disconnect between guidelines and practice would be to ensure that guidelines have a less dominant but essential role within our all-encompassing (and inescapable) mindlines, where all types of relevant knowledge can be melded and critiqued. But another more fundamental question remained in my mind: what was the logic behind trying to eliminate wider types of knowledge from the evidence used in the guidelines themselves?

During my work in the guidelines world, the term 'evidence' was so overused – a tendency that spread also to the wider world of evidence-based practice (EBP) – that it lost its meaning for me, and so I turned to epistemology to rediscover it at a philosophical level. My aim here is to show that useful evidence isn't what some EBM purists presumed it to be and that modern EBP has no choice but to embrace all kinds of evidence.

Objective evidence as a neutral arbiter

I think part of what caused EBM's problems in the first place was a failure to define what is meant by 'evidence'. Fortunately, this is a question that philosophers have grappled with, and they have suggested some possible answers that may help solve the difficulties I was seeing. Advances in knowledge during the scientific revolution were spurred by developing systematic evidence-assessment methods used across all sciences to determine universally observable public knowledge. This uncontroversial knowledge then served as a neutral arbiter for advancing theories. The desire for a neutral arbiter also spilled over to the philosophy that underpinned science, where 'natural philosophers' (as these scientists would have called themselves) created a propositional argument-based framework for settling disputes among scientific theories. They thought a linear logic-based structure could objectively represent the natural world for analysis without making any substantive claims of its own in the process (Williamson 2013). But logic frameworks are full of substantive claims dependent on linear, and 'hyperintellectualised' constraints of language and sentence structures that cannot accurately represent or derive objective knowledge. Despite such flaws, the EBM purists also adopted a logic-based framework to serve as a neutral arbiter to objectively transform clinical knowledge and reduce experiential errors and centred the movement on that logic while they de-emphasized clinical experience (EBM Working Group 1992)

Grading of Recommendations, Assessment, Development, and Evaluations

GRADE (Grading of Recommendations, Assessment, Development, and Evaluations) is a good example of the efforts made within EBM to provide objective facts and logic. It is a widely used transparent framework for grading the quality of evidence when making practice recommendations. GRADE members form international working groups of clinicians and epidemiologists to develop methodological guidance about topics such as how to incorporate equity into guidelines or how to assess the efficacy of diagnostics and prognostic factors. GRADE is also used in health technology assessments for market-access submissions to national regulatory agencies and in creating guidelines for how to manage diseases.

As part of GRADE's evidence-assessment framework, weak and strong recommendations rely on systematically reviewing the total body of published clinical studies, using the approach of the Cochrane Collaboration. The assessors then apply quality assessment factors (risks of bias, imprecision, inconsistency, indirectness, and publication bias), which allow them the option of decreasing their collective level of certainty by one or two levels (e.g., from high to moderate) (https://bestpractice.bmj.com/info/toolkit/learn-ebm/what-is-grade/).

Weak recommendations can result when the quality of evidence is low, the value of benefits over harm are unclear, and/or there is large variability in treatment-related patient values/preferences (Neumann 2016). When applying weak recommendations to an individual patient, clinicians need to share decision-making with him or her. For strong recommendations, clinicians are simply expected to apply them unless there is a strong reason not to. Notice that such statements are structured as immutable, often binary, judgements: "weak" "strong" "certain" "low quality" "desirable", etc. So, when moving from a weak to a strong recommendation, the value judgements flip (less to more, weak to strong, and low quality to high quality).

Policymakers created and spread guidelines around the world like wildfire, and similarly, GRADE has widely caught on. I think this rapid pace of guidelines dissemination was enabled by a combination of (1) easy transportation of the explicit step-by-step directions for how to apply the framework, including judgements that were simply translatable to binary decisions, and (2) underplaying the clinician's personal and collective experiences as to what determines the relevance and applications of the guidelines to practice. The results were there just to plug and play in any situation.

But how solid was the basis for this apparent objectivity? When I looked closely at guidelines, I realised they didn't stick to their own strictures of objective evidence. In fact, many of the strongly recommended guidelines were inadvertently based on clinical common-sense type knowledge! Although GRADE had set out to explicitly expose and score the degree to which guidelines relied on robust scientific knowledge, even guidelines rated highly by GRADE failed to do so. And in most cases, published literature comprising the body of knowledge for these guidelines only produced weak recommendations that required common sense to navigate the enormous grey area. Consider Table 12.1, where I summarise from GRADE papers the sources of evidence for several sets of guidelines.

The table shows that 36% of strong recommendations from the Endocrine Society should not strictly have been subjected to GRADE since they are good practice statements, whereas GRADE should only be applied to research evidence. Yet they were strong recommendations because the evidence is clinical common sense (or, perhaps, the collective mindline). Similarly, of the recommendations GRADEd as "strong" in WHO guidelines, 18% were based on good practice statements. Also, the Endocrine Society misused GRADE such that only 35/121 (29%) of strong recommendations with low certainty evidence were properly GRADEd. Only 25/160 (16%) of WHO strong recommendations with low certainty evidence were properly GRADEd. Moreover, although two-thirds of American College of Chest Physicians guidelines were weak recommendations, common sense still required clinicians to follow them (Neumann, Santesso, Akl et al. 2016). So we see that many strongly recommended guidelines are not derived from objective knowledge after all, but consist instead of clinical common sense, unnecessarily codified or inadequately supported by evidence. Perhaps fittingly, GRADE responded to this

TABLE 12.1 GRADE and the sources of evidence

Examples of the misuse of GRADE	*Guidelines not meant to be GRADEd*
Strong recommendations based on common sense evidence (Guyatt, Alonso-Coello, Schünemann et al. 2015)	• The percentage of guidelines based entirely on good practice statements (i.e., clinical common sense): • Endocrine Society Guidelines (2005–2011): 43/121 (36%) • World Health Organization (WHO) guidelines: 29/160 (18%)
Strong recommendations based on inadequate evidence (Neumann, Santesso, Akl, et al. 2016)	• Endocrine Society Guidelines: evidence for 121/357 (37%) strong recommendations were based on low/very low certainty, of which 35 (29%) satisfied GRADE assessment criteria • WHO guidelines: 160/456 were strong based on low/very low certainty; 25/160 (16%) of the strong recommendations were appropriately GRADEd

excess-of-guidelines crisis with more guidance. First, GRADE recommended not formally assessing good practice statements (Guyatt, Alonso-Coello, Schünemann et al. 2015). Shortly afterwards, GRADE provided another guidance statement that guideline panels should seldom make good practice statements (Guyatt, Alonso-Coello, Schünemann et al. 2016).

Common sense and the avoidance of infinite regress

Arguably, EBM has been guilty of committing what is called "infinite regress", which occurs across all disciplines that rely on untethered ivory-tower, logic-based frameworks. Infinite regress refers to the endless justification of propositions that themselves require further justification to support them, which continues infinitely. To avoid that trap, the 18th-century philosopher Thomas Reid proposed a grounded logic in which a foundation of common sense serves as the grounding where a belief no longer requires further justification; at that point, the logic is either believed or refuted (Reid 1997/1764). In this vein, aspects of EBP that rely on practitioners' experience, such as common sense and natural evidence sources, must serve to ground the untethered generalisations embodied in centralised guidelines.

Yet EBM purists were likely trying to circumvent this practical, common-sense grounding because they thought it biased the purity of their view of knowledge. So once the systematic review and guidelines evidence-assessment frameworks were prescribed, the 'evidence-based' movement was in danger of falling off a cliff, leaving practitioners with the demoralising conundrum of how to transform logic-based products into actionable practices without the anchor of their (now de-emphasised) practice-based skills and without using any of their (supposedly biased) experience and abilities. Were EBM purists abandoning the common-sense baseline that would have not only stopped the infinite regress of their logic but also at the same time shown them the limitations of guidelines?

Like EBP, the practice of law also needs to contextualise universal logic-based rules for practical applications to unique settings. How does the law deal with the perils of infinite regress? Legal-theory philosopher HLA Hart boiled the law down to "the union of primary and secondary rules... primary rules universally prescribe what citizens can and cannot do irrespective of context; secondary rules can change the primary rules, adjudicate disputes about these rules, and even interpret what the rules of a legal system really mean" (Hart 1994). Of course, rules upon rules are an ideal setting for infinite regress to flourish; however, these secondary rules are baseline "social rules" that draw upon "common sense and public weal" to interpret and apply the primary rules (Shapiro 2007 quoting Tennessee Valley Authority v. Hill 1978 p. 196). They specify the way in which the primary rules may be "conclusively ascertained, introduced, eliminated, varied, and even justifiably violated" (Hart 1994). Much like the problems encountered when trying to apply centralised guidelines to local clinical settings, in law it is impossible to propose standards of conduct that settle every contingency in advance. Guidance by precedent is imperfect because one cannot stipulate a standard of similarity between the two cases. Although common sense will tell you when a standard does not apply, there will always be a healthy number of conflicting standards that will seem more or less reasonable (Shapiro 2007). Hence, deciding which to apply inevitably relies on expertise about the subject matter, preferably agreed upon collectively.

Such expertise sounds a lot like collective mindlines. So, perhaps modern EBP can follow the same path as the law and create secondary rules that restore clinicians' autonomy by emphasising how clinical expertise is required to modify and apply guidelines and codified knowledge to local settings. Collective mindlines would be a main source of effective practical solutions; strengthening their role within practice would be a valuable target for modern EBP to focus on. And perhaps, as in the legal sphere, some secondary rules could be created to explicitly predicate the use of codified knowledge with practical expertise and the wisdom of collective mindlines, which would also avoid infinite regress.

The need for 'other evidence', collective mindlines, and evidentness

In practice, as Greenhalgh, Potts and Wong et al. (2009 p. 763) describe, "[C]linical work [is] less about decision-making than about addressing the ongoing, local question, what to do next? (Garfinkel 1967), and since health care work is personalised, filled with exceptions, and context bound," there are rarely external knowledge sources that can instantaneously provide useful evidence to help with quick answers for many issues. Such context-relevant, and less labour-intensive, types of justified beliefs come from common sense and collective mindlines, which purist EBM cannot allow for. As Gabbay and le May (2011) described, such collective mindlines meld the breadth of evidence that practitioners draw upon, not only many types and sources of knowledge, including experience, but also the expertise of a wide variety of professionals and others with whom the clinicians regularly interacted and who helped them develop the collective mindlines that enable them to get through fast-moving situations.

How, though, can clinicians justify such mindlines? They could do so through (a) individual introspection, memory, and reasoning about immediate observable and external evidence, or (b) iterative discussions with colleagues that enable the collective mindlines of community wisdom-based beliefs to emerge. Unlike the explicitly controlled step-by-step 'rules' found in systematic reviews and guideline development, both these processes of justification can only be sparsely described, leaving details to be filled in at the community level where much of the evaluation of the evidence is guided by 'hard to explain' common sense. This reliance on many kinds of evidence combined with common sense, leads me to my ultimate question: How can we epistemically unite pluralistic evidence sources in a justifiable way that modern EBP can run with and not be left behind?

One answer is suggested by a contemporary philosopher, Patrick Rysiew (2011). He has taken Thomas Reid's common-sense philosophy a step further by proposing that information only becomes evidence when it helps spark 'evidentness' (Rysiew 2011). By this term, he means that which makes something appear to be manifestly true. In the context of clinical practice that would be the 'aha' moment needed to proceed with the clinician's ongoing 'what to do next' decisions. In this way, evidence contributes to evidentness only insofar as it meets clinical practice's need for an actionable form of knowledge. Evidence can be internal, external, apparent through senses/intuition, or derived by logic, etc., so long as it helps to catalyse evidentness. Rysiew's model suggests that common sense – in this case, professional collective wisdom – can serve as a guide for the evidentness of pluralistic evidence (Rysiew 2011). Evidentness may occur where new evidence relates to existing expertise or past experience within a present context to advance knowledge or beliefs. Collective mindlines allow such evidentness to be confirmed as the vehicle transferring expert knowledge to the practitioner. And like scientific knowledge, common-sense evidentness is explicitly public because it can be recognised and used by others who are similarly situated and informed, but it is also open to them to refute the apparent evidentness if they can.

Similarly, collective mindlines developed among colleagues are often explicit agreements on what evidence is acceptably 'evident', whatever its source. The steps for creating these collective mindlines are surely a superior way to spark evidentness within the clinician's own mindlines than mere reliance on guidelines. Collective, relatively formal mindline-building activities like meetings, grand rounds, and other educational sessions are an added guarantee of evidentness. There are, of course, potential drawbacks like the echo-chamber/groupthink phenomenon, but perhaps these are the kinds of things that modern EBP should explicitly address to optimise clinician skills and judgement.

My reason for writing this chapter is to recommend that this view of collective evidentness be the arbiter for what comprises evidence in EBP. Not only does evidentness avoid the naïve infinite regress of evidence, but it also fits perfectly within how mindlines operate; it means that regardless of the evidence source, clinicians' actions are not determined externally through inert codified knowledge that ignores practitioners' collective and individual wisdom.

Most who now work in EBP – and especially in knowledge mobilisation – have advanced beyond the stale, old-hat arguments between implicit/tacit processes and explicit science-like methods as the basis for practice. Those who have examined practice point to the many crucial aspects of care that are beyond anything that scientific evidence can help with, whereas mindlines and common sense are quite capable of guiding rational actions that take account of research findings. A modern version of EBP would enable and facilitate pluralistic evidence sources to be brought back into practice. And foregrounding implicit thought processes, using abstract concepts like mindlines and evidentness, provides a useful scaffold to collectively identify, examine, validate, and nurture these internal "inspiring, hopeful, and profoundly satisfying" (Kirtane 2020 p.119) aspects of clinical practice. Art-like skills that inspire people to be clinicians in the first place include developing experience for how to determine and apply evidence (Worsham & Anupam 2019), contextual applications of decontextualised evidence (Saunders 2000), holistic treatments (Kirtane 2020), and caring/comforting (Goldman & Schafer 2011). Without these common-sense guided qualities – these aspects of collective professional wisdom – the application of research-based evidence to practice is "suboptimal, ineffective, or even detrimental" (Goldman & Schafer 2011).

I hope I have shown why it is perhaps time for those of us working to produce guidelines to recognise the practical and philosophical power of drawing on internalised, experiential, and other types of common sense at all stages of evidence-based clinical practice. Decision-making can be more robust when based not merely on science-based guidelines, but on the collective mindlines they inform. Collective mindlines are the means to restore autonomous clinical judgement within local contexts and away from centralised decision-making. Pluralistic evidence sources have far more practical value than purely research-based knowledge, and guideline producers must surely continue to acknowledge and capitalise on this insight.

Summary

- For modern EBP to continue its path towards serving clinicians and patients, it needs to further understand, legitimise, and build on the pluralistic evidence-based methods used to optimise good decision-making in practice.
- It is helpful to define evidence as whatever sparks evidentness, which is what makes something appear to be manifestly true. Evidentness is a contextually relative yet all-encompassing concept essential to decision-making.

- In order to optimise evidentness, EBP needs to build on explicit methods that help us understand and elaborate internal processes that render evidence usable, including the development of individual and collective mindlines.
- EBP will hopefully in the future support the strengthening of the role of collective mindlines and recognise their value as the source of community wisdom.
- This may require recognising and building on the notion of common sense as a guide to internal evidence assessments towards evidentness (perhaps like a personalised tacit/implicit version of the GRADE framework).

Acknowledgements

This work was funded by a grant from NMBU Norway (Norwegian University of Life Sciences). The author wishes to thank Dr Rani Lill Anjum for her philosophy support and Dr Samantha Copeland for help with early outline development.

References

Evidence-Based Medicine Working Group. 1992. 'Evidence-based medicine: a new approach to teaching the practice of medicine'. *JAMA*, 268(17): 2420–2425.

Gabbay J, le May A. 2011. *Practice-based evidence for healthcare – clinical mindlines*. New York, NY: Routledge.

Garfinkel H. 1967. '"Good" organizational reasons for "bad" clinic records', in H. Garfinkel (Ed.) *Studies in ethnomethodology*. Englewood Cliffs, NJ: Prentice-Hall, 186–207. (quoted in Greenhalgh, Potts, Wong et al.)

Goldman L, Schafer AI. 2011. *Approach to medicine, the patient, and the medical profession: medicine as a learned and human profession*. Cecil Medicine: Elsevier Health Sciences.

Greenhalgh T, Potts HWW, Wong G, Bark P, Swinglehurst D. 2009. 'Tensions and paradoxes in electronic patient record research: a systematic review using the meta-narrative method'. *Millbank Quarterly*, 87: 729–788.

Guyatt G, Alonso-Coello P, Schünemann HJ, Djulbegovic B, Nothacker M, Lange S, Murad MH, Akl EA. 2015. 'Guideline panels should not GRADE good practice statements'. *Journal of Clinical Epidemiology*, 68: 597–600.

Guyatt G, Alonso-Coello P, Schünemann HJ, Djulbegovic B, Nothacker M, Lange S, Murad MH, Akl EA. 2016. 'Guideline panels should seldom make good practice statements: guidance from the GRADE Working Group'. *Journal of Clinical Epidemiology*, 80: 3–7.

Hart HLA. 1994. *The concept of law*, Eds., P Bulloch and J Raz. Oxford: Clarendon Press.

Kirtane AJ. 2020. 'Practicing art in clinical medicine'. *Circulation: Cardiovascular Quality and Outcomes*, 13, e006457. https://doi.org/10.1161/CIRCOUTCOMES.119.006457

Neumann I, Santesso N, Akl EA, Rind DM, Vandvik PO, Alonso-Coello P, Agoritsas T, Mustafa RA, Alexander PE, Schünemann H, Guyatt GH. 2016. 'A guide for health professionals to interpret and use recommendations in guidelines developed with the GRADE approach'. *Journal of Clinical Epidemiology*, 72: 45–55.

Reid T. 1997. *An inquiry into the human mind on the principles of common sense*. [1764] Ed., D R Brookes, Edinburgh: Edinburgh University Press.

Rysiew P. 2011. 'Making it evident: evidence and evidentness, justification and belief', in, T Dougherty (Ed.) Evidentialism and its discontents. Oxford: Oxford University Press, 207–225.

Saunders J. 2000. 'The practice of clinical medicine as an art and as a science'. *The Journal of Medical Ethics and Medical Humanities*, 26: 18–22.

Shapiro, SJ. 2007. The Hart-Dworkin debate: a short guide for the perplexed. In: Public Law and Legal Theory Working Paper Series no. 77. University of Michigan Law School.

Williamson T. 2013. *Modal logic to provide structural cores for metaphysical theories*. Modal Logic as Metaphysics. Oxford: Oxford University Press.

Worsham C, Anupam BJ. 2019. 'The art of evidence-based medicine'. *Harvard Business Review*. https://hbr.org/2019/01/the-art-of-evidence-based-medicine

13

KNOWLEDGE TRANSFORMATION AMIDST THE 2020 COVID-19 SURGE

Report from New York City

Edward Suh and Peter C Wyer

Introduction

The spring 2020 COVID-19 surge in New York City (NYC) was devastatingly disruptive of normal healthcare services. It led to a dynamic interplay between rapidly accumulating information from research and the day-to-day exigencies of the evolving healthcare crisis. This was uncharted territory for which new mindlines were swiftly developed, we suggest, because that dire, urgent need led to widespread adoption of practices associated with the concept of learning healthcare systems. Researchers, guideline developers, and communities of practitioners communicated amongst themselves and with each other at a pace never seen before, allowing the generation and regeneration of mindlines that directly impacted on patient care. That terrible time taught us potential lessons that may apply to the organisation and conduct of clinical care during more normal periods, to maximising fruitful interaction between research communities and those engaged in healthcare delivery, and to the interchange between guidelines and mindlines.

In March of 2020, as the World Health Organisation (WHO) officially designated COVID-19 a global pandemic, hospitals in NYC were bracing themselves for what would emerge as the North American epicentre of the disease. This was a previously unknown virus, SARS-CoV-2, and standards for management of the illness did not exist. Clinical guidelines and protocols had to be developed based only on preliminary observations. Yet these were all the more necessary given the unprecedented surge of critically ill patients and localised depletion of healthcare resources and had to be formulated in the context of a highly polarised social and political environment that impeded coordination of the organised response.

In this chapter, we relate first-hand experience from within a major NYC healthcare system as experienced by one of us (ES), supplemented by narrative

DOI: 10.4324/9781003158721-13

inputs from other centres and reflective commentary. We paint a picture of how information from published research, recommendations from guideline developers, and reports of clinical experience from abroad were filtered and adapted through the day-to-day clinical experience and rapidly evolving clinical challenges. We also portray how new social frameworks formed within healthcare institutions and extended via social media (SM) networks generated novel channels for mindline development. We perceive that the experience embodies the principle of transformation of knowledge through practice. We furthermore propose that it encompasses potential lessons pertaining to the effectiveness of interactions between the guideline community and the realities of clinical practice in the future.

Prodrome

To me (ES) and most other emergency medicine physicians in New York City, the news of a novel coronavirus outbreak in Wuhan in the first week of 2020 was a distant and theoretical concern. Many were not aware of it at all. Over the course of the month, images of the disaster unfolding in China reached the virtual front pages. Still, few thought to familiarise themselves with the disease as clinicians, and it would have been nearly impossible to do so anyway from afar. Indeed, interested laypeople were perhaps likely to know just as much about the new illness. My mother related to me a video clip she had seen linked on Facebook of a man supposedly dying of COVID after collapsing while ambulating down a city street. At the time, I dismissed it as being implausible, inconsistent with the clinical course of an infectious respiratory illness.

By February, concern was increasing but there was still hope of containment. Just as we had approached earlier international outbreaks, quarantine measures and isolation of cases would keep the threat at bay. Although this began to be challenged with the emergence of outbreaks in Iran, South Korea, Italy, and even Seattle, and though anxiety about the spreading epidemic was rising, there were no signs of an outbreak in our city. Our hospital epidemiologists produced a flowchart for emergency department (ED) use that instructed us to ask about travel and isolate those who had recently been in affected areas. Otherwise, it was 'business as usual' – but this would soon change.

Reflection

For almost 20 years, following the Severe Adult Respiratory Syndrome (SARS) outbreak of 2003, the global health community had been warning that a worldwide contagion on the scale of the 1918 Spanish Flu was almost certain to occur. So even before WHO declared COVID-19 a pandemic in early March of 2020, the progressively distressing developments abroad raised public fears about this outbreak. One conduit of information for those keeping abreast of the latest stories was SM platforms. For healthcare professionals, these would soon prove to be not only important funnels and filters of news and personal opinions but extended modes of medical-knowledge communication and mindline development as well. Whereas during the SARS outbreak the internet had been used to send information from one point to another in a manner described by one author as an electronic "Pony Express" (Griffith, Antonio and Ahuja 2003), SM platforms fostered the rapid assembly of huge networks of medical professionals (Shekar and Aravantagi 2020). These modified virtual communities of practice would prove to be enormously influential on front-line clinicians (Ouyang 2020a).

Inception

In the first week of March, a middle-aged man in our hospital was placed on extracorporeal membrane oxygenation to treat an unusually aggressive pneumonia. The ICU team's request that he be tested for SARS-CoV-2 was initially denied as he did not meet the US Centers for Disease Control's exposure criteria. When a COVID test was finally returned positive for SARS-CoV-2, it was clear that NYC was not fully prepared for all the implications of that result. Hospital leadership started regular status updates and virtual physician 'huddles' began within our department. Other meetings were soon suspended as the hospital swung into preparation for a crisis. The first huddles were focused on operational readiness and conservation of personal protective equipment. An updated algorithm was produced by hospital epidemiologists that continued to focus on identifying possible COVID based on exposure.

By the second week of March, this approach was obsolete. Patients were pouring into the ED with concerning symptoms, and while only a minority 'qualified' for COVID testing, those who did were nearly all testing positive. Daily, more staff were being placed on quarantine or becoming symptomatic. In the process of tracking all the clinician exposures, the physician who led quality assurance in the ED noted some troubling trends. A few patients were being diagnosed with COVID after complaining of only gastrointestinal symptoms, or after being found incidentally febrile in the context of some seemingly unrelated chief complaint. Vignettes of these cases were distributed over the department email LISTSERV, as a warning to encourage vigilance in using personal protective equipment and raising clinicians' awareness of the variable presentations associated with this disease. It raised our awareness as well of quite how little we really knew about this novel illness in those first weeks.

The number of patients presenting with COVID continued to rise rapidly. Soon, every physician in the ED had seen cases. We shared our experiences with one another – on shift, between shifts, over group messaging chats that sprung up amongst the rank-and-file ED physicians. We shared stories of patients who had presented with mild illness and were discharged home and then returned soon after in severe distress and of patients who appeared initially well undergoing precipitous decompensation in the ED. In one particularly memorable and frequently shared case, a middle-aged man presented with moderate severity respiratory symptoms. As he sat in the ED waiting for an inpatient bed, he asked to be disconnected from the low-flow oxygen he was receiving to go to the bathroom. He was found a few minutes later, cyanotic and unresponsive, having died sitting in his chair. Testing was not yet available in real time, but clinicians were becoming familiar with the patterns of this disease. Yet simultaneously, as the increase in demand placed on us by COVID patients outpaced the growth in our ability to treat them, many felt an acute longing for clinical direction and coordination.

Reflection

Facing tremendous surge conditions, hospitals across the city assembled teams for the purpose of organising, updating, and redirecting clinical and logistical efforts day-to-day. These varied greatly between institutions; some of the variation reflected socioeconomic differences between healthcare systems and even individual sites (Uppal, Silvestri, Siegler In et al. 2020, Muscarella, Moran-Atkin et al. 2020, Dinesh, Mallick, Arreglado et al. 2021). Some municipal hospitals lacked the ability to make platforms for virtual meetings routinely available to clinical departments or individuals. In one such case, the emergency room (ER) became a venue for in-person interdepartmental and multidisciplinary meetings at each change of shift. This enabled coordination and knowledge sharing between leadership and clinicians across several clinical departments, with nursing and support service representatives. Close conversation between various disciplines was in many cases identified as an effective part of institutional responses (Goldman and Xyrichis 2020). We posit that these collaborations provided a fertile ground for the emergence of COVID-specific mindlines that crossed individual disciplines and accelerated the process of knowledge transformation.

Crisis

As hospitals throughout the city overflowed with COVID, it was clear this was a true crisis. The leadership of the hospital system convened a working group of emergency medicine physicians, including ES, to develop internal pathways for the care of COVID patients. Practice to that point had been relatively ad hoc, informed by general clinical experience. We sought to produce guidelines based on evidence.

There was a scant amount of peer-reviewed clinical literature to work with at that point, so we looked at all of it. We decided to defer questions of pharmacotherapeutics to the infectious-disease specialists working to standardise care after hospital admission. Our focus became diagnostic evaluation and admission thresholds. We had all seen versions of what I recalled from the video that my mother had described: COVID patients suddenly deteriorating, discharged patients returning to the ED in respiratory arrest. We realised that though we did not have a good way to determine which patients were at risk for sudden deterioration, we could not admit them all. The literature did give us some data on risk factors. It was clear that underlying medical conditions and very strikingly, age, were strongly correlated with morbidity. But this by itself was not enough to guide management; many patients with risk factors were doing well and others without them did poorly.

Two documents, both of which we would never have come across during a standard search, stood out in their disparate perspectives and impacts on our group. One, an English translation of Chinese guidelines compiled by Chinese billionaire business magnate Jack Ma and announced via Twitter, focused on resource-intensive approaches that were out of reach given our context. The other, a 13-page document produced by the Italian Society for Infectious and Tropical Diseases (2020) had been run through Google Translate and uploaded onto an obscure section of the American College of Emergency Physicians website. We found out about it via a Facebook group post. This document addressed issues of clinical management in a more analogous context.

While the bulk of the Italian guideline addressed medications, it also included some suggested pathways for making disposition decisions. Buried in one complex diagram was a suggestion that oxygen saturation measured with exertion could be used as part of a triage stratification scheme. This caught the eye of the guideline group. We had each noted that O_2 *saturations seemed to drop in some patients with minimal activity; that explained the many instances of patients, who appeared to be in only minimal distress while sitting in a stretcher, collapsing with mild effort. Testing it on a few patients on my next shift it seemed to have some discriminatory value. I recalled learning about exercise challenge of pulmonary function in the paediatric emergency medicine literature (Pan, Stiell, Clement et al. 2009; Ali, O'Connell, Kass et al. 2011); another team member was aware of a "six-minute walk test" used by pulmonologists for COPD (Rasekaba, Lee, Naughton et al. 2009). Perhaps measuring oxygen on exertion would allow us to identify the highest-risk group and reduce the load on the hospital. As the magnitude of our resource constraints deepened over the few days that the working group met, exertional saturation found its way as a major decision point in the pathway that was released that fourth week of March. It quickly became part of standard practice across the EDs of our hospital system.*

Reflection

One of the medical themes that was a focus of mainstream news media coverage in the early weeks of the US COVID-19 epidemic was the shortage of reliable polymerase chain reaction tests. In NYC EDs, the issue of diagnosis turned out to be short-lived. Initial guidance by public health authorities and hospital epidemiologists had been focused on potential exposure to COVID-19 based on travel or close contacts, an approach based on the assumption that COVID-19 was not in circulation in the local community. Hospital guidance for isolation of patients and use of our limited personal protective equipment supply followed the same lines. It became clear to clinicians that these standards were inadequate, as many staff became sick or had to go out on quarantine. In response, some staff began to treat every patient with viral symptoms as if they had COVID-19, and that initial disobedience to hospital policy quickly became the norm for the group as they suggested that approach to one another. The decision to treat every patient as a possible COVID-19 patient also resolved the testing question – without any particular therapies to offer or any specific approaches to management, making a formal diagnosis added little. SARS-CoV-2 quickly became by far the most common cause of respiratory viral syndrome; hospital visits by patients with other acute health needs plummeted (Lange, Ritchey, Goodman et al. 2020). By then, many patients with mild illness were being instructed by public health authorities to self-isolate at home. In that context, individual clinicians quickly developed illness scripts (Schmidt, Norman and Boshuizen 1990) that recognised the phenotype of severe COVID-19, with its peculiar extreme hypoxia and characteristic course. What had begun in China as a previously unknown syndrome calling for advanced diagnostics had been transformed into the commonplace. That combination of local conditions and individual expertise drove continued iteration of diagnostic mindlines that allowed efficient assignation of diagnostic likelihood.

Diagnosis, therefore, was no longer an issue for the NYC emergency medicine clinical-pathway team. Rather, the way they drew on the Italian COVID-19 guideline highlights the way that local context, clinical knowledge, and social processes within a community of practice evolve guidelines as they are adapted for use. Indeed, the suggestion regarding consideration of oxygen desaturation in the Italian document had been almost parenthetical. It was identified because the New York team's personal experience attuned them to the concept and reinforced it as they integrated it with their existing clinical knowledge.

It should be stressed that incorporating this approach into the COVID-19 pathway in no way constituted a validated strategy such as would have been expected in less dire circumstances. In the context of the crisis, the team needed to rely on provisional guidance, subject to empiric validation in real practice. Indeed, both the Chinese and Italian guidelines documents themselves constituted products of health systems under siege rather than being typically developed, structured healthcare recommendations.

In that volatile and uncertain early phase of the pandemic, 'research' findings were being rapidly released and often presented contradictory results. This did not completely negate the potential value of such inputs. At a recent conference in New York on the challenges to clinical guidance posed by the pandemic, a representative of the Canadian Thoracic Society described how that organisation abandoned its usual rigorous approach to guideline development, which characteristically requires 2 years to complete, in favour of a more fluid approach of releasing 'position papers', which were not as definitive but tailored to emerging needs (Gupta 2021).

An illustrative feature of the New York experience was that it demonstrated how expert clinicians acquire new knowledge when faced with the unfamiliar. They turn not only to 'official' sources of information but seek out and share clinical experience with their peers. The sharing we observed was not limited to local interpersonal networks. Rather, online communities and SM networks greatly amplified the reach of any individual's related experience and allowed patterns that might have previously been hidden to come to light, even when individual communications were direct and private (Ouyang 2020b).

Sharing of cases was a powerful method of reinforcing key findings. For example, obesity had not been reported as a risk factor in initial observational studies (Shi, Yu, Zhao et al. 2020). Yet across the United States, front-line clinicians were able to observe that a disproportionate number of patients with severe illness were obese. While it would be weeks before observational data was published confirming the association, this awareness led to the inclusion of obesity as a risk factor from the beginning (Suh, Bodnar, Melville et al. 2020). Features of COVID-19 such as thrombotic manifestations and cardiac effects were also discussed on SM in advance of formal confirmation (Aggarwal, Alasnag and Mamas 2020). Indeed, some healthcare-focused SM networks contained posts with enough detail to reconstruct patient-level data that in aggregate provided enough clinical data to approximate a formal observational study (Sun, Chen and Viboud 2020). In the Facebook groups the authors were involved in, there were constant posts sharing specific clinical circumstances and soliciting advice. The comments and replies doubtless informed many physicians, both active and passive participants, directly contributing to mindline formation.

Even when it came to formal recommendations or data, interpersonal networks and SM played an important role. While they were used extensively by organisations as a distribution channel for official information, the ability to re-tweet or re-post on many platforms allowed individuals to shape the receipt of non-anecdotal information – whether news reports, published literature, pre-prints, local protocols, or perhaps most significantly Free Open Access Medical Education (FOAM) posts (Gai, So, Siddiqui et al. 2021). This brought to the forefront of the conversation those things that resonated most with clinicians.

"How many vents are left?"

At the height of the surge, ventilator availability was a major news topic. In that context, the idea of 'awake prone positioning' had great appeal. The physiological concept was simple – patients whose lungs were not drawing in enough oxygen, because they were filling up with fluid and inflammatory debris, would be placed prone on their abdomens, which would allow the posterior parts of the lungs greater expansion and improve the pattern of blood flow as well. It had been known for decades as a technique for patients who were already on ventilators but had not been really used otherwise. Heretofore, if a patient's lungs were so dysfunctional, they would be directly placed on a ventilator.

A FOAM post from 2016 had suggested the idea that awake prone positioning might be an option for some patients with severe lung injury who could not be intubated (Farkas 2016). It was now being discussed by ER doctors all across the city on various SM channels and within local groups. As we reviewed the evidence, the anecdotes, and our own clinical experience, the potential benefit seemed to outweigh the potential harms. Within days, a protocol was put in place (Jiang, Lebaron, Bodnar et al. 2020).

Elsewhere in the hospital, practice teams independently interpreted and adapted research reports to their specific contexts. Pulmonary critical care specialists reported having developed a protocol for determining need for mechanical ventilation from preliminary publications. Specifically, if a non-ventilated patient could maintain an oxygen level of 95% in the prone position for at least one hour, intubation could be deferred (Thompson, Ranard, Wei et al. 2020). Though it was unclear if this manoeuvre ultimately improved survival in individual patients, the inpatient teams realised that effectiveness in the context of exhaustion of resources is a complex issue. Even transient postponement of ventilation for some patients might well have saved the lives of others.

The ventilator shortage led us to make another discovery. A concept that circulated widely earlier in the year was the idea that using non-invasive ventilation or high-flow nasal cannula oxygenation would only delay an inevitable intubation, and physicians discouraged each other from using these tools. However, as we began to delay intubation to spare devices, some patients with severe disease were hanging on days after being on the precipice of respiratory failure. Other patients who had heard that being put on the ventilator was uniformly fatal were refusing intubation despite medical advice to the contrary and were surviving their admission. Studies would subsequently suggest the utility of a delayed approach to intubation. Fortunately, by late April, a rapid decline in COVID cases was well underway, so this would not be implemented into practice until the next surge in cases began in the late fall.

Reflection

The initial COVID-19 surge in NYC was a wrenching experience for all concerned as both patients and healthcare workers fought for their lives. At the height of the outbreak, up to 800 patients a day were dying of the disease, and healthcare workers had begun to succumb to the stress of the emergency. We have described how that extreme experience provided a context within which the transformation of externally generated knowledge and the role of socially situated clinical practice rubrics, or mindlines, emerged in an enhanced way as critically necessary adaptations. At the same time, within this 'abnormal' period, the underlying cognitive and social processes by which clinicians acquire and evolve knowledge were still the 'normal' ones, and, from this standpoint, we detect several salient lessons for the future.

The surge experience was characterised by a fluid state in which clinical demands, logistics of providing care, external medical knowledge, hospital protocols, guideline-community outputs, and governmental responses at every level were changing and evolving. In that context, these dimensions were intensely interconnected with one another and to actual clinical practice. Although all recommendations and decisions were necessarily provisional, the time frames of preliminary research reports, clinical recommendations, and practice were in synchrony. In contrast, clinical research findings often face significant barriers to uptake even when the evidence is strong (McGlynn, Asch, Adams et al. 2003). Some of this is likely due to the time required for new research to be incorporated into standard guideline recommendations, which may be four years or longer. For this timeframe to meaningfully interact with the clinical-practice domain, the latter would need to be static and unchanging, which is in fact never the case (Greenhalgh 2020).

The Surviving Sepsis Campaign guidelines (see Box 13.1), for example, advocated for the initiation of a complex and invasive protocol of haemodynamic optimisation for patients who presented to the EDs with sepsis. The implementation of that protocol was out of the reach of most EDs. However, the research that the protocol was based on, which indicated that early treatment saves lives, had already led to a shift in practice towards the earlier recognition and prompt fluid resuscitation of sepsis patients, which led to improvement in patient outcomes. It took over ten years for the guidelines and clinical practice to become aligned.[1] Had these domains intersected and interacted earlier, the disparate realms of guidelines and mindlines might have reinforced, rather than contradicted, each other, and many more patients might have benefited. The COVID-19 experience suggests that these gaps do not need to be quite so wide if the research, guidelines, and practice communities can each adjust.

BOX 13.1 SEPARATE WINDING PATHS OF GUIDANCE AND PRACTICE – THE EXAMPLE OF SEPSIS

In 2004, an ad hoc committee made up largely of academic specialists and researchers in critical care titled themselves the Surviving Sepsis Campaign and published a guideline for emergency and intensive care management of patients with severe sepsis (Dellinger, Carlet, Masur et al. 2004). (See also Chapter 8) The guideline was based largely upon a single randomised trial which had reported an impressive improvement in survival when patients were treated in the ED using a complex protocol for haemodynamic optimisation (Rivers, Nguyen, Havstad et al. 2001). This protocol was widely disseminated and had significant impact on clinical practice but not necessarily in the fashion that its authors had envisioned. Previously, a prevailing attitude toward patients with severe sepsis was that their mortality was so high that treatment was unlikely to change their outcome, but the Rivers trial changed that perception. However, the protocol advocated by the Surviving Sepsis Campaign required placing central venous catheters for invasive monitoring and specified complex interventions triggered by strictly defined haemodynamic thresholds. As a result, very few EDs embraced the full protocol. Nevertheless, there was a broad shift towards prioritising the early recognition of sepsis and widespread adoption of a more aggressive approach towards intravenous fluid resuscitation and antibiotic treatment. The potential usefulness of using just these components of the Surviving Sepsis Campaign approach had been suggested by some experts in the literature (Marik, Raghunathan and Bloomstone 2013) and was indirectly validated by a systematic review done by practising emergency practitioners (Jones, Brown, Trzeciak et al. 2008). The latter summarised data on the effectiveness of multifaceted treatment protocols for patients with severe sepsis over the previous several decades across many trials and suggested that earlier initiation of treatment accounted for the effectiveness of interventions rather than particular monitoring techniques or haemodynamic optimisation protocols. Eventually, large multicentre trials demonstrated that there was indeed no benefit to the full protocol beyond early resuscitation and antibiotics (Yealy, Kellum, Huang et al. 2014). Only in 2017, more than 15 years after the publication of the initial trial, did an update of the Surviving Sepsis guideline acknowledge these developments (Rhodes, Evans, Alhazzani et al. 2017).

Specifically, we suggest that, even in non-crisis conditions, the guidelines community needs to acknowledge the importance of less definitive, more adaptive, products that can address the immediate needs of clinical practice well before the results of longer-term and more definitive research become available. It also needs to appreciate the complexity of the process through which research information and recommendations ultimately inform practice.

During the COVID-19 surge, various organisations introduced products that moved in this direction. The US National Institutes of Health, for example, convened a panel of experts to produce continuously updated guidelines and recommendations for various aspects of COVID-19 evaluation and management; they used established principles from the guideline community such as structured searches, transparency in methods and evaluation of the strength of research evidence to give influential recommendations easily accessible on a website (COVID-19 Treatment Guidelines Panel 2020). The largest professional society for emergency medicine, the American College of Emergency Physicians, established a "field guide" that provided a channel for invited organisations and groups to present tools and approaches that had been used at their own institutions, making practice data available well ahead of the usual timeline of publication and dissemination (American College of Emergency Physicians 2020). We suggest that the guideline community might learn from this that a timely and relevant word can be more useful than final or definitive guidance, particularly when there is an immediate clinical demand. Leaders in guideline development can pivot towards tools that more explicitly allow for local and individual knowledge and experience to inform practice and acknowledge limitations that are inherent to medical knowledge.

Reciprocally, the practice community needs to create and maintain social and administrative frameworks and processes conducive to fluid and adaptive incorporation of transformed external inputs into daily workflow. During the COVID-19 surge, not every organisation was equally positioned to rapidly implement new knowledge in an effective way. Such organisations and systems might benefit from the formation of roles and groups having expertise in adaptation of guidelines to local environments. Such consortiums of potential knowledge transformation might serve to level the playing field in this respect. The other side of that coin is developing expertise in collecting, interpreting, and applying local practice data. The ability to understand how external data correlates to local experience and how locally generated data can be properly gathered and rigorously analysed deserves to be recognised as an emerging sentinel capability applying not only to emergent crises such as COVID-19 but also to the ongoing delivery of healthcare.

As a final point, we suggest that published responses to the COVID-19 pandemic on the part of advocates of the evidence-based-medicine movement, while valuably emphasising the price potentially paid for poor quality research and while defending the need for scientific rigour (Glasziou, Sanders and Hoffmann 2020; Djulbegovic and Guyatt 2020) have at times seemed to miss the nascent significance of the dynamic relationships between researchers and practitioners that arose and of the imminence of the need for guidance on the part of on-the-ground practitioners. As an example, weak preliminary data and an absence of other options led to widespread use of agents such as hydroxychloroquine and ivermectin early in the pandemic. While they have now been proven ineffective, for too long there was an absence of rigorous and definitive trial data, especially when compared to the extensive clinical experience that had rapidly accumulated. Though careful analysis of the data eventually emerged that showed the enthusiasm for these medications to be unwarranted, unnecessary delay, as well as the lack of conclusive findings, left physicians and patients susceptible to agitation and advocacy by proponents and disseminators of mis-information. We suggest that leaders and funders in the world of clinical research need to recognise the need to develop research streams that are driven by the evolution of clinical practice and that can address questions that are directly and immediately germane to patient care, even if they are only able to offer provisional guidance. Rigour in research design and interpretation needs to move closer to the clinical problems that are affecting patients.

A construct that captures many of the most useful features of the responses of the NYC healthcare community to the first COVID-19 surge is that of the 'learning health system' (Institute of Medicine (United States) and National Academy of Engineering (United States) Roundtable on Value & Science-Driven Health Care 2011). The COVID-catalysed transformation of individual institutions into alignment with this concept has been recognised in the literature (Stefan, Salvador and Lagu 2021). The challenge posed by this experience is whether such change can be sustained in non-emergent settings. A full elaboration of this matter is beyond the scope of this chapter, but we consider that an important point of departure for exploring the inter-relationship between the concept of clinical mindlines and organisational learning is provided by the work of the Japanese organisation theorists Nonaka and Takeuchi as previously summarised by Gabbay and le May (2011) and discussed in Chapter 5 of this book. We suggest that the COVID-19 experience may have given us a glimpse of how it might be possible for Nonaka and Takeuchi's elegant construct, the SECI cycle, to emerge and take root within and between existing healthcare organisations under circumstances of crisis in healthcare as well as beyond.

Summary

- The crisis caused by the COVID-19 surge in NYC during March of 2020 forced healthcare systems and clinicians to develop and rely upon new, silo-breaking networks of communication.
- These new communities of practice facilitated both knowledge creation and dissemination.
- Clinicians' tremendous perceived need for guidance, and guideline developer's lack of usual data sources from which to make them, forced those groups to work hand in hand.
- Clinical teams transformed published recommendations and the interpretation of research findings in ways that addressed the immediate patient care needs they faced during the pandemic surge, a context-bound process that epitomised the mindlines model in clinical practice.
- Lessons from this extraordinary time can catalyse the process of knowledge creation, integration, and transformation within more normal healthcare contexts.
- Research, clinical guideline, and clinical practice communities all need to make adjustments that would allow closer communication and collaboration also under stable healthcare circumstances.

Note

1 [It is interesting to note the subtle differences between the US and Scottish interpretation of these same scientific findings on sepsis and how they affected practice (Chapter 8) – a good example of the mindlines model in action! *Editors*].

References

Aggarwal NR, Alasnag M, Mamas MA. 2020. 'Social media in the era of COVID-19'. *Open Heart*, 7(2): e001352. doi: 10.1136/openhrt-2020-001352. PMID: 32994354; PMCID: PMC7526301.

Ali SS, O'Connell C, Kass L, Graff G. 2011. 'Single-breath counting: a pilot study of a novel technique for measuring pulmonary function in children'. *Am J Emerg Med*, 29: 33–36.

American College of Emergency Physicians. 2020. '*ACEP COVID-19 field guide* [online]'. *American College of Emergency Physicians*. Available: https://www.acep.org/covid19-field-guide [Accessed 11/1/2021].

Covid-19 Treatment Guidelines Panel. 2020. *Coronavirus disease 2019 (covid-19) treatment guidelines* [online]. National Institutes of Health. Available: https://www.covid19 treatmentguidelines.nih.gov/ [Accessed 11/1/2021].

Dellinger RP, Carlet JM, Masur H, Gerlach H, Calandra T, Cohen J, Gea-Banacloche J, Keh D, Marshall JC, Parker MM, Ramsay G, Zimmerman JL, Vincent JL, Levy MM. 2004. 'Surviving sepsis campaign guidelines for management of severe sepsis and septic shock'. *Crit Care Med*, 32: 858–873.

Dinesh A, Mallick T, Arreglado TM, Altonen BL, Engdahl R. 2021. 'Outcomes of Covid-19 admissions in the New York City public health system and variations by hospitals and Boroughs during the initial pandemic response'. *Front Public Health*, 9: 570147.

Djulbegovic B, Guyatt G. 2020. 'Evidence-based medicine in times of crisis'. *J Clin Epidemiol*, 126: 164–166.

Farkas J. 2016. 'PulmCrit Wee- Proning the non-intubated patient'. *PulmCrit* [online]. Available from: https://emcrit.org/pulmcrit/proning-nonintubated/ [Accessed 21 September, 2016].

Gabbay J, le May A. 2011. *Practice-based evidence for healthcare: clinical mindlines*. London: Routledge Taylor & Francis.

Gai N, So D, Siddiqui A, Steinberg BE. 2021. 'Dissemination of anesthesia information during the coronavirus disease 2019 pandemic through Twitter: An infodemiology study'. *Anesth. Analg.*, 133: 515–525.

Glasziou PP, Sanders S, Hoffmann T. 2020. 'Waste in Covid-19 research'. *BMJ*, 369, m1847.

Goldman J, Xyrichis A. 2020. 'Interprofessional working during the COVID-19 pandemic: sociological insights'. *Journal of Interprofessional Care*, 34: 580–582.

Greenhalgh T. 2020. 'Will Covid-19 be evidence-based medicine's nemesis?' *PLoS Med*, 17: e1003266.

Griffith J, Antonio G, Ahuja A. 2003. 'SARS and the modern day pony express (the World Wide Web)'. *AJR Am J Roentgenol*, 180: 1736.

In H, Muscarella P, Moran-Atkin E, Michler RE, Melvin WS. 2020. 'Reflections on the coronavirus disease 2019 (COVID-19) epidemic: The first 30 days in one of New York's largest academic departments of surgery'. *Surgery*, 168: 212–214.

Institute of Medicine (US) and National Academy of Engineering (US) Roundtable on Value & Science-Driven Health Care. 2011. *Engineering a learning healthcare system: a look at the future: workshop summary*, Washington, DC: National Academies Press.

Italian Society for Infectious and Tropical Diseases. 2020. Guidelines for the treatment of people with COVID-19 disease Edition 2.0, 13 March 2020. Available: https://www.acep.org/globalassets/images/italian-guidelines-for-covid-19-google-translate.pdf.pdf [Accessed 6 June 22].

Jiang LG, Lebaron J, Bodnar D, Caputo ND, Chang BP, Chiricolo G, Flores S, Kenny J, Melville L, Sayan OR, Sharma M, Shemesh A, Suh E, Farmer B. 2020. 'Conscious proning: An introduction of a proning protocol for nonintubated, awake, hypoxic emergency department COVID-19 patients'. *Acad Emerg Med*, 27: 566–569.

Jones AE, Brown MD, Trzeciak S, Shapiro NI, Garrett JS, Heffner AC, Kline JA. 2008. 'The effect of a quantitative resuscitation strategy on mortality in patients with sepsis: A meta-analysis'. *Crit Care Med*, 36: 2734–2739.

Lange SJ, Ritchey MD, Goodman AB, Dias T, Twentyman E, Fuld J, Schieve LA, Imperatore G, Benoit SR, Kite-Powell A, Stein Z, Peacock G, Dowling NF, Briss PA, Hacker K, Gundlapalli AV, Yang Q. 2020. 'Potential indirect effects of the Covid-19 pandemic on use of emergency departments for acute life-threatening conditions – United States, January-May 2020'. *MMWR Morb Mortal Wkly Rep*, 69: 795–800.

Marik PE, Raghunathan K, Bloomstone J. 2013. 'Rebuttal from Dr Marik *et al*'. *Chest*, 144: 379–380.

McGlynn EA, Asch SM, Adams J, Keesey J, Hicks J, Decristofaro A, Kerr EA. 2003. 'The quality of health care delivered to adults in the United States'. *N Engl J Med*, 348: 2635–2645.

Ouyang H. 2020a. '"At the front lines of coronavirus", Turning to Social Media'. *The New York Times*, 18 March 2020.

Ouyang H. 2020b. 'I'm an E.R. doctor in New York. None of us will ever be the same'. *The New York Times*, 17 April 2020.

Pan AM, Stiell IG, Clement CM, Acheson J, Aaron SD. 2009. 'Feasibility of a structured 3-minute walk test as a clinical decision tool for patients presenting to the emergency department with acute dyspnoea'. *Emerg Med J*, 26: 278–82.

Rasekaba T, Lee AL, Naughton MT, Williams TJ, Holland AE. 2009. 'The six-minute walk test: a useful metric for the cardiopulmonary patient'. *Intern Med J*, 39: 495–501.

Rhodes A, Evans LE, Alhazzani W, Levy MM, Antonelli M, Ferrer R, Kumar A, Sevransky JE, Sprung CL, Nunnally ME, Rochwerg B, Rubenfeld GD, Angus DC, Annane D, Beale RJ, Bellinghan GJ, Bernard GR, Chiche JD, Coopersmith C, De Backer DP, French CJ, Fujishima S, Gerlach H, Hidalgo JL, Hollenberg SM, Jones AE, Karnad DR, Kleinpell RM, Koh Y, Lisboa TC, Machado FR, Marini JJ, Marshall JC, Mazuski JE, Mcintyre LA, Mclean AS, Mehta S, Moreno RP, Myburgh J, Navalesi P, Nishida O, Osborn TM, Perner A, Plunkett CM, Ranieri M, Schorr CA, Seckel MA, Seymour C W, Shieh L, Shukri KA, Simpson SQ, Singer M, Thompson BT, Townsend SR, Van Der Poll T, Vincent JL, Wiersinga WJ, Zimmerman JL, Dellinger RP. 2017. 'Surviving sepsis campaign: International guidelines for management of sepsis and septic shock: 2016'. *Intensive Care Med*, 43: 304–377.

Rivers E, Nguyen B, Havstad S, Ressler J, Muzzin A, Knoblich B, Peterson E, Tomlanovich M. 2001. 'Early goal-directed therapy in the treatment of severe sepsis and septic shock'. *N Engl J Med*, 345: 1368–1377.

Schmidt HG, Norman GR, Boshuizen HP. 1990. 'A cognitive perspective on medical expertise: theory and implication'. *Acad Med*, 65: 611–621.

Shekar S, Aravantagi A. 2020. 'Are social media groups the novel physician lounges to combat Covid times?' *J. Gen. Intern. Med.*, 35: 3355–3356.

Shi Y, Yu X, Zhao H, Wang H, Zhao R, Sheng J. 2020. 'Host susceptibility to severe covid-19 and establishment of a host risk score: findings of 487 cases outside Wuhan'. *Crit Care*, 24: 108.

Stefan MS, Salvador D, Lagu TK. 2021. 'Pandemic as a catalyst for rapid implementation: How our hospital became a learning health system overnight'. *Am J Med Qual*, 36: 60–62.

Suh EH, Bodnar DJ, Melville LD, Sharma M, Farmer BM. 2020. 'Crisis clinical pathway for COVID-19'. *Emerg Med J*, 37: 700–704.

Sun K, Chen J, Viboud C. 2020. 'Early epidemiological analysis of the coronavirus disease 2019 outbreak based on crowdsourced data: a population-level observational study'. *Lancet Digit Health*, 2: e201–e208.

Thompson AE, Ranard BL, Wei Y, Jelic S. 2020. 'Prone positioning in awake, nonintubated patients with Covid-19 hypoxemic respiratory failure'. *JAMA Intern Med*, 180: 1537–1539.

Uppal A, Silvestri DM, Siegler M, Natsui S, Boudourakis L, Salway RJ, Parikh M, Agoritsas K, Cho HJ, Gulati R, Nunez M, Hulbanni A, Flaherty C, Iavicoli L, Cineas N, Kanter M, Kessler S, Rhodes KV, Bouton M, Wei EK. 2020. 'Critical care and emergency department response at the epicenter of the Covid-19 pandemic'. *Health Aff (Millwood)*, 39: 1443–1449.

Yealy DM, Kellum JA, Huang DT, Barnato AE, Weissfeld LA, Pike F, Terndrup T, Wang HE, Hou PC, Lovecchio F, Filbin MR, Shapiro NI, Angus DC. 2014. 'A randomized trial of protocol-based care for early septic shock'. *N Engl J Med*, 370: 1683–1693.

14

THE MINDLINES MODEL

An update

John Gabbay and Andrée le May

In this chapter, we try to update where the mindlines model has got to since we first suggested it. To do this, we will draw on around a thousand publications that we have looked at to see what people have said about our findings. Readers will be relieved to know that we will not attempt a comprehensive review here, but merely try to convey an overall impression while picking out some interesting examples. Our aim is simply to shed some light on these questions:

- *Is the mindlines model misleading?* (Has anyone disputed our findings or suggested that we have somehow got things wrong?)
- *Have things changed?* (Does the mindlines model need to be revised? For example, has the role of mindlines changed or diminished since we did our fieldwork, due to the rise of easily accessed online information?)
- *How have people transformed and/or used it?* (How has the mindlines model been interpreted or altered when people cite it, and how have people used it in practice?)

Is the mindlines model misleading?

As we reviewed all the citations, we were particularly seeking studies that might fundamentally contradict our findings. We found none. The face validity of the mindlines model seems to have been accepted and has persisted. Nor were there any critiques that questioned our methods, apart from one paper pointing to the lack of clinical data to justify our conclusions, such as details of the variations in prescribing (Ibargoyen-Roteta, Mateos del Pino, Gutiérrez-Ibarluzea et al. 2018). Indeed, several publications cited the mindlines study as an example of the value of ethnography in health and social care research (e.g., Allen 2010; Colling, McNinch & Lighthizer 2011; Draper 2015).

DOI: 10.4324/9781003158721-14

Have things changed?

We were also keen to check whether the original mindlines model might have been markedly affected by the expansion of potential Web-based influences and the ease of consulting guidelines online during a consultation. A recent study of hospital doctors in the USA helped to answer this question. Lander and Balka (2019) followed two teams and found – very similarly to what we saw some 15 years ago – that

> as team members gained experience, they increasingly incorporated [different kinds of] evidence into their mindlines. Evidence was often blended together to arrive at shared understandings and approaches to patient care that included ways to filter evidence.
>
> *(Lander & Balka 2019)*[1]

The only significant change from our findings was, as one would expect, that junior hospital physicians in the USA relied even more these days on online sources such as "UpToDate®" than those we had observed. Of particular interest, though, was Lander and Balka's carefully quantified confirmation not only that the physicians rarely consulted guidelines directly, but that as they progressed from novice to expert, they increasingly relied on the experience they were building into their mindlines.

A study of advanced nurse practitioners came to similar conclusions (King, Sanders & Todd 2021). Their ethnography in a UK emergency department found the nurses, who were making hard decisions that involved blurred boundaries with the doctors, needed to mobilise knowledge in ways that were multifarious, complex, and "messy". When deciding whether they could discharge a patient, they used many shortcuts in seeking out what they needed to know and used a similar range of knowledge sources to those that we had observed – which included often turning to senior colleagues. The only key difference from what we had found was the use of smartphone apps to give them rapid, easy access to guidance. However, the more experienced the nurses were, the less they needed to consult such sources. So, again, the general picture is of the practitioners accumulating knowledge from many sources, especially colleagues, and melding those sources as they learnt the ropes until they were able to quickly make complex and time-pressured decisions by drawing increasingly on their internalised and collectively reinforced knowledge.

In a leading article called "Mindlines in a Digital Age" Cunningham and Shirley (2015) reviewed how Dutch and Australian doctors consult the internet; the authors also used the results to suggest a model of online learning and knowledge construction. They found – not surprisingly – that doctors do look things up online much more than they used to; they look for answers to queries in 15%–20% of consultations, but for more difficult problems they prefer to consult a colleague. When they do so, "near colleagues are still of great importance, but social media and networks are allowing access to a much wider set of peers". The authors conclude that doctors are still developing, sharing, and using mindlines. Again, nothing has changed in principle. But the practical implications of the new, internet-mediated collective mindlines are manifold and require better training in methods for critically appraising such sources, and for enabling clinicians to make better use of digital media when socially constructing and sharing the knowledge embedded in their mindlines. These findings echo those of an earlier Australian study of the use of electronic decision support tools in primary care. Their paper, "New Tools for an Old Trade...", concluded, "[E]lectronic support systems ... that are inconsistent with these mindlines may be viewed [by the practitioners] as irrelevant and potentially even untrustworthy" (Peiris, Usherwood, Weeramanthri et al. 2011). Mindlines, they argue, are mediated through social processes and that "it is only through appreciation of the socio-technical dimensions of these tools that we will be able to understand their broader implications". Some who are in the business of developing such tools have similarly recognised the need to consider mindlines in the development of "context aware" decision support systems (Tawfik & Anya 2015).

Wieringa, Engebretsen, Heggen and Greenhalgh (2018) did a digital ethnography – in essence, monitoring three online virtual networks of ~35 000 doctors in the UK, Norway, and (mostly) the Netherlands, focusing on their online chats about statins and cholesterol. This proved to be a fruitful way to explore how mindlines are disclosed and developed. They found "sparse" explicit references to evidence and guidance; rather, the tendency was to share and discuss anonymised cases as a way of developing their knowledge and interpreting their views of best practice. Often this focussed on unusual "outlier" patients, where presumably the existing guidelines – or even the local collective mindlines – were not easily applicable, or on patients where, e.g., national guidance or reimbursement rules were at odds with individual circumstances. The online posts included a good deal of "not-so-explicit knowledge" closely resembling the collective sensemaking we had observed in our ethnographies, much of which helped to collegially reinforce the doctors' knowledge while building up a collective view of appropriate practice and encouraging a sense of cohesion and social solidarity. In short, what they found online in 2018 was very similar to what we and others had previously observed in the flesh – the main difference being an understandably reduced emphasis on the more personal and local aspects of patient stories, which would not be comprehended by geographically remote online colleagues.

Finally, and also suggesting that little has changed even as recently as 2021, a UK study used a mindlines lens to interpret their findings about the influences on general practitioners' (GPs) management of hypertension in older patients with multimorbidity. They found that the difficult decision to deprescribe antihypertensives, although recommended in the available guidance, was influenced by the GPs' own experience and that of their colleagues:

> Where the evidence base on the need to deprescribe was perceived to be clearer, such as in response to a trigger event, GPs' mindlines were well developed. In other scenarios, however, mindlines tended to emerge more readily only among those physicians who have been practising longer.
>
> *(Kuberska, Scheibl, Sinnott et al. 2021)*

The conclusion from these and other studies is that while the detail of how people access external written knowledge sources may have shifted towards online media, the information accessed in that way is just one more source that feeds into the practitioners' mindlines. Our own anecdotal conversations with, and informal observations of, practitioners also suggest that it is now much more common than it was to look online for guidance while formulating a decision, even during a consultation. However, such activities still appear to take place within the context of drawing upon, and developing, their mindlines both individually and collectively.

How have people transformed and/or used the mindlines model?

It follows from the mindlines model that you, the reader, will have already formulated your own interpretation of what you have read and heard about it. Some aspects may have rung bells and reinforced your existing understanding; some aspects you may have rejected, ignored, or modified to make the model more relevant to your own context and experience. If you talk about it with others, your ideas will probably shift again. As we have seen in Chapter 2, such transformation is the inevitable consequence of the social life of knowledge. Being reflexive about this, it has been interesting to review how others have quoted or used our research findings on mindlines.

To ascertain what resonated the most among those who cited the mindlines model in their publications, we noted on a spreadsheet all the relevant accessible passages in the nearly 800 publications to which we have been alerted by ResearchGate, an online service that sends its members an email each time their work is cited. This exercise did not include a other ~200 publications we had accessed by other means. It was not a systematic review, nor were we aiming to update Wieringa and Greenhalgh's systematic review of mindlines (2015). Ours was unashamedly an expedient sample intended simply to get a general impression as to what proportion of publications said what about our findings. On the spreadsheet we, therefore, noted whenever a publication mentioned a particular facet of the mindlines model (e.g., the role of social interaction, multiple sources of evidence, tacit knowledge, context, complexity, use of guidelines, and so on). Citations are of course made for a host of reasons, so this is far from a foolproof way of ascertaining the conceptual impact of the mindlines model. Nevertheless, despite being an inexact measure, this exercise did highlight the extent to which the different facets of the mindlines model hit home with the authors concerned. Most of the citations were what Wieringa and Greenhalgh (2015) call 'nominal', i.e., simply referring to our research because it resonated with a point the authors were making. Usually, this was done briefly in passing, but sometimes more extensively (e.g., Salter & Kothari 2016).

Poor practice?

We had worried that – because the title of our original paper had, in retrospect, perhaps misleadingly contrasted mindlines and guidelines – many would suggest mindlines as a likely cause of poor care because they enable practitioners to ignore guidelines. We were relieved to find that even though around a third of all the publications emphasised that clinicians tend not to explicitly follow guidelines, most authors seemed to recognise the more nuanced conclusion that mindlines were a way of adapting guidelines to the contextual complexity of practice. Many of them cited our work in support of the need to rethink how best to optimise evidence-based practice, or to highlight how circumstances so often militate against following guidance (e.g., Lange, Mwisongo & Mæstad 2014; Ingvarsson, Augustsson, Hasson et al. 2020). In short, the mindlines model has not been used to attack or defend evidence-based practice, but usually to suggest ways of improving it.

Only around 1 in 20 linked mindlines explicitly to an increased risk of poor care, mostly with a nominal citation that added no detail. Very few were explicit; one example was in a book on patient safety and pointed to some of the perverse (pecuniary) incentives underpinning mindlines that we also witnessed in our USA ethnography (Gabbay & le May 2011, p. 167). They described mindlines as

> collective "rules-based" errors which institutionalise inappropriate care in certain communities of practice. Many inappropriate investigations and interventions are perpetuated by mindlines in the face of new information that renders the practices out-dated and/or less risk- or cost-effective.
>
> *(Runciman & Lunby 2009, p. 201)*

Another example, in a paper on individual nursing decisions and judgement, stated that once guidance becomes

> part of the healthcare professional's own frame of reference … [s]uch internalised information is notoriously unreliable when used in judgements and decision making.
>
> *(Thompson, Aitken, Doran et al. 2013)*

One of the co-authors of this statement reveals elsewhere that he has equally little faith in mindlines that entail group decisions (Mannion & Thompson 2014). As a final example, a recent paper from the Mayo Clinic on cognitive bias refers to the "mental shortcuts" entailed in mindlines as "having the potential … to prevent evidence-based decisions". (Having listed the potential pitfalls of such shortcuts, the authors go on to advocate three sets of "debiasing strategies" for avoiding them and then – with no hint of irony – state that "there is no evidence for the effectiveness" of most of these debiasing strategies in a medical context") (Dobler, Morrow & Kamath 2019).

We can only hope that another apparent criticism was not intended, nor a Freudian error:

> [C]linicians rarely accessed and used evidence from research or guidelines but rather relied on 'mindless' [*sic*], personal guidelines collectively, reinforced by their own experience, interactions with colleagues, opinion leaders, patients, business and system constraints.
>
> *(Gildenhuys, Lee & Isbister 2009)*

Multiple sources of evidence

It is of course well recognised that evidence-based practice needs to rely on

> the conscientious, explicit and judicious use of current best evidence, in combination with the physician's clinical expertise and the preferences and situation of the patient in making decisions about the care of individual patients.
>
> *(Dawes, Summerskill, Glasziou et al. 2005)*

So, it is not surprising that a substantial proportion of publications that mention mindlines focus on where and how that clinical expertise comes into the process. Well over a quarter (>200) of the ResearchGate publications that we reviewed stressed the multiplicity of evidence sources that clinicians use, and a substantial proportion of those specifically highlighted experience. A fifth of all the citations referred to the importance of tacit knowledge. We found many variations in how researchers have described and categorised the many types of evidence that feed into mindlines or clinical decisions, but none that casts any doubt on the principle that mindlines incorporate and meld all sorts of evidence of which research is but one. As the illustrative Table 14.1 suggests, there are many ways to cut the cake, but all of them confirm that clinicians and related professions draw upon many types of evidence for their knowledge-in-practice-in-context. Some of these authors focus also on the *processes* by which so many forms of evidence are brought together, such as Risør (2017) who gives a blow-by-blow account of the way that interns process all the information that shapes their clinical decisions, a process he likens to a musical "jam session", and two studies that describe the many ways in which healthcare commissioners process knowledge as they arrive at their context-bound decisions (Wye, Brangan, Cameron et al. 2015a, 2015b and Gabbay, le May, Pope et al. 2020; Nicolini, Bharatan, Gkeredakis et al. 2022). Hurst's approach to elucidating how practice is embodied in the moment-to-moment application of mindlines (Hurst & Greenhalgh 2019) is further developed in Chapter 4.

The views of patients are an important part of the mindlines model, but surprisingly few publications, fewer than 10%, made even a passing mention of their role in influencing mindlines (illustrative Table 14.2). Among those that do, two have chapters in this book. Cowdell (Chapter 5), having worked to understand

TABLE 14.1 Examples of publications that refer to the mindlines model and emphasise the many categories of knowledge sources that practitioners draw upon

Publication	*Focus*	*Summary of categories of evidence linked to mindlines*
Trevithick (2008)	Social work	• Theoretical knowledge (or theory) • Factual knowledge (including research) • Practice knowledge (including practice/practical/personal knowledge and experience)
Barley, Pope, Rupatharshini et al. (2009)	UK consultant psychiatrists	• Acquired • Interpreted • Individual experience • Contextual Each of these can be 'self' or 'others', and 'personal' or 'scientific'
Boshoff (2014)	Science communication in general	• Procedural knowledge (codified and uncodified or tacit) • Personal knowledge • Factual and potentially factual knowledge • Opinion and belief All continually refined
Sedig, Parsons, Naimi et al. (2015)	Clinical cognition in general	• Mental structures (e.g., internalised knowledge) • Communicated (information from others) • Artifact (e.g., from documents)
Wye, Brangan, Cameron et al. (2015a, 2015b)	UK NHS commissioners	• People-based (e.g., local contacts, experience, and data) • Organisation-based (e.g., best practice, guidance, info tools)
Risør (2017)	Danish medical interns	• Context • Relationships • Information • Action Clinical decision-making is like a "jam session" that brings these four together

(Continued)

TABLE 14.1 (Continued)

Publication	*Focus*	*Summary of categories of evidence linked to mindlines*
Wong, Job and Anstey (2020)	Welsh clinical students	• Colleague and patient stories • Continuing professional development • Experience and judgement • Research and guidelines
Hurst and Mickan (2017)	'Knowledge encounters' across all healthcare	• Codified knowledge • Individualised codified knowledge • Procedural knowledge • Process or policy knowledge • Experiential knowledge • Product or service knowledge Analyses with whom and where encounters took place
King, Sanders and Todd (2021)	UK A&E nurses	• Education and courses • National and local guidelines • Smartphone apps • Colleagues • Patient notes and records • Patients/carers • Tacit knowledge
Nicolini, Bharatan, Gkeredakis et al. (2022)	UK NHS commissioners	• Expertise-based (Providers, colleagues, patients, families, and carers) • Local (Patient profile, activity, finance, contracting, outcomes, observation) • Trans-local (Examples of practice from other sites, including new pathways) • Universal (NHS reports, NICE guidance and guidelines, right care, public health)

TABLE 14.2 Examples of publications that referred to patients' influence on mindlines

Publication	*Focus*	*Indicative statement*
Griffiths, Anto, Chow et al. (2007)	UK patients with diabetes	"[R]elying on internalized guidelines. These may be based on evidence but are reinforced by their experience and what others say, including colleagues and patients. … The importance of involving the patient in deciding on how far they should adhere to guidelines has also been highlighted".
Booth, Tolson, Hotchkiss et al. (2007)	Scottish gerontological nurses	"[T]he identification and synthesis of nurses' tacit knowledge, and the experiences of patients, as a legitimate form of evidence complementary to research-based knowledge".
Oduro-Mensah, Kwamie, Antwi et al. (2013)	Ghanaian maternal and newborn health services	"[C]are decision making of frontline providers was influenced by clinical guidelines, 'mindlines' or tacit knowledge and 'client-lines' or client influences related to the preferences and pressures of the client and the wider family and community, including social, religious and cultural values and beliefs".
Cowdell (2018, 2019) and Chapter 5	UK Primary care management of eczema	"[E]thnographic study of the influence of lay mindlines on eczema self-management in primary care in the UK".
Wong, Job and Anstey (2020)	Welsh clinical students	"[W]e endeavour to further highlight the importance and relevance of patients' stories in healthcare curriculum and to issue a clarion call to encourage patients' involvement at all stages in the development and ongoing support of healthcare practitioners" – described as the "complex wisdom" of mindlines.
Locock, Graham, King et al. (2020)	UK multidisciplinary staff groups, focusing on how patient experience data can help improve care	"Gabbay and le May acknowledge that clinical mindlines 'may seem to be a dangerous shortcut', in that they may fail to engage with known research evidence. The same may be true of patient-centred improvement if it fails to engage with patients' actual needs and preferences, and reinforces continued staff assumptions that they 'know what their patients think'".

(*Continued*)

TABLE 14.2 (Continued)

Publication	*Focus*	*Indicative statement*
Blanco-Mavillard, Parra-García, Fernández-Fernández et al. (2020)	Spanish hospital ward staff	"[O]ptimal decisions would require the integration of such evidence with clinical experience together with patient involvement in shared decision-making, shaping and coproducing practice 'mindlines'".
Ladds, Rushforth, Wieringa et al. (2021)	UK healthcare workers with long COVID	"Alongside professional contacts, many participants reported the support offered by patient developed Mindlines developed from the experiences of unwell colleagues or through social media communities".
Næss (2021)	Norwegian doctors in primary and secondary care	"[P]hysicians' referral practice is contextual and relies profoundly on interactions with patients, the way patients present their unique concerns and experiences, and how these are interpreted by physicians in conjunction with national guidelines, previous experience (both their own and their associates in the medical community), and the organizational structures framing their practice".
Beckett, Deave, McBride et al. (2022) and Chapter 3 of this book	UK Trauma services, study involving patients, researchers, and practitioners	"[P]rimary intent was to develop and test a new method to enhance practitioner mindlines/practice, other stakeholders" by enabling patients and other key players to contribute their perspectives.

patients' as well as practitioners' mindlines about the treatment of childhood eczema (Cowdell 2018, 2019) has used the findings to develop more effective ways to alter the uptake of, e.g., steroid creams in the care of children with eczema. Beckett and her colleagues (2022) used novel ways to allow patients and a wide range of practitioners to expose and understand each other's mindlines, which brought about changes not only in attitudes and behaviours but also in the kinds of psychological support systems being offered by those working with people who have been injured in accidents (Chapter 3). This was a clear example of how co-production, bringing together the users and the providers of a service, can – through sharing and comparing mindlines – have an impact on care.

Guidelines and mindlines

Before reviewing what has been published about mindlines and guidelines, it is worth returning briefly to the 15 interviews that we held with scholars who have engaged with the mindlines model (see Chapter 2). They revealed that a major appeal of the mindlines model has been the legitimation of well-grounded evidence from sources other than research, but without denigrating formal scientific knowledge. One senior clinical academic told us how he had finally felt vindicated by our findings; he had long contested the hierarchy of evidence espoused by the EBM movement (systematic reviews of randomised controlled trials at the top, clinical case reports at the bottom), and advocated a more open-minded approach. Another declared that the model "helps escape the hegemony of EBM", while another academic, who is influential in the world of health and social-care policy, described it as helping "prevent 'epistemicide'", by which he meant the tendency to use scientific research to extinguish all other ways of knowing. A leading medical educator who has made much use of mindlines in his work invoked a telling metaphor: just as dumpling soup requires both the dumplings and the soup around it, he argued, making a clinical decision requires both solid scientific knowledge and other – more fluid, less tangible but equally necessary – types of knowledge (Launer 2012). His hope – and that of most of our other interviewees – was that an understanding of clinical mindlines would reverse the increasing polarisation between the scientific knowledge, emphasised by guidelines, and other types of legitimate knowledge. We need better melding of the two: he calls it "bothness", and also used the analogy of a Möbius strip comprising both evidence-based practice and practice-based evidence, a continuum that looks superficially as though it has two sides. Finally, a senior nurse-researcher, well known for developing methods for implementing research in the world of practice, told us how she had welcomed our explanation of the inevitable incorporation of many kinds of evidence into practitioners' decisions. In short, it seems that the melding of different ways of knowing appears to have been a well-accepted facet of the mindlines model, and one that strongly appeals to practitioners because (as a national GP leader put it) "it reminds people of why they became GPs, of the role of clinical wisdom" and (as a leading GP trainer put it) "it gives GPs permission to use their professional skills and knowledge".

Almost all the authors who describe the different types of evidence within mindlines have done so at least partly to critique the naïve view that scientific evidence – which is usually the dominant evidence within guidelines – always trumps other sources (e.g., Swayne 2012; Schulte 2020). Wyer and Loughlin (2020), for example, argue strongly that much harm has come from the false dichotomy between objective and subjective knowledge and the misleading hierarchies of evidence promulgated by EBM. Walach and colleagues have likewise argued against the hegemony of research-based evidence (Walach, Falkenberg, Fønnebø et al. 2006). But does that mean research-based guidelines are unhelpful? No. We have always believed they play a vital part in evidence-based practice but would be more useful if those who are developing, producing, and implementing guidelines had a better understanding of how people incorporate them into their mindlines. When reviewing the publications, we were therefore on the lookout for how others had interpreted the implications of mindlines for guidelines.

Not surprisingly, a substantial proportion of the papers discussed the role of guidelines, and to our relief, none of them used the notion of mindlines to reject them in principle. However, many of them cited mindlines in support of the view that guidelines are not always fit for purpose and/or their use needs further thought. Illustrative Table 14.3 gives examples, among which are both theoretical analyses and empirical studies. The table does not include any of the large number of publications that simply mentioned how guidelines are (or rather are not) used in practice. Some authors also raise important questions about the guideline-writing process (e.g., Wieringa, Engebretsen, Heggen et al. 2021) – a theme that Wieringa, Hughes, and Matovinovic develop in Chapters 10–12. These and many other publications lead to the inescapable conclusion that guidelines should take more account of mindlines.

Mindlines and fidelity to guidelines

One consequence of the melding of evidence into mindlines is the almost inevitable transformation of guidelines as they are incorporated into daily practice. This poses difficulties for those wishing to use compliance with guidelines as a way of performance-managing practitioners. It is also potentially problematic in medico-legal cases: does one assess practice against the guideline or the collective mindline and, if so, how does one reliably ascertain the latter? The practitioner may have read the guideline and it may have influenced their mindline, but what they eventually agree to do with the patient in front of them may appear not to follow that guideline. Who is to say they are wrong? There is no independent final arbiter – not authoritative bodies like guidelines committees, who know little of the local context, and not the local groups with their collective mindlines, who may unwittingly have transformed the original findings beyond what is scientifically valid. We were therefore surprised to find – other than in a long and comprehensive review of every conceivable aspect of clinical guidelines (Boon 2006) – almost no explicit reference to this important consequence of mindlines. An exception that briefly touched upon it was Møller, who asked, in her PhD about Danish social workers,

> If we accept the concept of mindlines as a way of conceptualizing processes of professional knowledge use and development, this leads to a pressing question: What kinds of social processes, organizational structures and routines enable continuous checking and qualification of professional mindlines, and according to whose standards?
>
> *(Møller 2018 p. 32)*

The social life of mindlines

Around 15% of all the publications mentioned how mindlines help to deal with the complexity of clinical decisions (e.g., Hurst 2019), and a similar number highlighted the importance of context. What seems to have most often struck a chord,

TABLE 14.3 Examples of publications discussing the role of guidelines in relation to mindlines

Publication (including short title)	*Focus*	*Synopsis of the role of guidelines in relation to mindlines*
Swinglehurst (2005) *Evidence-based guidelines: The theory and the practice*	Review of the nature and production of guidelines	Mindlines mean that guidelines are no replacement for clinical expertise or complex clinical decision-making, but are still useful.
Greenhalgh and Russell (2009) *Evidence-based policy-making: a critique*	Political theory: e.g., socio- linguistics and argumentation theory	The mindlines model is one of four examples of interpretivist and critical (*vs* positivist) models of evidence use.
Smith and Alderson (2012) *Guidelines in anaesthesia: support or constraint?*	Editorial review of the role of guidelines in anaesthesia	"For many of the moment-to-moment decisions, there is no directly applicable research evidence, and our work [anaesthetics] points to an individual anaesthetic 'mindline' constructed for each individual case. In other words, we are thrown back on our experience and professional intuition".
Launer (2015) *Guidelines and mindlines*	"Reflection" on the socially constructed nature of clinical knowledge	Advocating more awareness of the place of the mindlines "paradigm" and how mindlines work alongside guidelines.
Oyebode, Patrick, Walker et al. (2016) *The ghost in the machine? The value of expert advice in the production of evidence-based guidance…*	The kinds of evidence appropriate for the production of evidence-based guidance (NICE panel members)	Advocating a role for practice-based evidence in guideline production.
Gené-Badia, Gallo, Caïs et al. (2016) *The use of clinical practice guidelines in primary care: professional mindlines and control mechanisms*	Catalonian primary care teams	GPs – and especially nurses – do and should use their "midlines" [*sic*] when using guidelines, which are most helpful when not a bureaucratic requirement.
Elwyn, Wieringa and Greenhalgh (2016) *Clinical encounters in the post-guidelines era*	An analysis of the use of knowledge tools, using an exemplar case	There are "potential benefits of fast and frugal knowledge tools", alongside the way clinicians use their mindlines.

(Continued)

TABLE 14.3 (Continued)

Publication (including short title)	*Focus*	*Synopsis of the role of guidelines in relation to mindlines*
Wyer (2018) *From MARS to MAGIC: The remarkable journey through time and space of the GRADE initiative*	Analytical critique of the Grading of Recommendations Assessment, Development and Evaluation initiative	The mindlines model does not justify rejection of guidelines but does suggest that excessive attempts to complexify them may be counterproductive. Efforts might better be directed towards strengthening the social processes.
Brichko, Mitra, and Cameron (2018) *When guidelines guide us to harm*	Australian emergency medicine (editorial)	Collectively reinforced approaches, or "mindliness" [*sic*], should be encouraged when using guidelines, which can otherwise cause harm.
English, Tickle, das Nair et al. (2020) *Consensus-based good practice guidelines for clinical psychologists…*	Delphi study of staff to develop guidance that will help them enable sexual expression in people with intellectual disabilities	The mindlines model was used to underpin the Delphi process, which therefore used experience-based clinical vignettes to supplement the guidelines being reviewed. Similar methods should help incorporate practice-based evidence in future guidelines.
Copeland (2020) *The guidelines challenge*	Philosophically informed analysis of the problems with guidelines	There is a need to be transparent about the limitations of guideline creation and implementation, and the necessary place for mindlines.
Bierbaum, Rapport, Arnolda et al. (2020) *Clinicians' attitudes and perceived barriers and facilitators to cancer treatment clinical practice guideline adherence:*	Systematic review of qualitative and quantitative literature on clinical practice guidelines (CPGs)	"It is important that cancer treatment CPG implementation strategies … [take]… into account the social and organizational structures that influence implementation, and ensuring that they are tailored to the local context".
Wyer and Loughlin (2020) *Person centered healthcare and clinical research…*	Philosophical analysis of the nature of clinical knowledge	Mindlines are a practical way to blend different types of knowledge that have been subjected to a false dichotomy and misleading hierarchy.
Pilbeam, Tonkin-Crine, Martindale et al. (2022) *How do healthcare workers 'do' guidelines?…*	How COVID-19-related policy decisions and guidelines impacted on healthcare workers. Longitudinal interview study	Guidelines "fell short": to be enacted they needed to be more adaptable to context and complementary with mindlines.

however, was the *social* nature of knowledge; nearly half of all the publications referred to it (see Figure 14.1).

Many of these citations dwell on the role that interactions with colleagues play in bringing different forms of knowledge together. For example, the author of a Norwegian study of accident and emergency nurses concludes their "triage mindlines" were interactively constructed as the nurses consulted each other and their senior colleagues while developing their skills (Johannessen 2017). The important role of colleagues when formulating mindlines has similarly been described not only in primary care clinicians in the UK, but also in Denmark (Le, Lykkegaard, Pedersen et al. 2017), Australia (Pickles, Carter, Rychetnik et al. 2016), Spain (Labrador 2009), and the US (Epling, Mader & Roseamelia 2015), as well as social workers (Møller 2018), psychiatrists (Barley, Pope, Chilvers et al. 2008), Canadian cancer surgeons (Gagliardi, Wright & Anderson 2007), advanced nurse practitioners (King, Sanders & Tod 2021), occupational therapists (Clarke & Ryan 2017), physiotherapists (Thille, Frank & Sudmann 2020), public health teams (Meagher-Stewart, Solberg & Warner 2012), health-service managers (Nicolini, Powell & Korica 2014; Bresnen, Hodgson, Bailey et al. 2017), healthcare commissioners (Wye, Brangan, Cameron et al. 2015a, 2015b; Gabbay, le May, Pope et al. 2020), and many others. The notion that one's colleagues play an important part in formulating one's mindlines seems widely to have struck a chord (Figure 14.1).

Some of these accounts explored in detail the collective nature of the knowledge used. For example, Locock, Graham, King et al. (2020, p. 63) found that among teams of practitioners working alongside patients to improve services, a change of practice

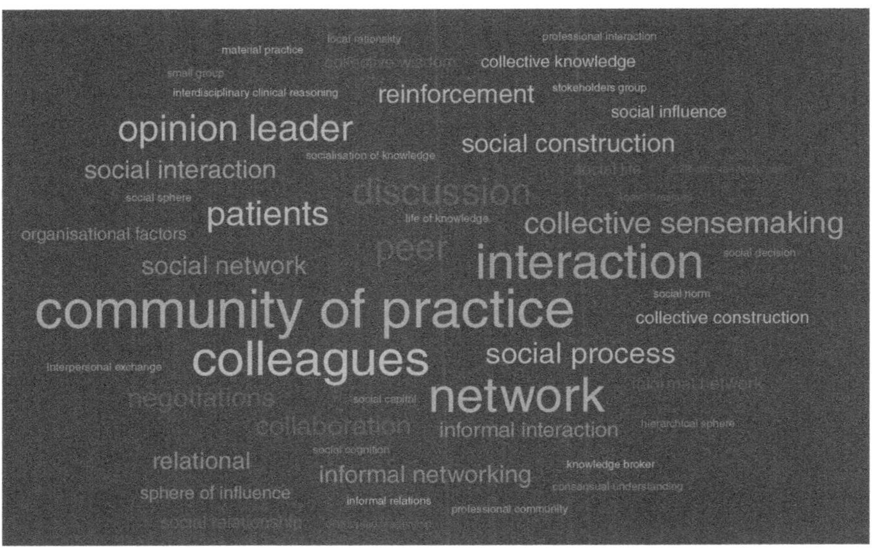

FIGURE 14.1 Word cloud based on 550 mentions of social interaction in relation to mindlines.

was a slow "process of illumination, a gradual dawning rather than the flicking of a switch". They suggested that the accumulated staff wisdom – shared and developed between ward clerks, the healthcare assistant, the patient experience officer, the staff nurse, the ward manager, and the consultant and, ideally, the patient and their family – may sometimes be the most reliable guide to action. This "team mindline", in which new data was absorbed and melded with existing, often non-clinical knowledge was a form of sensemaking that was able to markedly strengthen quality-improvement initiatives. It altered the collective mindline and became what the authors called "team-based capital", a collective form of professional capital (Locock, Graham, King et al. 2020, p. 96). The idea of mindlines as a form of intellectual or professional capital (e.g., also Vagnoni 2018) was rarely mentioned among the publications we reviewed.

In an ethnographic study to try and explain the variation of prescribing in general practices, Grant, Sullivan and Dowell (2013) identified two sets of decisions, the macro (local prescribing policy) and the micro (prescribing for the individual patient). Both were mediated by mindlines based on many types of evidence such as experience; interactions with colleagues, including local consultants; pharmacists; and drug reps. Macro decisions, however, were shaped more by external influences such as the health board and audit reports and, above all, internal meetings. The primary care teams that performed better against most external criteria were the ones who made the space, e.g., at practice meetings, to develop macro-prescribing policies by collectively discussing their mindlines.

The question of making sufficient time and space for colleagues to talk together about their practice was highlighted also in several of the many studies that cited the development of mindlines as an essential route to better practice. One example is a study of Danish primary care (Le, Lykkegaard & Pedersen 2017), which concluded that the practices that held frequent meetings to discuss their care performed better than those that did not. Another is Epling, Rockwell, Miller et al. (2021), who found that diabetic care improved when four US primary care teams were each explicitly offered meetings in which to discuss their diabetes mindlines, including how they handled the barriers to good care. However, such discussions may be impeded by the hierarchical relationships between the participants (Oborn & Dawson 2010; Swennen, van der Heijden, Boeije et al. 2013). As Carrier found when studying practice nurses, the development of one discipline's mindlines (those of the nurses) can be heavily curtailed by another discipline (the doctors) if care is not taken to moderate the power-relations within the groups that formulate practice mindlines. As a result of this and other, largely organisational influences, the practice nurses that she observed "lacked collective mindlines for the more complex cases and conditions they were increasingly presented with" (Carrier 2020).

Communities of practice and networks

The aforementioned observations highlight how important it is to give the room needed – not just in terms of space and time but also intellectual and emotional space – for colleagues to talk in ways that help to develop their collective and individual mindlines. In our own recent practical work to help implement research in practice, we have stressed the importance of facilitating what we call "respectful critical conversations" to enable practitioners (preferably alongside patients) to improve care; this plays a crucial part in their sharing and developing aspects of their differing mindlines that might otherwise go unnoticed and unchallenged (bit.ly/impartgallery). In that work, we have made extensive use of communities of practice. One of the key features of successful community of practices (CoPs) is their ability to provide just such a space.

As the word cloud in Figure 14.1 suggests, alongside 'colleagues', the most commonly mentioned aspect of the social dimension of the mindlines model was 'community of practice'. Most of those citations are in publications advocating or evaluating communities of practice, often focusing on how they foster the sharing of knowledge, tacit or otherwise (see illustrative Table 14.4). Indeed, the term 'community of practice' appears to be regarded as a byword for collective learning (e.g., Soubhi, Bayliss, Fortin et al. 2010) through the productive exchange of stories, of personal and practical experiences, and of circumstantial understanding – all of which are ways of promoting the contextual adroitness embodied in a collective mindline.

Whiteford and Byrne, reporting a careful study of an accident and emergency working group concerned with alcohol services in Liverpool, point out, however, that the term 'community of practice' can be used too simplistically. Nevertheless, they conclude, communities of practice can play an important role – one that could be enhanced once their complexities and challenges are better understood (Whiteford & Byrne 2014). Also working in the North West of England, Kislov and colleagues studied the work of communities of practice deliberately set up between multi-professional primary-care teams to help improve services for people with chronic kidney disease. They observed that, although new knowledge was readily shared within the teams, strong inter-organisational boundaries impeded such sharing between the teams. They concluded that there is a need not only to understand much better the landscapes of such boundaries but also to carefully tailor a developmental approach – no easy task – if such 'engineered' communities of practice are to succeed (Kislov, Walshe & Harvey 2012).

Of course, not only communities of practice but also networks can provide a context for sharing and developing mindlines. Just over 5% of the papers we reviewed explicitly mentioned networks, rarely going beyond citing our work to support the view that clinicians rely on colleagues to develop their knowledge (and/or, more rarely, explicitly introducing the term 'mindlines' in that regard). Some authors, therefore, advocate – as Peiris and colleagues put it (Peiris, Usherwood, Weeramanthri et al. 2011) – "energising" networks to facilitate that process, though few say how to do so, whether in terms of virtual or in-person networks. One careful piece of research that examines the role of networks in developing mindlines is by Tooman (2019), who examined in Scotland how knowledge was interconnected and 'shepherded' across different domains to improve the care of sepsis (see Chapter 8).

TABLE 14.4 Examples of publications that mention discussing the role of CoPs in collectively developing knowledge related to mindline development

Publication	*Focus*	*Type of CoP*	*Explicit link to mindlines model*	*Indicative statement*
Jiwa, Deas, Ross et al. (2009)	Standards of practice among Australian GPs	CoP deliberately set up (15 GPs), facilitated and evaluated	"[F]ormal and informal networking as a key to conveying … the preference of clinicians for their own internal tacit guidelines"	"[P]ractitioners who participated in all aspects of the project substantially improved the quality of their referral letters".
Soubhi, Bayliss, Fortin et al. (2010)	Primary-care practice for patients with multimorbidity	None: Theoretical paper, advocating establishment and evaluation of CoPs	Suggests the mindlines study as one of the empirical strands underpinning the theoretical understanding of collective learning	"Clinicians in these communities would define common goals, cocreate care plans, and engage in reflective case-based learning. As community members manage their knowledge, gain insights, and develop new care strategies, they can improve care for patients with multiple conditions".
Ranmuthugala, Plumb, Cunningham et al. (2011)	Peer-reviewed empirical research on CoPs in the healthcare sector	Systematic review of the literature on CoPs in healthcare	No, but includes 2004 mindlines study as one of the few using multiple methods to study CoPs	"CoPs can have a role in … gaining competencies following completion of basic training; …; sharing information; reducing professional isolation; and facilitating the implementation of new processes and technology" But their cultivation "requires a greater understanding of how to establish and support CoPs to maximise their potential to improve healthcare".

Meagher-Stewart, Solberg, Warner et al. (2012)	Canadian public practitioners	Set up and facilitated via study team	Tacit knowledge – as fostered by CoPs – is the preferred source for evidence-informed decision-making	"CoP helped practitioners build relationships and community capacity, share and create knowledge, and build professional confidence and critical inquiry".
Ikioda and Kendall (2016)	UK health visitors	Existing online CoP	"[O]pportunities for practitioners to share and exchange stories of local, personal and practical experiences about best practice … as collective mindlines … in Communities of Practice"	"[T]he success of online CoPs as interventions to improve and transform healthcare practice around the six high impact areas is promising. … Participating in online discussion saved time and strengthened and improved support from peers that would otherwise be unavailable to geographically distributed practitioners".
Le, Lykkegaard, Pedersen et al. (2017)	Management of respiratory disease in Danish primary care practices	Survey of existing practice of 'knowledge implementation'	"The development of the questionnaire was primarily inspired by … mindlines"	"Interdisciplinary and GP meetings held on a weekly basis were significantly associated with a higher level of quality of care".
Lacasta Tintorer, Manresa Domínguez, Pujol-Rivera et al. (2018)	Online communication tool between primary and hospital care in Catalonia	Existing "community of clinical practice"	"[S]ocial interaction, which is one of the main channels through which healthcare professionals create their own tacit knowledge"	Some evidence that care improved thanks to this "collaborative tool that provides reliable, up-to-date information that is highly transferrable to clinical practice", but they had mixed user views. The system requires technical and organisational changes for it to function well.
Shaheen, Kothari, Conklin et al. (2021)	Network of 8,000 health professionals engaged in the care of older people in Ontario, Canada	Two existing CoPs for sharing knowledge	"In this way, CoP members not only share explicit (codified or written) knowledge acquired through training, but also tacit knowledge derived from their shared experiences"	"CoPs are a powerful strategy for supporting knowledge sharing" … but … "fostering a culture of change in a CoP operating in a complex system environment may be difficult to implement in practice".

Using mindlines to explain and improve practice

Have people applied the mindlines model deliberately to improve care? Certainly, the concept is now well embedded in the literature on implementation, knowledge mobilisation, and behaviour change in clinicians (e.g., Nutley, Walter & Davies 2007; Clark, Park & Burke 2013; Collier, Hodgins, Johnston et al. 2019; Weekes 2020; Greenhalgh & Wieringa 2011; Lamont 2019). But has it actually been used and if so how?

There are many potential – and closely interlinked – ways to apply the mindlines model besides actually using it to try and change practice and policy. It can also be used to explain why people practise as they do, as well as to influence people's modes of learning. Both can be steps towards improving practice.

Explaining practice

The mindlines model has been used to explain clinical behaviour in a range of studies whose findings could illuminate better ways to change practice (see illustrative Table 14.5). A particularly detailed example, although retrospective and therefore not aiming to influence practice, shows the potential of using the mindlines lens to understand the behaviour of a whole discipline that turned out to be seriously misguided. Ducey, Donoso, and Ross (2020) used the mindlines model to illuminate how pelvic surgeons adopted and then abandoned transvaginal synthetic mesh to treat vaginal prolapse. They found that, in the 1990s, the surgeons' collective mindline had at first a strong anatomical focus: mesh was seen quite simply as the best way to restore the original anatomy. The dominant surgical mindline relied partly on collective sensemaking that rendered it "almost unethical" for a surgeon to deny women the mesh repair. And although that claim was supposedly rooted in evidence that met the standards of EBM, it turned out in retrospect to be rather shaky. Moreover, whilst couched in terms of existing and ongoing trials of anatomical repair, it was also partly rooted in various commercial and financial interests. Despite mounting anecdotal evidence that – whatever the apparent anatomical benefits – the outcomes experienced by many patients could be dire, the dominant view was to discount that clinical evidence and await the results from further trials. Eventually, however, the surgical community found themselves forced to reconfigure their collective mindline from one embedded in an EBM/anatomical approach to a mindline based more on patient experience and functional outcome. By 2020, this had altered not only how and why surgeons practised but also how they regarded their own role and their duty as practitioners. This kind of analysis could well be used to influence similar aberrations of practice in future.

Directly changing practice

Fewer than 5% of the publications we reviewed considered in any detail the potential for using the mindlines model to bring about change, let alone gave examples of

TABLE 14.5 Examples of publications in which mindlines were used to help explain the behaviour of practitioners

Publication / methods	*Focus*	*Question addressed*	*Indicative quotation*
Williams, Skinner, Dowell et al. (2007) Focus groups and interviews	UK Primary care management of epilepsy	To try and understand a 'failure' to implement guidelines based on new research	"Our data may help clarify some of the organizational, social, and psychological variables and processes that create or maintain such mindlines".
Barley, Pope, Chilvers et al. 2008 Interviews	UK consultant psychiatrists	"[T]o identify potential barriers to the implementation of guidelines for the pharmacological management of schizophrenia"	"[T]he use of mindlines by these psychiatrists suggests that we need to reconsider how we can best ensure the transfer of research evidence into practice".
Elstad, Lutfey, Marceau et al. (2010) Interviews	US, UK, and German physicians' views on diabetes	Why physicians with greater experience may provide *poorer* quality care than their less experienced counterparts, as captured by various quality assurance measures	For "some of these subtle skills… or cognitive processes involved in clinical decision making… [i]n tune with Gabbay & le May's 'mindlines' … we found that physicians gained their experience in part through their professional interactions".
Löfgren, Silén and Alexanderson (2011) Questionnaire survey	Swedish physicians' sickness certification	How physicians with limited direct training can learn about sickness-absence certification	"The concept of mindlines appears useful in understanding how physicians have learned how to deal with sickness certification… However, learning mainly through participation is not inherently a 'positive' phenomenon, because it can also lead to passiveness or 'learned helplessness' … they also gain knowledge in the form of by-products of the learning situation, which can be called the 'hidden curriculum'".

(*Continued*)

TABLE 14.5 (Continued)

Publication / methods	*Focus*	*Question addressed*	*Indicative quotation*
Epling, Mader and Roseamelia (2015) Focus groups	Physicians in New York State	Why the practice of diagnosing and managing patients with low Vitamin D levels is so variable	"The findings detailed in this article reinforce the concept of 'mindlines'. …The overall impression of the formation of emerging practice concerning vitamin D is that it was often initiated by patient demand, but was then constructed and reinforced by incidental reading; brief, purposeful research; influence by physician champions; informal conversations with colleagues; results of consultations by specialists; and more patient demand".
Wye, Brangan, Cameron et al. (2015a, 2015b); Gabbay, le May, Pope et al. (2020) Case studies	UK NHS commissioners	How healthcare commissioners acquire and process the knowledge they need to make commissioning decisions	"The ways that commissioners treated knowledge were similar to the ways that multisectoral policy-making groups and clinical communities of practice treat knowledge in developing their 'mindlines'".
Farr and Cressey (2015) Interviews	UK NHS primary care staff	Views on performance and quality: how do staff know if they are doing a good job and what might motivate them?	"Whilst Gabbay and May [*sic*] highlight the use of 'clinical mindlines' in clinical decision making, that are based on internalised collective and tacit aspects of knowledge, this study extends this notion of the tacit and collective in the accounting for and understanding of performance and quality within health services".
Pickles, Carter, Rychetnik and Entwistle (2016) Interviews, grounded theory	UK and Australian GPs	How and why UK and Australian GPs differ in the use of prostate cancer screening	"Like the UK GPs, the Australian GPs' mindlines were developed and reinforced via similar processes of experience, repetition and interactions, but these occurred within local circumstances and macro systems that looked very different to the UK situation. It is likely that Australian GPs' mindlines vary considerably from one GP to the next as they navigate and interpret the changeable conditions".

Bresnen, Hodgson, Bailey et al. (2017) Interviews and observations	UK NHS hospital managers	How managers acquire and apply their management knowledge	"[T]his article has examined how managers in the NHS relate to different sources and forms of knowledge, drawing upon a socialized conception of knowledge mobilization".
Tooman (2019) and Chapter 8 Case study design	Knowledge network on sepsis care in Scotland and beyond	How knowledge about sepsis is mobilised within and between the research, policy and practice communities	"[T]his work extends the academic literature that explores the diversity, complexity, and interconnectivity of knowledge for practice by emphasising the role of social interactions in supporting knowledge networks; and the study demonstrates the successful use of Soft Knowledge Systems and Clinical Mindlines as a combined 'relational knowledge systems' lens to better understand knowledge mobilisation processes."
Everson, Hollingsworth, and Adler-Milstein (2019) Analysis of hospital performance data	USA non-federal acute care hospitals	How (and why) the performance of different groups of hospitals varies	"This idea is supported by the study of 'mindlines' in health care, which focuses on how providers that communicate with one another influence each other's behavior. We therefore sought to explore differences in the extent to which groups of hospitals under each method shared similar behaviors".
Ducey, Donoso, Ross et al. (2020) Interviews and documentary analysis	European and US pelvic-floor surgeons	Why surgeons adopted and then abandoned transvaginal mesh for prolapse repair	Mindlines, "a moral-epistemological way of knowing, feeling and acting" are "collective guides for what makes sense and what is responsible. Recognition of harms from transvaginal mesh reconfigured surgical mindlines" which were "not determined by the findings of EBM".
Brattgjerd (2021) Chapter 7 Case studies	Norwegian palliative care nurses	How nurses managed to adapt the use of a standardised care plan	Standardisation and nursing practice are characterised by two incompatible logics: the "rigid-rational order" of guidelines and the "value-rational order" of practice, which are resolved by "loose coupling" that involves mindlines.
Nathan, Gabbay, Boyle et al. (2021) Focus groups	Community and hospital teams	What influences clinicians' decisions to admit patients with acute psychiatric crises to hospital?	"The theoretical framework 'mindlines' may be a useful starting point to consider where these influences sit within the overall decision-making processes".

doing so. Yet, applying the mindlines model as a deliberate way to improve practice can be effective, as several of the contributions to this book demonstrate (see particularly Chapters 3 and 5).

An early application of an analysis of mindlines to bring about change was by Chandler and colleagues. They carried out an ethnography in Tanzania to try to understand why doctors were over-diagnosing malaria, which leads to the damaging and costly problem of misuse of antimalarial drugs across much of Africa. They found that multiple social influences were reducible to a set of mindlines that doctors had acquired at many stages of their training, and which the research team was able to summarise in a simplified form. This allowed the team to explain to the guideline writers and to the practitioners themselves why the practice in the field was so much at variance with the guidance. They concluded that, to bring mindlines and guidelines into closer alignment,

> [i]nterventions to change clinical decision-making need to focus on the influencing factors identified and need to use methods that address the collective nature of mindlines currently in use.
>
> *(Chandler, Jones, Boniface et al. 2008)*

Such insights allowed them to conduct controlled trials in which the interventions consciously involved attempts to understand and change mindlines through group discussions linked to targeted messaging. One such trial in Tanzania showed that the inclusion of such measures was associated with the near elimination of the over-prescribing of antimalarials (Chandler, Meta, Ponzo et al. 2014; Cundill, Mbakilwa, Chandler et al. 2015). A related study in Cameroon, also designed to test such methods, concluded that

> [e]nhanced clinician training, designed to translate knowledge into prescribing practice and improve quality of care, has the potential to halve overtreatment in public and mission health facilities in Cameroon.
>
> *(Mbacham, Mangham-Jefferies, Cundill et al. 2014)*

Another example of using mindlines to effect change was in the USA, where Epling and colleagues tested whether what they called "mindlines-producing conversations" in four primary-care practices would help implement evidence to improve diabetes control. In each location, they arranged and facilitated one-off, informal discussions aimed at the development of mindlines around evidence-based interventions. The research team "looked specifically for evidence of the participants in the meeting discussing and adapting the evidence and having the sorts of discussions that would help them develop the appropriate 'mindlines' (knowledge-in-practice-in-context) for diabetes care", and present many examples of such conversations in their data. Doctors, nurses, and administrative staff talked about what they did and why, suggested ways to do things more in line with the guidance, and reflected on possible solutions to the barriers that they were encountering. As a result, the researchers report, the practices were "adopting and adapting the evidence to suit their own needs and context. Performance metrics regarding diabetes control for the four practices improved after the intervention" (Epling, Rockwell & Miller 2021).

Andrews, working mainly in Wales, has blazed a trail in changing policy and practice by using the principle of mindlines in multisectoral communities of practice designed to share mindlines in the care of older people. This work has resulted in fundamental changes in Welsh national policies as well as the organisational policy of the care-home provider companies he was working with (Andrews, Gabbay, le May et al. 2020).

In Bristol, Wye, Cramer, Beckett et al. (2020) worked as, and evaluated, knowledge brokers across healthcare commissioning (i.e., policymaking) and academic communities to try to develop both "research-informed commissioning" and "commissioning-informed research". The latter turned out to be the more successful, but both communities noted changes in attitude, knowledge, skills, and confidence. Wye's team used a variety of methods such as embedding and "buddying-up" to foster respectful critical conversations within and between the commissioning and academic organisations, and did so explicitly using the principles of the mindlines model.

Finally, Langley and colleagues, in the UK, have demonstrated also the value of co-production, using a method that they developed by drawing on the notion of mindlines and the structured approach of codesign (Langley, Wassall, Geddis-Regan et al. 2022). They worked with groups from care homes to understand how best to develop a complex intervention that would enable the staff to provide daily oral care to elderly residents. Such care is the subject of a National Institute for Health and Care Excellence (NICE) guideline that care-home staff perceived to be of little practical value; it was "too general, passive, idealised and even patronising". But through the codesign process with the staff and residents, the team elicited a clearer mutual understanding of the context (e.g., lack of time and resource; the increasing proportion of residents with dementia), the challenges (e.g., dangerous "refusal behaviour"), and the potential solutions. This has led to a highly practical Care Home Oral Care Toolkit that enables the staff to implement the NICE guidance on oral care in ways firmly rooted in a shared understanding of the staff's knowledge-in-practice-in-context that recognises and enhances their contextual adroitness.

Changing practice through new ways of learning

Improved practice also comes about when mindlines develop as a result of changes in the way professionals are trained (Carrier 2019). We ourselves advocated in our 2011 book that more should be done to help train people to assess the robustness not just of research-based evidence – as is now routinely taught across healthcare thanks to the sterling efforts of the EBM movement – but also to develop ways to do so for the other types of evidence that help to form practitioners' mindlines. Later that year, we produced a first effort at doing that (le May & Gabbay 2011) (Table 14.6).

TABLE 14.6 Assessing the rigour of evidence – some initial elements for consideration

Research-based evidence	*Own experiences*	*Theoretical perspectives (non-research-based)*	*Clients'/patients'/carers' experiences*	*Role models'/experts' opinions*	*Policy directives*
Link between research and clinical situation Strengths and weaknesses of design in relation to aims of research Reliability and validity/credibility Appropriateness of findings to clinical issue Appropriateness of recommendations for practice How this research fits in with other findings Likelihood of transferability to practice setting Evidence of use elsewhere or evaluation of impact	Relevance to the clinical situation Frequency/uniqueness of experience Extent to which experience has been rigorously subjected to critical reflection/audit Extent to which experiences have been shared by others Extent to which other sources of evidence support experiences Extent of transferability of experiences to current situation	Link between theory and clinical situation Strengths and weaknesses of argument being presented What sources of evidence are used? Credibility/face validity How this theory measures up to other theories Appropriateness of theory to clinical issue Appropriateness of recommendations for practice Likelihood of transferability to practice setting Evidence of successful use elsewhere or evaluation of impact	Relevance to the current situation Frequency/uniqueness of experience Extent to which experiences have been shared by others Extent to which other sources of evidence support experiences Richness of the description Extent of transferability of experiences to current situation	Depth and breadth of expertise Credibility/ reputation Face validity of advice Reason for choice – what defines expertise? What sources of evidence are drawn upon to support knowledge? Relevance of advice to current situation Likelihood of transferability of evidence to practice setting Evidence of use elsewhere or evaluation of impact	Possible conflict of interest of policy makers vis-à-vis this clinical situation Type and strength of evidence used to support directive(s) Relevance to current situation or clinical issue Currency – date when last reviewed Likelihood of transferability to practice setting Evidence of use elsewhere or evaluation of impact

© le May and Gabbay: Evidence-based practice – more than research needed! In (eds.) Lewith G, Jonas W, Walach H (2011 p. 399) *Clinical research in complementary therapies*. Elsevier

More actively, there have also been courses developed that are informed by the mindlines model. In Chapter 9, Wijchen and Alme describe what we believe is currently the most radical educational use of the mindlines model, which they claim is leading to an improved professional ethos and competence among their Dutch cohort of physiotherapy students. In the UK, Reeve and colleagues have also been using the mindlines model to inform their educational approach to enable education and training methods to be more attuned to the needs of the 'expert generalism' of doctors working in primary care (Reeve, Dowrick, Freeman et al. 2013). The training scheme that they have designed explicitly sets out to help GPs to be "skilled and confident in the professional generation and use of 'knowledge-in-practice-in-context'". This includes working with "communities of action" and nurturing "networks of support" to enable GPs to learn from and with each other as they develop what the scheme calls the "clinical scholarship" that leads to "pragmatic wisdom" (Reeve 2018, 2022).

Besides these examples (and of course the principle of communities of practice discussed earlier) (see above), our review of publications found relatively few specifically educational applications of the mindlines model in training programmes. There were references to its relevance to the notion of 'learning organisations' (e.g., Crites, McNamara, Akl et al. 2009), or organisational knowledge management (e.g., Kennedy & Burford 2013), or the place of problem-based learning (Wyer 2019). Some authors have recognised the care needed to alter and improve "deeply-rooted" practices as part of the process of learning linked to mindlines (Björnsdóttir, Kristinsson & Hansen 2010; Petto & Hinds 2009). Others have stressed the time and effort needed to help practitioners unlearn and relearn the kind of embedded knowledge found in mindlines (e.g., Bate, Hutchinson, Underhill et al. 2012; Nilsen, Neher, Ellström et al., 2017). Papakostopoulou and Hurst (2018) also emphasise the need to take note of the mindlines model when designing dissemination strategies for research. There are, though, some who assume that the secret to improving mindlines is simply to use the standard techniques of EBM to instil the scientific evidence (Garrison, Dupras, Merry et al. 2011).

Topic-specific training, for example by promulgating research-based guidelines, is often regarded as a crucial part of helping practitioners practise in line with research evidence. This has sometimes been the responsibility of the guidelines producers, so we had conversations with several of the leading members of the implementation-support systems run by NICE, some of whom have published on this topic (Maskrey, Underhill & Hutchinson 2009a; Maskrey, Underhill, Hutchinson et al. 2009b, 2010). Although the NICE guidance on how to implement guidance (NICE Implementation Strategy Group 2022) makes no reference to mindlines or associated ideas, the concept of mindlines has influenced the thinking of these NICE key players. This came about because they had originally been tasked with trying to get guidelines into practice by using conventional means (newsletters, evidence summaries, local guidelines, lectures, training programmes, etc.) but had intuitively known that using such methods to persuade practitioners to change their habits would be an uphill struggle. Reading our work, they told us, had legitimated that perception; this encouraged them to build on that understanding rather than continue struggling against the grain. It also allowed them to argue the case for doing things in a different way that takes the mindlines model into account. The model is now included in the training of NICE Prescribing Associates, whose role is to help promote the uptake of prescribing guidance; as a result, they now increasingly work by setting up local communities of practice and networks to discuss new guidance (although current shortages among National Health Service (NHS) staff are making it difficult to find the necessary time and space for the discussions).

Those charged by NICE to help implement guidance in this way have done so by melding of the results of our research with many other sources of knowledge about clinical decision making (National Prescribing Centre 2011). These have included educational concepts about the difference between theoretical and practical learning (Sfard 1998), the work of Greenhalgh and colleagues on innovation diffusion (Greenhalgh, Robert, Macfarlane et al. 2004), Croskerry's accounts of the cognitive psychology of decision-making (Croskerry 2008, 2013), ideas about "information mastery" (Slawson & Shaughnessy 2005), and Tversky and Kahneman's dual-process theory (Bate, Hutchinson, Underhill et al. 2012; Maskrey, Underhill & Hutchinson 2009a), now widely popularised as "fast and slow" thinking (Tversky & Kahneman 1974; Kahneman 2012) (discussed below).

A large proportion of the papers that engaged with the mindlines model aligned and combined it with other theoretical frameworks and approaches. This was no surprise; it is exactly the kind of transformation that the model itself would predict. As the model is absorbed and melded with what people already know, it is bound to be transformed and used in a large variety of ways.

Philosophical questions

Our 15 scholar-interviewees often wanted to expound on the philosophical and social-psychological concepts that underpin the mindlines model, in particular the view that knowledge is socially constructed. Several of them stressed the importance of collective thinking and "connectivity" of clinical knowledge – how it grows by discussion and relies therefore on trusted and trusting relationships between colleagues. One, a psychology researcher, referred specifically to the relevance of 'socially extended cognition' and another, a social-work academic, went so far as to invoke the concept of 'ubuntu' – a term denoting that we are who we are, and we know what we know, only because of others around us – and linked this explicitly to mindlines.

The idea that discussions between people result in changes in how they all understand or act in the world, leads us to some philosophical conundrums. To what extent does any newly emergent shared knowledge exist as merely a set of individual thoughts? Or is it somehow a collectively held entity in its own right? Is the whole more than the sum of the parts? Or is the new knowledge perhaps not even an entity but a collectively constructed activity? We have no intention of tackling such centuries-old thorny problems here, having already broached them as far as we feel competent to do (Gabbay & le May 2011, Chapter 9). However, when writing about notions such as collective mindlines, some have amplified our suggestion that they may be a form of distributed cognition – the idea that knowledge is dispersed across social groups and across time, not just guidelines-in-the-head, but guidelines in the group of colleagues and/ or patients (Rapley 2008; Sedig, Parsons, Naimi et al. 2015; Bleakley 2021). This is compatible with the suggestion that mindlines have a collective existence that practitioners share through their dialogue. Such a view links also to the concept of polyphony – attributed to Bakhtin, the early 20th-century Russian thinker, who argued that true knowledge emerges from the interaction of multiple perspectives. This implies that a person's knowledge doesn't exist in itself, but in its relations with other people and things (Greenhalgh 2010) – again a view that is highly compatible with the concept of a collective mindline The influential work of the mid-20th-century Russian psychologist Vygotsky has been mentioned too in this context (Kennedy & Burford 2013). Its relevance here is that Vygotsky maintains that every high-level cognitive function emerges principally *between* people (i.e., as an 'inter-psychological process') and only later as an 'intra-psychological process', internal to each individual. The thinking embodied in mindlines also embraces Vygotsky's principle that learning cannot be separated from the culture and language in which it happens, nor divorced from the roles we play in society.

When referring to philosophical questions about the status of collective mindlines, we are reminded that we must always acknowledge Wittgenstein, for whom all knowledge is collective (Greenhalgh 2010, Greenhalgh & Wieringa 2011). Through a Wittgensteinian lens, the way that practitioners communicate the complex knowledge of mindlines can be seen as an example of a "language game". From that, it follows that mindlines are understood and communicated in terms that cannot have precise meanings, but only mutually accepted "family resemblances" that can only be understood in context, and only if one has been ' trained' in the implicit conventions and "rule following" of a "language-in-use" (Wittgenstein 1953). This perspective also plays a part in the work of Tsoukas and others who – drawing a distinction between propositional knowledge and narrative knowledge – investigate the latter in terms of distributed, complex knowledge that is mutually constituted at both the organisational and personal level (Tsoukas 2005). Finally, another epistemological avenue that has been linked to the mindlines model, and which draws on socio-materialist theories, is the idea that people's actions are inextricably bound up not only with their social but also their material world (e.g., Orlikowski 2007) – a process in which mindlines may play a crucial role (e.g., Hurst 2019 and see also Chapter 4).

System 1½ – slowly formed fast thinking?

One theoretical model that has been increasingly mentioned in connection with mindlines is Kahneman's highly influential work on "fast and slow" thinking (Kahneman 2012). Several of the publications citing mindlines appear to have conflated them with his (fast) "System-1" (intuition) thought processes, i.e., the immediate, automatic, and relatively effortless way that we all make the majority of our decisions thanks to instinct and experience. (Examples include Maskrey, Underhill & Hutchinson 2009a; Lucchiari & Pravettoni 2011; Te Pas, van Dijk, Bartelink et al. 2013; Thompson, Aitken, Doran et al. 2013; Mannion & Thompson 2014; Reach 2014; Dobler, Morrow & Kamath 2019) This may, however, be misleading. Individual mindlines are open to errors, of course, and collective mindlines are open to perpetuating them. But it would be a mistake to assume – as some of these authors do – that the remedies for error-prone System-1 thinking will also fix the defects of mindlines. The connections need to be explored more fully, but until that work is done, we would simply say that, in our view, the conflation is deceptive.

The chief similarity between mindlines and System-1 thinking is the 'fast and frugal' speed of decision-making – without which much of the day-to-day work of clinical practice would be nigh on impossible. However – as we have always stated – this does not mean that mindlines are equivalent to System-1 thinking, with the same error-prone heuristics and biases. On the contrary, mindlines seem to us to be a way of avoiding simple System-1 thinking whilst also, even when making very complex decisions, removing the need for the much slower rigours of Kahneman's (slow) "System-2" (reasoning) thought processes, for which there may be no time. System-2 processes are characterised by rational, logical, analytical thinking and information gathering that requires time and effort. Such thinking underpins a significant part of what becomes internalised over many years into mindlines. They are the result of practitioners reading, appraising, memorising, and constantly replenishing their knowledge through continuous professional development and thoughtful reflection on and in practice.

We, therefore, maintain that mindlines exemplify a kind of thinking that is characterised by neither System-1 nor System 2, but a simultaneous combination of both. The thought processes (let us tentatively call them System-1½) are an essential means of making swiftly the kinds of complex, time-pressured decisions so often required by clinical practitioners. Correcting errors due to System-1½ thinking will be a different order of (largely relational) activity quite different from the methods that might avoid or correct mistaken System-1 heuristics.

System-1½ is fast thinking that is slow and arduous to learn and continually update. That is why it is such a crucial part of the professional capital of the clinical practitioner: it takes years to acquire. Over the course of a clinical career, practitioners are continually condensing and packing a wealth of detailed System-2-based knowledge, alongside other forms of evidence, into their rapidly accessed mindlines. It may be that the better practitioners are those who make sure they are able to constantly seek out and critically deliberate upon new evidence as, with their colleagues, they absorb and embed it into ever more richly nuanced and evolving mindlines.

Summary

- We provide an update on the mindlines model, based on a narrative review of around 1,000 publications that cite the findings from our ethnographies, supplemented by 15 interviews with scholars who have engaged with the model.
- None of the publications has disagreed with our findings.
- Despite the advent of easily accessed online information since our fieldwork, there appears to be no fundamental change in the role that mindlines play in clinical practice.
- As the model itself would predict, people have modulated, selectively (often severely) truncated, or transformed our research findings as they have used them in their academic practice.
- Citations cover most of the facets of the mindlines model, with an emphasis on the "social life" of mindlines, the melding of multiple sources of evidence, and the relationship between mindlines and guidelines.
- A few studies suggest that when purposefully applied, mindlines can be used not only to explain practice but also to improve it, either directly or through mindlines-based approaches to education and training.
- Mindlines are complex and socially constituted, and are therefore not equivalent to the apparently intuitive, fast and frugal thinking described by Tverksy and Kahneman's dual-process theory; they are a slowly constructed form of fast thinking that is essential to clinical practice.

Note

1 As our citations are likely to be accessed mostly online, we will not provide the page number for quotations except for books, theses, and reports.

References

Allen D. 2010. 'Care pathways: An ethnographic description of the field'. *International Journal of Care Coordination International Journal of Care Pathways*, 14: 4–9. https://doi.org/10.1258/jicp.2009.009015

Andrews N, Gabbay J, le May A, Miller E, Petch A, O'Neill M. 2020. 'Story, dialogue and caring about what matters to people: Progress towards evidence-enriched policy and practice'. *Evidence and Policy*, 16:4 597–618. https://doi.org/10.1332/174426420X15825349063428

Barley M, Pope C, Chilvers R, Sipos A, Harrison G. 2008. 'Guidelines or mindlines? A qualitative study exploring what knowledge informs psychiatrists decisions about antipsychotic prescribing'. *Journal of Mental Health*, 17:1, 9–17. https://doi.org/10.1080/09638230701498358

Bate L, Hutchinson A, Underhill J, Maskrey N. 2012. 'How clinical decisions are made'. *British Journal of Clinical Pharmacology*, 74(4): 614–620. https://doi.org/10.1111/j.1365-2125.2012.04366.x

Beckett K, DeaveT, McBride T, le May A, Gabbay J, Kapoulas U, Long A, Warburton G, Wogan C, Cox L, Thompson J, Spencer F, Kendrick D. 2022. 'Using Forum Theatre to mobilise knowledge and improve NHS care: the Enhancing Post-injury Psychological Intervention and Care (EPPIC) study'. *Evidence & Policy*, 18(2): 236–264. https://doi.org/10.1332/174426421X16420902769508

Bierbaum M, Rapport F, Arnolda G, Easpaig BNG, Lamprell K, Hutchinson K, Delaney GP, Liauw W, Kefford R, Olver I, Braithwaite J. 2020. 'Clinicians' attitudes and perceived barriers and facilitators to cancer treatment clinical practice guideline adherence: a systematic review of qualitative and quantitative literature'. *Implementation Sci*, 15: 39. https://doi.org/10.1186/s13012-020-00991-3

Björnsdóttir I, Kristinsson KG, Hansen EH. 2010. 'Diagnosing infections: a qualitative view on prescription decisions in general practice over time'. *Pharm World Sci*, 32: 805–814. https://doi.org/10.1007/s11096-010-9441-6

Blanco-Mavillard I, Parra-García G, Fernández-Fernández I, Rodríguez-Calero MA, Personat-Labrador C, Castro-Sánchez E. 2020. 'Care of peripheral intravenous catheters in three hospitals in Spain: Mapping clinical outcomes and implementation of clinical practice guidelines'. PLoS ONE, 15(10): e0240086. https://doi.org/10.1371/journal.pone.0240086

Bleakley A. 2021. 'Re-visioning clinical reasoning, or stepping out from the skull'. *Medical Teacher*, 43(4): 456–462. https://doi.org/10.1080/0142159X.2020.1859098

Boshoff N. 2014. 'Types of knowledge in science-based practices'. *Journal of Science Communication* 13(3): A06. https://doi.org/10.22323/2.13030206

Boon HTK. 2006. 'Clinical practice guidelines: a critical review'. *International Journal of Health Care Quality Assurance*, 19(2): 195–220. https://doi.org/10.1108/0952686061065171

Booth J, Tolson D, Hotchkiss R, Schofield I. 2007. 'Using action research to construct national evidence-based nursing care guidance for gerontological nursing'. *Journal of Clinical Nursing*, 16: 945–953. https://doi.org/10.1111/j.1365-2702.2007.01773.x

Brattgjerd M. 2021. *Standardization of nursing; how is the practice of the profession affected? A qualitative study based on a standardized action plan for dying patients.* Nord University https://nordopen.nord.no/nord-xmlui/handle/11250/2770986

Bresnen M, Hodgson D, Bailey S, Hyde P, Hassard J. 2017. 'Mobilizing management knowledge in healthcare: Institutional imperatives and professional and organizational mediating effects'. *Management Learning*, 48(5): 597–614. https://doi.org/10.1177/1350507617718257

Brichko L, Mitra B, Cameron P. 2018. 'When guidelines guide us to harm'. *Emergency Medicine Australasia*, 30: 740–742. https://doi.org/10.1111/1742-6723.13189

Carrier J. 2019. 'Implementing evidence in local and global contexts'. *International Journal of Evidence-Based* Healthcare, 17: S22–S23. https://doi.org/10.1097/XEB.0000000000000182

Carrier J. 2020. 'An ethnographic exploration of the social organisation of general practice nurses' knowledge use: more than "mindlines"?' *Journal of Research in Nursing*, 25(6–7): 604–615. https://doi.org/10.1177/1744987120937411

Chandler CI, Jones C, Boniface G, Juma K, Reyburn H, Whitty CJM. 2008. 'Guidelines and mindlines: why do clinical staff over-diagnose malaria in Tanzania? A qualitative studys'. *Malaria Journal'* 7: 53. https://doi.org/10.1186/1475-2875-7-53

Chandler, CIR, Meta J, Ponzo C, Nasuwa F, Kessy J, Mbakilwa H, Haaland A, Reyburn H. 2014. 'The development of effective behaviour change interventions to support the use of malaria rapid diagnostic tests by Tanzanian clinicians'. *Implementation Science*, 9: 83. https://doi.org/10.1186/1748-5908-9-83

Clark F, Park DJ, Burke JP. 2013. 'Dissemination: bringing translational research to completion'. *American Journal of Occupational Therapy*, 67(2): 185–193. https://doi.org/10.5014/ajot.2013.006148

Clarke C, Ryan D. 2017. 'An exploration of occupational therapists' views and experiences of using evidence-based practice to develop professional knowledge in a local authority setting'. *Brighton Journal of Research in Health Sciences*, 3(1). *blogs.brighton.ac.uk/bjrhs/2017/07/03/an-exploration-of-occupational-therapists-views-and-experiences-of-using-evidence-based-practice-to-develop-professional-knowledge-in-a-local-authority-setting/*

Collier A, Hodgins M, Johnston B, Tieman J. 2019. Evidence-based palliative care: How can we account for the messy world of practice? *Palliative Medicine*, 33(7): 723–725. https://doi.org/10.1177/0269216319845977

Colling T, McNinch T, Lighthizer DR. 2011. Transportation research record: Journal of the Transportation Research Board, No. 2213. Transportation Research Board of the National Academies, Washington, DC. pp. 63–71. https://doi.org/10.3141/2213-09

Copeland S. 2020. 'The guidelines challenge', in R Anjum, S Copeland, E Rocca (Eds.) *Rethinking causality, complexity and evidence for the unique patient.* Cham: Springer. https://doi.org/10.1007/978-3-030-41239-5_6

Cowdell F. 2018. 'Knowledge mobilisation: an ethnographic study of the influence of lay mindlines on eczema self-management in primary care in the UK'. *BMJ Open*, 8(8):e021498. http://dx.doi.org/10.1136/bmjopen-2018-021498

Cowdell F. 2019. 'Knowledge mobilisation: an ethnographic study of the influence of practitioner mindlines on atopic eczema self-management in primary care in the UK'. *BMJ Open*, 9(7):e025220. http://dx.doi.org/10.1136/bmjopen-2018-025220

Crites GE, McNamara MC, Akl EA, Richardson WS, Umscheid CA, Nishikawa J. 2009. 'Evidence in the learning organization'. *Health Res Policy Sys*, 7: 4. https://doi.org/10.1186/1478-4505-7-4

Croskerry P. 2008. 'Achieving quality in clinical decision making: cognitive strategies and detection of bias'. *Academic Emergency Medicine*, 9(11): 1184–1204. https://doi.org/10.1197/aemj.9.11.1184

Croskerry P. 2013. 'From mindless to mindful practice—cognitive bias and clinical decision making'. *The New England Journal of Medicine*, 368:2445–2448.

Cundill B, Mbakilwa H, Chandler CI, Mtove G, Mtei F, Willetts A, Foster E, Muro F, Mwinyishehe R, Mandike R, Olomi R, Whitty CJM, Reyburn H. 2015. 'Prescriber and patient-oriented behavioural interventions to improve use of malaria rapid diagnostic tests in Tanzania: facility-based cluster randomised trial'. *BMC Med*, 13: 118. https://doi.org/10.1186/s12916-015-0346-z

Cunningham AM, Shirley A. 2015. 'Mindlines in a digital age.' *Education for Primary Care*, 26(5): 293–296. https://doi.org/10.1080/14739879.2015.1079010

Dawes M, Summerskill W, Glasziou P, Cartabellotta A, Martin J, Hopayian K, Porzsolt F, Burls A, Osborne J. 2005. 'Sicily statement on evidence-based practice'. *BMC Med Educ*, 5: 1–8. https://doi.org/10.1186/1472-6920-5-1

Dobler CC, Morrow AS, Kamath CC. 2019. 'Clinicians' cognitive biases: a potential barrier to implementation of evidence-based clinical practice'. *BMJ Evidence-Based Medicine*, 2019(24): 137–140. http://dx.doi.org/10.1136/bmjebm-2018-111074

Draper J. 2015. 'Ethnography: principles, practice and potential'. *Nursing Standard*, 29(36): 36–41. https://doi.org/10.7748/ns.29.36.36.e8937

Ducey A, Donoso C, Ross S, Robert M. 2020. 'From anatomy to patient experience in pelvic floor surgery: mindlines, evidence, responsibility, and transvaginal mesh'. *Social Science & Medicine*, 260: 113151. https://doi.org/10.1016/j.socscimed.2020.113151

Elstad EA, Lutfey KE, Marceau LD, Campbell SM, von dem Knesebeck O, McKinlay JB. 2010. 'What do physicians gain (and lose) with experience? Qualitative results from a cross-national study of diabetes'. *Social Science & Medicine*,70(11): 1728–1736. https://doi.org/10.1016/j.socscimed.2010.02.014.

Elwyn G, Wieringa S, Greenhalgh T. 2016. 'Clinical encounters in the post-guidelines era'. *BMJ*, 353: i3200. https://doi.org/10.1136/bmj.i3200

English B, Tickle A, das Nair R, Moore K. 2020. 'Consensus-based good practice guidelines for Clinical Psychologists to support care staff in enabling sexual expression in people with intellectual disabilities—a Delphi study'. *Journal of Applied Research in Intellectual Disabilities*, 33: 268–282. https://doi.org/10.1111/jar.12671

Epling JW, Mader EM, Roseamelia CA, Morley CP. 2015. 'Emerging practice concerning vitamin d in primary care'. *Qualitative Health Research*, 25(7): 1005–1012. https://doi.org/10.1177/1049732314554100

Epling JW, Rockwell MS, Miller AD, Carver MC. 2021. 'Socializing the evidence for diabetes control to develop "mindlines": a qualitative pilot study'. *BMC Family Practice*, 22: 177. https://doi.org/10.1186/s12875-021-01521-w

Everson J, Hollingsworth JM Adler-Milstein J. 2019. 'Comparing methods of grouping hospitals'. *Health Services Research*, 54: 1090–1098. https://doi.org/10.1111/1475-6773.13188

Farr M, Cressey P. 2015. 'Understanding staff perspectives of quality in practice in healthcare'. *BMC Health Services Research*, 15: 123. https://doi.org/10.1186/s12913-015-0788-1

Gabbay, J, le May A, Pope C, Brangan E, Cameron A, Klein JH, Wye L. 2020. 'Uncovering the processes of knowledge transformation: the example of local evidence-informed policy-making in United Kingdom healthcare'. *Health Res Policy Sys*, 18: 110. https://doi.org/10.1186/s12961-020-00587-9

Gagliardi AR, Wright FC, Anderson MAB, Davis D. 2007. 'The role of collegial interaction in continuing professional development'. *Journal of Continuing Education in the Health Professions*, 27(4): 214–219. https://doi.org/10.10020chp.140

Garrison GM, Dupras DM, Merry SP, Smith AJ. 2011. 'Clinical problem solving', in RE Rakel, DP Rakel (Eds.) *Textbook of family medicine* (8th ed.). Philadelphia: Elsevier Saunders.

Gené-Badia J, Gallo P, Caïs J, Sánchez E, Carrion C, Arroyo L, Aymerich M. 2016. 'The use of clinical practice guidelines in primary care: professional mindlines and control mechanisms'. *Gaceta Sanitaria*,30(5): 345–351. https://doi.org/10.1016/j.gaceta.2016.01.005

Gildenhuys, J, Lee, M, Isbister, GK. 2009. 'Does implementation of a paediatric asthma clinical practice guideline worksheet change clinical practice?' *International Journal of Emergency Medicine*, 2: 33–39. https://doi.org/10.1007/s12245-008-0063-x

Grant A, Sullivan F, Dowell, J. 2013. 'An ethnographic exploration of influences on prescribing in general practice: why is there variation in prescribing practices?' *Implementation Sci*, 8: 72. https://doi.org/10.1186/1748-5908-8-72

Greenhalgh T, Robert G, Macfarlane F, Bate P, Kyriakidou O. 2004. 'Diffusion of innovations in service organizations: systematic review and recommendations'. *The Milbank Quarterly* 82(4): 581–629. https://doi.org/10.1111/j.0887-378X.2004.00325.x

Greenhalgh T, Russell J. 2009. 'Evidence-based policymaking a critique'. *Perspectives in Biology and Medicine*, 52(2): 304–318. https://doi.org/10.1353/pbm.0.0085

Greenhalgh T. 2010. 'What is this knowledge that we seek to "exchange"?' *The Milbank Quarterly*, 88: 492–499. https://doi.org/10.1111/j.1468-0009.2010.00610.x

Greenhalgh T, Wieringa S. 2011. 'Is it time to drop the "knowledge translation" metaphor? A critical literature review'. *J R Soc Med*, 104: 501–509. https://doi.org/10.1258/jrsm.2011.110285

Griffiths F, Anto N, Chow E, Manazar U, van Royen P, Bastiaens H. 2007. 'Understanding the diversity and dynamics of living with diabetes: a feasibility study focusing on the case'. *Chronic Illness*, 3: 29–45. https://doi.org/10.1177/1742395307079194

Hurst D, Mickan S. 2017. 'Describing knowledge encounters in healthcare: a mixed studies systematic review and development of a classification.' *Implementation Sci*, 12: 35. https://doi.org/10.1186/s13012-017-0564-1

Hurst D. 2019. 'Practice, complexity and evidence-based practice'. *Br Dent J*, 227: 12–14. https://doi.org/10.1038/s41415-019-0423-3

Hurst D, Greenhalgh T. 2019. 'Knowing in general dental practice: anticipation, constraint, and collective bricolage'. *J Eval Clin Pract.*, 25: 921–929. https://doi.org/10.1111/jep.13051

Ibargoyen-Roteta N, Mateos del Pino M, Gutiérrez-Ibarluzea I, Benguria-Arrate G, Rada-Fernández de Jauregui D, Domingo-Rico C, Regidor Fuentes I, González Santisteban R, Armendáriz Cuñado M, Jaio Atela N. 2018. 'Variability in the prescription of drugs with uncertain effectiveness. The case of SYSADOA in the Basque Country'. *GMS Health Technol Assess*, 14(Doc01). https://doi.org/10.3205/hta000130

Ikioda F, Kendall S., 2016. 'Transformation of health visiting services in England using an Online Community of Practice'. *Health Policy and Technology*, 5(33): 298–306. https://doi.org/10.1016/j.hlpt.2016.02.006

Ingvarsson S, Augustsson H, Hasson H, Nilsen P, von Thiele Schwarz U, von Knorring M. 2020. 'Why do they do it? A grounded theory study of the use of low-value care among primary health care physicians'. *Implementation Science*, 15: 93. https://doi.org/10.1186/s13012-020-01052-5

Jiwa M, Deas K, Ross J, Shaw T, Wilcoz H, Spilsbury K. 2009. 'An inclusive approach to raising standards in general practice: working with a "community of practice" in Western Australia'. *BMC Med Res Methodol*, 9: 13. https://doi.org/10.1186/1471-2288-9-13

Johannessen LEF. 2017. 'Beyond guidelines: discretionary practice in face-to-face triage nursing'. *Sociology of Health & Illness*, 39(7): 1180–1194. https://doi.org/10.1111/1467-9566.12578

Kahneman D. 2012. *Thinking fast and slow*. London: Penguin Books.

le May A, Gabbay J. 2011. 'Evidence-based practice – more than research needed!', in G Lewith, W Jonas, H Walach (Eds.) *Clinical research in complementary therapies* (pp. 391–405). London: Elsevier.

Löfgren A, Silén C, Alexanderson K. 2011. 'How physicians have learned to handle sickness-certification cases'. *Scandinavian Journal of Public Health*, 39(3): 245–254. https://doi.org/10.1177/1403494810393301

Kennedy M, Burford S. 2013. 'A comparative analysis of conceptions of knowledge and learning in general and public sector literature 2000–2009'. *International Journal of Public Administration*, 36(3): 155–167, https://doi.org/10.1080/01900692.2012.749279

King R, Sanders, T, Todd A. 2021. 'Shortcuts in knowledge mobilization: an ethnographic study of advanced nurse practitioner discharge decision-making in the emergency department'. *Journal of Advanced Nursing*, 77: 3156–3167. https://doi.org/10.1111/jan.14834

Kislov R, Walshe K, Harvey, G. 2012. 'Managing boundaries in primary care service improvement: A developmental approach to communities of practice'. *Implementation Sci*, 7: 97. https://doi.org/10.1186/1748-5908-7-97

Kuberska K, Scheibl F, Sinnott C, Sheppard JP, Lown M, Williams M, Payne RA, Mant J, McManus RJ, Burt J. 2021. *British Journal of General Practice*, 71(708): e498–e507. https://doi.org/10.3399/bjgp21X714305

Labrador JRR. 2009. 'Identificación y modulación del comportamiento sistemáticamente irracional en medicina y salud pública'. *Rev Esp Salud Pública*, 2009(83): 43–57.

Lacasta Tintorer D, Manresa Domínguez JM, Pujol-Rivera E, Beneyto SF, Tuduri ZM, Saigí-Rubió F. 2018. 'Keys to success of a community of clinical practice in primary care: a qualitative evaluation of the ECOPIH project'. *BMC Fam Pract*, 19: 56. https://doi.org/10.1186/s12875-018-0739-0

Ladds E, Rushforth A, Wieringa S, Taylor S, Rayner C, Husain C, Greenhalgh T. 2021. 'Developing services for long COVID: lessons from a study of wounded healers'. *Clinical Medicine*, 21(1): 59–65. https://doi.org/10.7861/clinmed.2020-0962

Lamont T. 2019. '*Making research matter: steps to impact for health and care researchers'*. Bristol: Policy Press.

Lander B, Balka E. 2019. 'Exploring how evidence is used in care through an organizational ethnography of two teaching hospitals'. *J Med Internet Res*, 21(3): e10769. https://doi.org/10.2196/10769

Lange S, Mwisongo A, Mæstad O. 2014. 'Why don't clinicians adhere more consistently to guidelines for the Integrated Management of Childhood Illness (IMCI)?' *Social Science and Medicine*, 104: 56–63. https://doi.org/10.1016/j.socscimed.2013.12.020

Langley J, Wassall R, Geddis-Regan A, Watson A, Verey A, McKenna G, Brocklehurst P, Tsakos G. 2022. 'Putting guidelines into practice: Using co-design to develop a complex intervention based on NG48 to enable care staff to provide daily oral care to older people living in care homes'. *Gerodontology*. https://doi.org/10.1111/ger.12629

Launer J. 2012. 'Dumpling soup'. *Postgraduate Medical Journal*, 88: 243–244.

Launer J. 2015. 'Guidelines and mindlines'. *Postgrad Medical Journal*, 91(1081): 663–664. http://dx.doi.org/10.1136/postgradmedj-2015-133766

Le JV, Lykkegaard J, Pedersen LB, Riisgaard H, Nexøe J, Lemmergaard J, Søndergaard J. 2017. 'Are formalised implementation activities associated with aspects of quality of care in general practice? A cross-sectional study'. *Brit J Gen Prac Open*, 1(2). https://doi.org/10.3399/bjgpopen17X100737

Locock L, Graham C, King J, Parkin S, Chisholm A, Montgomery C, Gibbons E, Ainley E, Bostock J, Gager M, Churchill N, Dopson S, Greenhalgh T, Martin A, Powell J, Sizmur S, Ziebland S. 2020. 'Understanding how front-line staff use patient experience data for service improvement: an exploratory case study evaluation'. *Health Serv Deliv Res*, 8(13). https://www.journalslibrary.nihr.ac.uk/hsdr/hsdr08130/#/abstract

Lucchiari C, Pravettoni G. 2011. 'Cognitive balanced model: a conceptual scheme of diagnostic decision making'. *Journal of Evaluation in Clinical Practice*, 18(1): 82–88. https://doi.org/10.1111/j.1365-2753.2011.01771.x

Mannion R, Thompson C. 2014. 'Systematic biases in group decision-making: implications for patient safety'. *International Journal for Quality in Health Care* 26(6): 606–612. https://doi.org/10.1093/intqhc/mzu083

Maskrey N, Underhill J, Hutchinson A. 2009a. 'Getting a better grip on research: the comfort of opinion'. *InnovAiT (RCGP)*. https://doi.org/10.1093/innovait/inp085

Maskrey N, Underhill J, Hutchinson A, Shaughnessy A, Slawson D. 2009b. 'Getting a better grip on research: a simple system that works'. *InnovAiT (RCGP)*. https://doi.org/10.1093/innovait/inp106

Maskrey N, Underhill J, Hutchinson A, Shaughnessy A, Slawson D. 2010. 'Getting a better grip on research: the maze of the most busy life'. *InnovAiT (RCGP)*. https://doi.org/10.1093/innovait/inp108

Mbacham WF, Mangham-Jefferies L, Cundill B, Achonduh OA, Chandler CIR, Ambebila JN, Nkwescheu A, Forsah-Achu D, Ndiforchu V, Tchekountouo O, Akindeh-Nji M, Ongolo-Zogo P, Wiseman V. 2014. 'Basic or enhanced clinician training to improve adherence to malaria treatment guidelines: a cluster-randomised trial in two areas of Cameroon'. *The Lancet Global Health*, 2(6): e346–e358. https://doi.org/10.1016/S2214-109X(14)70201-3

Meagher-Stewart D, Solberg SM, Warner G, MacDonald J, McPherson C, Seaman P. 2012. 'Understanding the role of communities of practice in evidence-informed decision making in public health'. *Qualitative Health Research*, 22(6): 723–739. https://doi.org/10.1177/1049732312438967

National Prescribing Centre. 2011. Making decisions better. *MeReC Bulletin* 2011, 22(1): 1–8. http://www.carerightnow.co.uk/wp-content/uploads/2015/08/MAKING-DECISIONS-BETTERmerec_bulletin_vol22_no11.pdf

Møller AM. 2018. *Organizing knowledge and decision-making in street-level professional practice: A practice-based study of Danish child protective services* PhD thesis, University of Copenhagen. https://www.researchgate.net/publication/325780927_Organizing_knowledge_and_decision-making_in_street-level_professional_practice_A_practice-based_study_of_Danish_child_protective_services#fullTextFileContent [accessed May 2022].

Næss SCK. 2021. 'CPP or not, that is the question: physicians' work with activating CPPs'. *Qualitative Health Research*, 31(11): 2084–2096. https://doi.org/10.1177/10497323211020708

Nathan R, Gabbay M, Boyle S, Elliott P, Giebel C, O'Loughlin C, Wilson P, Saini P. 2021. 'Use of acute psychiatric hospitalisation: a study of the factors influencing decisions to arrange acute admission to inpatient mental health facilities'. *Frontiers in Psychiatry*, 12. https://doi.org/10.3389/fpsyt.2021.696478

NICE Implementation Strategy Group. 2022. *Into practice guide: Practical steps to improving the quality of care and services using NICE guidance.* https://www.nice.org.uk/about/what-we-do/into-practice/resources-help-put-guidance-into-practice (last accessed June 2022)

Nicolini D, Powell J, Korica M. 2014. 'Keeping knowledgeable: How NHS Chief Executives mobilise knowledge and information in their daily work'. *Health Serv Deliv Res*, 2(26). https://www.ncbi.nlm.nih.gov/books/NBK259958/

Nicolini D, Bharatan I, Gkeredakis E, Manning R, Swan J. 2022. 'From evidence use to evidencing work: towards a processual view of the role of evidence in commissioning policy-making' in N Burgess, Currie G (Eds.) *Sustainable healthcare*. London: Palgrave McMillan.

Nilsen P, Neher M, Ellström PE, Gardner B. 2017. 'Implementation of evidence-based practice from a learning perspective'. *Worldviews on Evidence-Based Nursing*, 14(3): 192–199. https://doi.org/10.1111/wvn.12212.

Nutley S, Walter I, Davies HTO. 2007. *Using evidence: how research can inform public services* Bristol: Policy Press.

Oborn, E, Dawson S. 2010. 'Knowledge and practice in multidisciplinary teams: Struggle, accommodation and privilege'. *Human Relations*, 63(12): 1835–1857. https://doi.org/10.1177/0018726710371237

Oduro-Mensah E, Kwamie A, Antwi E, Amissah Bamfo S, Bainson HM, Marfo B, Coleman MA, Grobbee DE, Agyepong IA. 2013. 'Care decision making of frontline providers of maternal and newborn health services in the greater Accra region of Ghana'. PLoS One,8(2): e55610. https://doi.org/10.1371/journal.pone.0055610

Orlikowski WJ. 2007. 'Sociomaterial practices: exploring technology at work'. *Organization Studies*, 28(9): 1435–1448. https://doi.org/10.1177/0170840607081138

Oyebode O, Patrick H, Walker A, Campbell B, Powell J. 2016. 'The ghost in the machine? The value of expert advice in the production of evidence-based guidance: a mixed methods study of the NICE interventional procedures programme'. *International Journal of Technology Assessment in Health Care, 32*(1–2): 61–68. https://doi.org/10.1017/S0266462315000690

Papakostopoulou M, Hurst D. 2018. 'Disseminating research evidence: what matters to general dental practitioners?' *Br Dent J*, 225: 413–417. https://doi.org/10.1038/sj.bdj.2018.737

Peiris D, Usherwood T, Weeramanthri T, Cass A, Patel A. 2011. 'New tools for an old trade: a socio-technical appraisal of how electronic decision support is used by primary care practitioners'. *Sociology of Health & Illness*, 33(7): 1002–1018.

Petto P, Hinds P. 2009. 'Out with the old, in with the new: new findings replacing previous care practices'. *Cancer Nursing*, 32(5): 343–344. https://doi.org/10.1097/NCC.0b013e3181b38f3b

Pickles K, Carter SM, Rychetnik L, Entwistle V. 2016. 'Doctors' perspectives on PSA testing illuminate established differences in prostate cancer screening rates between Australia and the UK: a qualitative study'. *BMJ Open*, 6: e011932.

Pilbeam C, Tonkin-Crine S, Martindale A, Atkinson P , Mableson H, Lant S, Solomon T, Sheard S, Gobat N. 2022. 'How do healthcare workers 'do' guidelines? Exploring how policy decisions impacted uk healthcare workers during the first phase of the COVID-19 pandemic'. *Qualitative Health Research*, 32(5): 729–743. https://doi.org/10.1177/10497323211067772

Ranmuthugala G, Plumb JJ, Cunningham FC, Georgiou A, Westbrook JI, Braithwaite J. 2011. 'How and why are communities of practice established in the healthcare sector? A systematic review of the literature'. *BMC Health Serv Res*, 11: 273. https://doi.org/10.1186/1472-6963-11-273

Rapley T. 2008. 'Distributed decision making: the anatomy of decisions-in-action'. *Sociology of Health & Illness*, 30: 429–444. https://doi.org/10.1111/j.1467-9566.2007.01064.x

Reach G. 2014. 'Clinical inertia, uncertainty and individualized guidelines'. *Diabetes & Metabolism*, 40(4): 241–245. https://doi.org/10.1016/j.diabet.2013.12.009

Reeve J. 2018. 'Scholarship-based medicine: teaching tomorrow's generalists why it's time to retire EBM'. *British Journal of General Practice*, 68(673): 390–391. https://doi.org/10.3399/bjgp18X698261

Reeve J. 2022. 'Championing and cultivating the pragmatic wisdom and clinical scholarship at the heart of modern general practice.' *Wise GP Website*. https://sapc.ac.uk/article/gp-scholarship-wise-gp-programme (Accessed June 2022)

Reeve J, Dowrick C, Freeman GK, Gunn J, Mair F, May C, Mercer S, Palmer V, Howe A, Irving G, Shiner A, Watson J. 2013. 'Examining the practice of generalist expertise: a qualitative study identifying constraints and solutions'. *JRSM Short Rep.*, 4(12). https://doi.org/10.1177/2042533313510155

Risør T. 2017. 'Trail blazing or jam session? Towards a new concept of clinical decision-making'. *Anthropology & Medicine*, 24(1): 47–64. https://doi.org/10.1080/13648470.2016.1239695

Runciman WB, Lunby J. 2009. 'Regulating clinical practice', in J Healy, P Dugdale (Eds.) *Patient safety first* (pp. 181–210). Oxford and New York: Routledge.

Salter KL, Kothari A. 2016. 'Knowledge "translation" as social learning: negotiating the uptake of research-based knowledge in practice'. *BMC Medical Education*, 16: 76. DOI https://doi.org/10.1186/s12909-016-0585-5

Sedig K, Parsons P, Naimi A, Willoughby K. 2015. 'Reconsidering healthcare evidence as dynamic and distributed'. *International Journal of Evidence-Based Healthcare*, 13(2): 43–51. https://doi.org/10.1097/XEB.0000000000000030

Sfard A. 1998. 'On two metaphors for learning and the dangers of choosing just one'. *Educational Researcher*, 27: 2. https://doi.org/10.3102/0013189X027002004

Shaheen Q, Kothari A, Conklin J, Sibbald S. 2021. 'Supporting successful communities of practice for older adults: a qualitative secondary analysis'. *Educational Gerontology*, 47(5): 207–221. https://doi.org/10.1080/03601277.2021.1907899

Schulte MC. 2020. 'Knowledge does not equal evidence — what to do with what we have evidence for?', *Evidence-based medicine – a paradigm ready to be challenged?* (pp. 75–106). Stuttgart: JB Meltzer. https://doi.org/10.1007/978-3-476-05703-7_4

Slawson DC, Shaughnessy, AF. 2005. 'Teaching evidence-based medicine: should we be teaching information management instead?' *Academic Medicine*, 80(7): 685–689. https://doi.org/10.1097/00001888-200507000-00014

Smith A, Alderson P. 2012. 'Guidelines in anaesthesia: support or constraint?' *British Journal of Anaesthesia*, 109(1): 1–4. https://doi.org/10.1093/bja/aes149

Soubhi H, Bayliss EA, Fortin M, Hudon C, van den Akker M, Thivierge R, Posel N, Fleiszer D. 2010. 'Learning and caring in communities of practice: using relationships and collective learning to improve primary care for patients with multimorbidity'. *The Annals of Family Medicine*, 8(2): 170–177. https://doi.org/10.1370/afm.1056

Swayne J. 2012. 'The problem with science-the context and process of care: an excerpt from remodelling medicine'. *Glob Adv Health Med.*, 1: 78–87. https://doi.org/10.7453/gahmj.2012.1.1.014

Swennen MHJ, van der Heijden GJMG, Boeije HR, van Rheenen N, Verheul FJM, van der Graaf Y, Kalkman CJ. 2013. 'Doctors' perceptions and use of evidence-based medicine: a systematic review and thematic synthesis of qualitative studies'. *Academic Medicine*, 88(9): 1384–1396. https://doi.org/10.1097/ACM.0b013e31829ed3cc

Swinglehurst D. 2005. 'Evidence-based guidelines: the theory and the practice'. *Evidence-Based Healthcare and Public Health*, 9(4): 308–314. https://doi.org/10.1016/j.ehbc.2005.05.012

Tawfik H, Anya O. 2015. 'Evaluating practice-centered awareness in cross-boundary telehealth decision support systems'. *Telematics and Informatics*, 32: 486–503.

Te Pas E, van Dijk N, Bartelink MEL, Wieringa-De Waard M. 2013. 'Factors influencing the EBM behaviour of GP trainers: A mixed method study'. *Medical Teacher*, 35(3): e990–e997. https://doi.org/10.3109/0142159X.2012.733044

Thompson C, Aitken L, Doran D, Dowding D. 2013. 'An agenda for clinical decision making and judgement in nursing research and education'. *International Journal of Nursing Studies*, 50(12): 1720–1726. https://doi.org/10.1016/j.ijnurstu.2013.05.003

Thille P, Frank AW, Sudmann TT. 2020. 'Finding the right track: Embodied reflecting teams for generous physiotherapy' in DA Nicholls, KS Groven, EA Kinsella, RL Anjum (Eds.) *Mobilizing knowledge in physiotherapy: critical reflections on foundations and practices*. London: Routledge.

Tooman TR. 2019. Shepherding knowledge: a case study of social interactions that support knowledge mobilisation for sepsis care in Scotland. PhD Thesis, University of St Andrews. https://research-repository.st-andrews.ac.uk/handle/10023/19246

Trevithick P. 2008. 'Revisiting the knowledge base of social work: a framework for practice'. *The British Journal of Social Work*, 38(6): 1212–1237. https://doi.org/10.1093/bjsw/bcm026

Tsoukas H. 2005. *Complex knowledge: studies in organizational epistemology*. Oxford: Oxford University Press.

Tversky A, Kahneman D. 1974. 'Judgment under uncertainty: heuristics and biases'. *Science*, 185: 1124–1131 (Reprinted in eds. D Kahneman, P Slovic, A Tversky) 1982, *Judgment under uncertainty: heuristics and biases*. Cambridge and New York: Cambridge University Press.

Vagnoni E. 2018. 'Intellectual capital in the context of healthcare: does it matter?', in J Guthrie, J Dumay, F Ricceri, C Nielsen (Eds.) *The Routledge companion to intellectual capital*. London: Routledge.

Walach H, Falkenberg T, Fønnebø V, Lewith G, Jonas WB. 2006. 'Circular instead of hierarchical: methodological principles for the evaluation of complex interventions'. *BMC Med Res Methodol.*, 6: 29. https://doi.org/10.1186/1471-2288-6-29

Weekes LM. 2020. 'Theoretical bases of interventions to improve use of medicines and tests', in L Weekes (Ed.) *Improving use of medicines and medical tests in primary care* (pp. 29–58). Singapore: Springer. https://doi.org/10.1007/978-981-15-2333-5_2

Whiteford M, Byrne P. 2014. 'Talking about alcohol: communities of practice and patient pathways'. *Journal of Research in Nursing*, 20(1): 12–25. https://doi.org/10.1177/1744987114548744

Wieringa S, Engebretsen E, Heggen K, Greenhalgh T. 2018. 'How knowledge is constructed and exchanged in virtual communities of physicians: qualitative study of mindlines online'. *Journal of Medical Internet Research*, 20(2): e34. https://doi.org/10.2196/jmir.8325

Wieringa S, Engebretsen E, Heggen K, Greenhalgh T. 2021. 'Clinical guidelines and the pursuit of reducing epistemic uncertainty. An ethnographic study of guideline development panels in three countries'. *Social Science & Medicine*, 272: 113702. https://doi.org/10.1016/j.socscimed.2021.113702

Wieringa S, Greenhalgh T. 2015. '10 years of mindlines: a systematic review and commentary: Implementation'. *Science*, 10: 45. https://doi.org/10.1186/s13012-015-0229-x

Williams B, Skinner J, Dowell J, Roberts R, Crombie I, Davis, J. 2007. 'General practitioners' reasons for the failure of a randomized controlled trial (The TIGER Trial) to implement epilepsy guidelines in primary care'. *Epilepsia*, 48: 1275–1282. https://doi.org/10.1111/j.1528-1167.2007.01057.x

Wittgenstein L. 1953. *Philosophical investigations* (Trans. GEM Anscome, R Rhees, 1976 edition). Oxford: Basil Blackwell.

Wong KY, Job C, Anstey S. 2020. 'Patients' stories in healthcare curricula: learning the art of healthcare practice with patients'. *Journal of Further and Higher Education*, 44, 6: 729–738. https://doi.org/10.1080/0309877X.2019.1596234

Wye L, Brangan E, Cameron A, Gabbay J, Klein J, Pope C. 2015a. 'Knowledge exchange in health-care commissioning: case studies of the use of commercial, not-for-profit and public sector agencies'. *Health Serv Deliv Res*, 3(19). https://doi.org/10.3310/hsdr03190

Wye, L, Brangan, E, Cameron, A, Gabbay J, Klein JH, Pope C. 2015b. 'Evidence based policy making and the "art" of commissioning – how English healthcare commissioners access and use information and academic research in "real life" decision-making: an empirical qualitative study'. *BMC Health Serv Res*, 15: 430. https://doi.org/10.1186/s12913-015-1091-x

Wye L, Cramer H, Beckett K, Farr M, le May A, Carey J, Robinson R, Anthwal R, Rooney J, Baxter H. 2020. 'Collective knowledge brokering: the model and impact of an embedded team'. *Evidence & Policy*, *16*(3): 429–452. https://doi.org/10.1332/174426419X15468577044957

Wyer PC. 2018. 'From MARS to MAGIC: The remarkable journey through time and space of the grading of recommendations assessment, development and evaluation initiative'. *J Eval Clin Pract.*, 24: 1191–1202. https://doi.org/10.1111/jep.13019

Wyer PC. 2019. 'Evidence-based medicine and problem based learning a critical re-evaluation'. *Adv in Health Sci Educ*, 24: 865–878. https://doi.org/10.1007/s10459-019-09921-5

Wyer PC, Loughlin M. 2020. 'Person centered healthcare and clinical research: the necessity of an evolutionary hierarchy of knowing and doing'. *European Journal for Person Centered Healthcare*, 8:2. http://dx.doi.org/10.5750/ejpch.v8i2.1847

15

POSTSCRIPT

Does the mindlines model apply beyond healthcare?

John Gabbay and Andrée le May

Branching out

Is the mindlines model exclusive to the clinical and caring professions? And if it is, then what makes their practice so different? Astute readers who are familiar with our work will have noticed that we no longer use the term "clinical mindlines". This postscript explains why we suspect that other walks of life also have similar needs for rapid access to their complex, hard-won, internalised wisdom. This was first highlighted for us when, after a long workshop with clinicians, a member of the IT support staff, who had been operating the equipment in the lecture theatre enthused, as he retrieved our lapel microphones, that he could see "exactly the same thing" within his own profession. Subsequently, as we reviewed the literature, we were surprised to find that journalists (Kantola & Harju 2021), engineers (Bârsan & Bondreia 2015), teachers (Bruce 2017, p. 2; Cain, Brindley & Brown 2019), and researchers in tourism (Fennell 2022) were using or referring positively to the mindlines model. That led us to strike up conversations with people from a range of different professions and trades, exploring whether mindlines may feature in occupational practices beyond the world of health and social care.

Our aim was exploratory. We must stress (a) this was not in any way a pucka piece of qualitative research, and (b) we make no claim these respondents are representative of their trades or professions. They speak as individuals. The conversations were relatively short and informal – 15–40 minutes – and were with people we happen to know. The ages ranged from four respondents in their early 30s to five in their 70s, the latter who had retired and were looking back over long careers. Some drew upon more than one occupation (e.g., a headmaster who became a schools inspector, a lawyer who since retirement has volunteered on a helpline, a

DOI: 10.4324/9781003158721-15

butcher who was also trained as a mechanic). We outlined very briefly for them the mindlines model (some of them had an inkling already from earlier conversations we had had) and then asked them to reflect on how far they felt this resonated with their own experience.

The discussions were unstructured and free-flowing, but we also used a variety of prompt questions such as "How did you learn to be a good [whatever occupation]?" or "Talk me through a situation where you were faced with doing something difficult that doesn't quite conform to what you were taught or to the instructions, guidance or protocols you are expected to follow". When they responded, we used follow-up probing questions, such as "Do you/did you discuss this kind of problem with colleagues/work mates?", or (if they mentioned an initial course about, say the theory and practice of their profession or trade) "Looking back now, how important to your development would you say the course was?" Apart from the barrister and the jazz musician, where the conversations were serendipitous, we told them it was for this book, and they gave permission for us to take notes. It was not appropriate to record the conversations – this was not a research project – but we always gave them the usual key research-ethics assurances that they would be anonymised and that they could withdraw at any stage. We present here snippets of the conversations to illustrate how the accounts compared with key facets of clinical mindlines. These snippets are not verbatim but reconstructed from our notes to represent as accurately as possible what we recall they said.

We will largely let them speak for themselves and give only the occasional commentary. Many of the snippets could exemplify more than one facet of the mindlines model, so there are cross-references and repetitions between them. Not all aspects of mindlines were explored in any depth, so an apparent lack of examples on any one of them should not be over-interpreted. And neither, of course, should it be forgotten that we have selected snippets to illustrate the potential of this route of inquiry, not to suggest anything more. This is simply an early sketch of this territory. It is for you the reader to judge (perhaps by putting yourself in the frame) how far and why the various facets of the mindlines model do or do not apply beyond the world of health and social care. So, having got the caveats out of the way, what did we find?

Exploring the features of mindlines in varied occupations

Each of the occupational roles appeared to show echoes of at least some, if not all, of the features of the mindlines model. The overlap with clinical mindlines was most apparent in those walks of life requiring the ability to make complex and contextually flexible decisions, often very quickly. But all the occupations, even those without strong time pressures, revealed aspects of mindlines that helped in handling situations where many – possibly conflicting – considerations must be handled within certain professional, organisational, and social norms. In the rest of this chapter, we give some illustrative examples, many of which could have been included under several headings. Some, therefore, appear in more than one of the following sections, which are arranged according to the main features of the mindlines model described in Chapter 2:

- formal knowledge *vs* knowledge-in-practice-in-context,
- accumulating multiple sources of (sometimes tacit) evidence while learning through practice,
- collective learning/communities of practice: sharing (or not) knowledge and experience,
- the part played by clients in formulating decisions about practice,
- the role of context,
- contextual adroitness, and
- that formal knowledge, when put into practice, is transformed by all these influences.

Formal knowledge vs knowledge-in-practice-in-context

All the discussions revealed the need not just for practical knowledge and skills but also for knowledge-in-practice-in-context. For some, this raised doubts about the benefits of formal courses and such resources as instructions and guidance. However, this is not to say that such resources have no value – one of our findings when observing clinicians in practice was that they were more reliant on deeply embedded formal knowledge than they might have conveyed in the kind of casual conversation we are reporting here.

Courses

1. (Butcher) *There was an in-house course for apprentices, but I mostly learnt by working alongside the butcher.*
2. (District judge) *After I'd been in legal practice for many years, the Queen 'was minded to appoint me', as they put it, to the judiciary. So I went on a two-day residential course, (which we subsequently have to do every year to keep up), where among other things they teach you 'judgecraft'. That's one of the few parts of the course that involve working in groups, rather than hearing lectures from eminent judges and academics. Judgecraft is not about black-letter law; it's about practical things. The sessions are demanding – you deal with role-play situations and you feel very exposed. To be honest it's a minor part of the course and not particularly valuable.*
3. (Pharmacist) *Most of my university course, back in the day, was hard science and gave us no training whatsoever for actually being a pharmacist. (Fortunately, courses are more practical now, I believe.) I learned to read and dispense while working first as a hospital pharmacist.*
4. (Roofers) *D: I went to college at 16. The lads all laugh at me for that – you don't need books to be a roofer, they say. But I did learn a lot, but I've also learnt from the thousands of roofs I've done since.*

R: *Yeah. At college, every roof is even and straight and all nice and then when you get to the old Victorian houses they never are.*

D: *(laughs) Yeah. You come across all sorts of variations that they never taught you about and you learn to deal with them. That little splinter of wood I chipped off the batten to put under that slate? They didn't teach me that in college! But you soon learn when it's needed. Like how I ditched those four slates before choosing this next one coz I had to check the thickness so it matches the slate I've just laid. If you don't do that then it comes out all uneven.*

5. (Armoured-vehicle second-in-command (2ic)) My job was to drive the tank, fix it if needed, and various other things. Most of it you learned through experience, which was absolutely key. When you're fresh from training you really don't know what you're doing; it takes you about six months in the tank to become proficient.

Instruction manuals and guidance

6. (Motor mechanic) *There are manuals four-inches thick to tell you how to strip an engine. But they assume it's on the bench and it's a new car. It's never actually like that.*
7. (Fishmonger) *The fish processing company I worked for bought this incredible piece of kit designed to fillet 50 plaice a minute. No chance. Our engineer went to the manufacturers to learn how to do it and we still couldn't get it anywhere near that rate. It was an interesting time! Eventually – and between us we had to work it out for ourselves – we learnt that the secret was to sort the fish into eight different sizes beforehand. We got it to 60/minute.*
8. (Architect) *We have the RIBA "Job Book" that takes you through every stage of a job, mostly around managing different stages of the process, what you need to do when. It's detailed and plodding, and I do refer to it sometimes. But actually, things have moved on in the way contracts are organised, so although I refer to it from time to time, I do always have to adapt it to suit.*
9. (Armoured-vehicle 2ic) *Instructions are like a framework. They set the boundaries of what you should and should not do. They're the guidelines within which you work because you always have to be responsive to the circumstances.*
10. (Head teacher) *There are lots of policies, of course, because they get inspected, but they rarely apply in real situations.*
11. (Butcher) Health and safety ... *We conform – and get all our certificates and everything – but not quite how it's laid down.*

Formalised knowledge vs practice

Formalised knowledge can take many forms besides courses and guidance.

12. (Project evaluator) *I wrote a long and in-depth guidance on how to design interventions, manage them, and monitor and evaluate them. I suspect not even the senior management team read it, at most glancing through the executive summary. Then if they*

are like me, they probably don't remember it – certainly not recommendation 24b from a 100-page report.

13. (Jazz musician) "*I love the maths side of music, but the way you're gonna know what people are doing is by using your ears and listening. So it's where the scientific approach meets a more aural organic approach. The early jazz musicians, who were at the forefront of trying to think how to do extensions and alternative scales over chords, would learn by ear. They would hear something and respond to it harmonically but then afterwards sit down at the piano, playing around and exploring why it had sounded good, rather than the other way round, which is learning the theory of it then trying to get used to the sound*". [transcribed quote]

Accumulating multiple sources of (sometimes tacit) evidence while learning through practice

Multiple sources of evidence

We did not specifically explore this question, but there were many hints of its relevance.

14. (Project evaluator) "*There are a huge number of influences on what people actually do. A vague intuitive sense of what is 'right', past experience, pressure from senior management, lessons taught in school and university, not wanting to look silly by doing something new, the culture of the organisation, and more. Our recommendations are just a small part of this*". [quote from email]
15. (Cabinet maker) *Maybe because I'm also a retired medic and theoretical chemist, I use all sorts of knowledge. For example, when I am doing inlay work, the techniques are not so very different from dissection with a scalpel or stitching! But I find myself using all sorts of things including old-fashioned maths and geometry, an ability to think in three dimensions, an ability I have to judge angles and straight lines to within a 16th of an inch in something as large as a sash window, a tactile sense of the wood, a good memory for all sorts of properties of different woods, understanding just by looking at it how the grain will look if I cut it in different ways, knowing who are the best suppliers of which type of wood. Most of these might have been innate, which is why I was attracted to cabinet making as a hobby in the first place, but otherwise, I have no idea where I got this repository of lots of different kinds of knowledge. It's just built up over many years.*

Learning through practice (in context)

16. (Butcher) *I mostly learnt by working alongside the butcher. See it, do it. After a week of watching how to bone out, you'd have a go and he'd comment. Then you'd begin to develop your own quicker ways of doing it.*
17. (Hospital discharge coordinator) *Our job – which is a new role introduced during COVID – is to smooth the way for patients to go home from hospital. It was hard to learn all the pathways. My background was as a chef, then working with a mental health*

charity, and then 18 months as a care assistant in a dementia care home. So when I got this job it was hard. A lot of crying and frustration if I'm honest. I thought I'd never learn to manage it.

18. (Pharmacist) *Some of the learning (which was mostly about drug interactions) was from what the computer flagged up, some was from experience. … As for learning how to run the business – I picked up shop-management training while working for Boots for a while, and from a business management course I had attended [in another country aimed at another industry]. And we get a lot of support from the national bodies. Then you just learn as you go.*
19. (Armoured-vehicle 2ic) *It's all about building up experience, for example during exercises and manoeuvres where you encounter a range of different scenarios and develop the skills to deal with them. After two years, I knew how to fix a tank. But what I didn't know was what to do when it throws a track in the middle of an exercise in a muddy field. You watch others who have done it before and you learn fast. You also learn a lot from trying to understand what went wrong.*
20. (Classical musician) *[Knowing whether to disagree about how to interpret a piece of music] is a tricky decision that you have to learn to make, and it needs you to take account of things like the period of the piece, the kinds of people you're working with, the likely audience expectations, the available rehearsal time, and so on. All sorts of considerations.*

Experience and tacit knowledge

21. (Fishmonger) *We had a quality control department who would grade the fish – cooking and testing it using the Torry test score. But I'd been working with fish for years, and I could always tell just by the colour and the eyes; they'd often ask me to confirm the grade when they weren't sure. We'd talk about it a lot.*
22. (Investment banker) *It's all so heavily controlled that as a portfolio manager you really only have room to be creative when deciding where to invest, and once that decision is made, you learn to buy and sell slowly enough so as not to alert others in the market.*
23. (Pharmacist) *You build up experience about which prescriptions to query – you'd never get anything else done if you queried everything.*
24. (Cabinet maker) *I can't tell you what a piece will look like till I'm doing it. I design as I go along. It depends on the feel of the wood and all sorts of things. And experience is all about knowing what to do when it's cocked up, so when it's finished no one can see!*
25. (District judge) *Over the years you come across situations you've seen time and time again and that guides you. You pick up little things along the way, and they form into a solid collection of things that mean you're a better judge than you were when you started – for example, how to speed things up, how to make it easier for claimants to hear and understand your judgement, or how to make sure they understand the appeals procedure.*
26. (Classical musician) *You need a lot of experience to know and understand these things (see item 20) and take them into account.*

27. (Head teacher) *Unlike safeguarding, one area that lacks lots of training and protocols for you to follow is how to deal with teachers and parents when things get difficult. Usually you only get help from the personnel people when it's too late and situation is already dire. So it's very much a matter of experience and seat of the pants.*
28. (Roofer) *You can feel it and tell by the weight. It's just something you learn. You also need to know good slates (see item 4).*
29. (Hospital discharge coordinator) *You learned, for example, who you needed to liaise with to organise occupational therapy and physio for a patient leaving with multiple fractures and how to get funding for carers. And with patient after patient having similar issues, you learnt who meets what criteria for which agency, which discipline, which care costs to access, and you learnt how to help stressed relatives. How to do that last one is just something you learn from experience. After a while, I gradually realised that when people were asking me questions, I was thinking "Hey! I know that!!"*

Collective learning/communities of practice: sharing (or not) knowledge and experience

30. (Motor mechanic) *There's loads of little tricks you learn that you pass on – especially at the race track when you're under time pressure. We tend to pool our brain power. Like when we developed a way of using hooks and counterweights to do a job next to the track without it springing up and knocking your head off. And you see some guy who's made a simple but amazing adaptation to a tool to get into a space you can never reach, and you think "how does that even happen?" I would never have thought of it.*
31. (Fishmonger) *When I started running my own stall it was very scary – you're spending a grand on fish that won't ride more than a couple of days. Lots of sleepless nights. I picked the brains of a few people who'd been doing it longer than me. I learnt from them that I just have to get to know what my customers want, and always pay more for top-quality stock or I'll soon lose them. It took me a couple of years to gauge it right.*
32. (Butcher) *We're always picking up new ways of doing things from each other; even from customers who've seen some new cut, so you go and check it out online and then try it out, work out how to do it better.*
33. (Fishmonger) *They'd often ask me to confirm the quality grade of the fish when they weren't sure. We'd talk about [grading fish] a lot (see item 21). ... Eventually – and between us we had to work [the filleting machine] out for ourselves – we learnt that the secret was to sort the fish into eight different sizes beforehand. We got it to 60/minute (see item 7).*
34. (Cabinet maker) *I apprenticed myself unofficially to a cabinet maker when I was at school just because I was interested. He would get me to make, say, a dovetail box and then criticise how I did it. And he drummed into me a lot of key principles like "measure ten times, cut once".*
35. (Head teacher) *You learn via the process of being a head, learning from mistakes, sometimes taking advice from governors. There was no forum to discuss these things with other heads, but there is now at least a mentoring scheme for new heads. However, you would tend to meet people at conferences who you got on with and who you could call.*

We'd kind of mentor each other, sometimes for hours on the phone and you'd learn a lot from that – often very unstructured – conversation that would help you next time, even if it was just giving you confidence that you hadn't done the wrong thing. Often it was a case of "well, this worked (or didn't work) for me in a similar situation".

36. (Armoured-vehicle 2ic) *The army isn't a great environment for talking! A lot of dark humour and that's about it. But we are always working as a team. In a battle, you know what the entire company is doing. We're in constant touch, constantly responsive to each other. Everyone knows. You're listening in to the radio, all learning together.*
37. (Helpline volunteer) *You learn first as a probationer, learning by doing, reflecting, hearing lots of helpful feedback from your mentor and others. Then once qualified, we have lots of ongoing training – a lot of it through role play, and we're positively encouraged to listen to our partners on the phone in the ops room. I often pick up little helpful phrases that I begin using myself. And they are doing likewise I suppose.*
38. (Architect) *Nowadays on a large project, there's a lot more use of specialists like structural engineers and mechanical and electrical, etc., and sometimes we all have access to the same computerised drawing, which makes communication easier; you pick up a lot of useful information that way. But not on smaller projects. Some small practices have informal support groups to overcome isolation.*
39. (Solicitor) *Would we chat about cases? No of course not. We had a computer that records every six minutes of our time and if you're sitting around chatting, you're not earning money! And neither would we swap hints or share local information with people from other companies at social gatherings. We're rivals.*
40. (Architect) *continuing professional development is all about technical things, very little about design – which is actually the most important and interesting thing. No one wants to talk about developing design skills because maybe they feel it's too difficult, they'd be exposing themselves, they feel they know it all anyway, they learnt it at undergraduate level, or even, sometimes, they'd be giving too much away.*
41. (District judge) *I have no idea if my fellow judges do the same. We don't talk about such things. And we can't discuss cases informally – no one else has read all the hundreds of pages in the papers and assessed the witnesses for hours as they give their evidence, so how could anyone give you any valid advice? That would be unsafe and unprincipled. Every judge has to take responsibility for their own decisions, and if you get it wrong, the appeal will tell you why; you can learn from that, and it's all in the public domain.*

    It's only in the group work on the annual two-day courses that anyone assesses and comments on your performance [see item 2]. Besides the judgecraft sessions, there are always a couple of 90- to 120- minute sessions when groups of four or five of us address "syndicate exercises". These are problems sent out in advance where you're supposed to have prepared for "what would you do here, and why" questions. There's a syndicate leader who has all the answers.
42. (Pharmacist) *We had little chance to chat to other pharmacists; we were quite isolated really. But at meetings (e.g., sponsored by pharma), we would take the opportunity to check out for example how people were coping with new regulatory requirements like having to write Standard Operating Procedures for everything. Soon after that rule came*

along, we were sharing them. And you'd learn who was good at what and occasionally call them for advice, but there were loads of times when I couldn't run something past someone else though I'd have liked to. You'd never call anyone (or help them out) if they were rivals in your own territory.

43. (Hospital discharge coordinator) *It was hard to learn all the pathways, but we worked in a team alongside trained nurses, and it was a new role (see item 17) that we were all learning. The five of you in the team might all have different opinions, and you all brought different backgrounds, skills, and specialisms, but you'd bounce suggestions off each other and learn a lot from that. I'd say 80% of what I learned I learned from them. We have discussions twice a day and lots of to-ing and fro-ing in between.*

Negotiation and social construction of knowledge

44. (Classical musician) *In an orchestra, those decisions are up to one person, the conductor, and we all quickly learn if we disagree to shut up and not waste everyone's time arguing. … But when you're playing chamber music, then these have to be group decisions, and quartets, for example, who play together for a long time choose like-minded members, who agree and learn to play together in a way that they stick with because it's successful. If you're new to a chamber group, you need to know just how much to voice an opinion. … All sorts of considerations. … And it's an instant, spur-of-the-moment decision. Get it wrong and you won't be asked back.*
45. (Investment banker) *… there are people constantly trying to push the boundaries. And the regulators find it hard to keep up. Both sides are learning all the time; the regulations have to keep changing.*
46. (Armoured-vehicle 2ic) *If a tank modification comes through, it's not something you can negotiate. Except for agreeing when it will be most convenient for each of the 12 tanks in your squadron, you just get on and do it.*

Making room for discussion/respectful critical conversations

47. (Butcher) *It's very different in different shops. The owner here wants you to show him things and we all want to learn and show off to each other. Other places I've worked weren't so open. They were hierarchical, restrictive – "Just do it". You don't learn, and you're not keen to do more.*
48. (Investment banker) *We work as a team making portfolio investment decisions; we deliberately have people who bring very different backgrounds and skills, so we have learned to question each other and avoid groupthink. Even though some are real experts, they sometimes make some basic mistakes but, in the end, however arrogant they are, they have no choice other than to take the comments on board and quietly accept when they have got things wrong. And they don't do it again.*
49. (Head teacher) *In dealing with EBD [Emotional and Behavioural Difficulties] I deliberately formed a team that was non-hierarchical so anyone could give anyone advice about a difficult problem. I had no problem when a teaching assistant made a suggestion, and I'd let her take on the situation if I was struggling. What I found as an inspector later*

was that hierarchical schools ran into difficulties on that score, leaving people to struggle. Common-room conversations in such places tended to be unhelpful and subversive, not helpful.

The part played by clients in formulating decisions about practice

50. (Butcher) *We're always picking up new ways of doing things from each other; even from customers who've seen some new cut, so you go and check it out online and then try it out, work out how to do it better.*
51. (Classical musician) *You need to be able to work with these things (e.g., differently tempered instruments – see also items 20 and 67) to please any given audience who might be expecting a different sound (e.g., vibrato or no vibrato?) from the one you prefer. We're judged by them, so we're influenced by them. No point being whacky if it doesn't go down well.*
52. (Architect) *Although there's a lot more use of specialists like structural engineers and mechanical and electrical, etc., we nowadays all have access to the same computerised drawing, so it makes communication easier. It's much more of a design team nowadays, often including the client.*

The role of context

There are many aspects of context, only some of which were explored in our conversations.

Local context

53. (Butcher) Health and safety? *We follow the HACCP [Hazard Analysis and Critical Control Point], but it's really designed for big stores where the staff, who aren't trained like us, might easily get it wrong. We just know when things aren't safe, like making sure there's nothing dripping onto the lamb in the fridge. And we've worked out ways to chill cooked meats very fast – in line with HACCP – without knackering our display fridge, which the regulations would make us do. If we did exactly what it says, we'd need to buy a new display fridge every couple of years. We conform – and get all our certificates and everything – but not quite how it's laid down.*

Speed and urgency of decisions

54. (Classical musician) *[whether to discuss interpreting the music. See item 20] is an instant, spur-of-the-moment decision. Get it wrong and you won't be asked back.*
55. (Architect) *If you are asked to make an on-site decision quickly, the advice is always not to do it then and there, but to go away and think about it. But I have learnt that sometimes that causes confusion and a loss of momentum. So I sometimes do make the decision, but if, having spoken to someone else or even just slept on it, I realised it might be wrong, I would have no hesitation changing my mind.*

56. (Barrister) *I don't think I ever have to use mindlines because I can take my time, looking up everything I need to with no time pressure to make an immediate decision. So I don't have to have that instant recall of knowledge and information that a doctor does.*

Professional identity, culture, and motives

57. (Armoured-vehicle 2ic) *Looking back, there was a lot of almost brainwashing. "Be the best". Encouraging us to be very competitive – at every level: army vs navy, your regiment, your company, your squadron, being better than all the others. Having specific emblems, ways of wearing your uniform, mascots, proud colours from battles hundreds of years ago. You come to fall in with that culture, and that's bound to impact on how you approach any situation.*
58. (Roofers) *R: Naah. I don't use a slate hammer. D will tell you it's useful for cutting slates the old-fashioned way and for making nail holes. Not many of us use them. He says it makes him a proper roofer! (laughs). I use a claw hammer, but they're heavier, more awkward. A slate hammer's better ergonomically. I'd quite like one but I don't do as much roofing; more general stuff, like all that excellent pointing I did yesterday (laughs again).*
    D: *Yeah but If we swapped tools, it'd be like having a foreign body in your hand. Useless.*
59. (Investment banker) *You need a carrot to motivate that kind of [investment team] group behaviour, and for us the carrot is money. If we get the investments right, we all maximise our bonuses. In another life, I am in a group working with artists that also functions well collectively, but the motive there is friendship and a shared vision, not money.*

Contextual adroitness

60. (Pharmacist) *You build up experience about which prescriptions to query – you'd never get anything else done if you queried everything you're technically supposed to. Some of the learning (which is mostly about drug interactions) was from what the computer flags up, some is from experience. For example, I might know that the patient had been on these drugs for a long time with no problems, or that the experienced local psychiatrist sometimes broke the golden rule about not combining certain anti-depressants, but they knew when to do that without any serious problems, even when the computer was jumping off the table saying not to do it. So you learned not to query that prescription.*
61. (Roofer) *The last job we did, the builder supplied the slates. We knew they was crap but the builders insisted. It was a nightmare. And we get the blame for doing a bad job. We knew straight off they wouldn't work, but he gave us no choice. And yes it was a bad job, but if anyone else had done it, it would have been a lot worse.*
62. (Investment banker) *You're working in a highly regulated environment where your every move is watched but where there are people constantly trying to push the boundaries.*
63. (Armoured-vehicle 2ic) *Yeah, it can be a problem when you move to another base. It takes about six months to learn your way around. But the army made sure that you*

worked with lots of different regiments in different places – even to the extent of some of our lads working as foot soldiers for a while – so that when the chips were down, whatever unit you were working with, you had already experienced lots of different scenarios and adapted to their different ways of doing things.

64. (Cabinet maker) *I can't tell you what a piece will look like till I'm doing it. I design as I go along. It depends on the feel of the wood and all sorts of things. And experience tells you what to do when it's cocked up so when it's finished no one can see.*
65. (Jazz musician) "*If you hear a piano player or soloist starting to play a different scale over a G7th, for example, you know it* can *work just to carry on playing a normal G7 line in C, but it's also really great if you can pick up on what people are doing, hear what they're playing and fit your harmony around it, like using a B-flat 7th tritone substitution, or a Mixolydian scale in B flat*".[transcribed quote]
66. (Architect) *Yes there are building regulations and so on. They used to be very prescriptive (use this material in this way), but now they are more about the end outcome (ensure this load-bearing capacity). They can be interpreted differently; e.g., different inspectors will accept different ways of solving the need to have fire-door protection for the third floor of a house. The increasing use of private building inspectors means you need to be very aware of that.*

Transformation of formal knowledge

67. (Classical musician) *You have to do what the score says, but quietly trying to be different from what everyone else does with it. You try to take the research on board. For example, the period instruments were tuned with different intervals compared to, say, a modern piano. They were tempered differently. What sounded right to them, and maybe to me, might not sound right to someone else and you have to adapt to that. ... You also need quite a lot of research into the different editions. For example, fingerings may have been made by an exceptional musician who had an unusual instrument, impossible for anyone else to fathom, but still persisting in print. (Editors get no credit for providing simple, obvious fingering!) You need a lot of experience to know and understand these things and take them into account.*
68. (Architect) *[Building regulations] can be interpreted differently. ... The increasing use of private building inspectors means you need to be very aware of that, especially since the Grenfell disaster, which shows that not everyone is honourable about how they interpret the regulations about building materials, for example. And that gets even more complicated because the chain of legal responsibility gets obscured when contracts move along the chain as the project develops.*

Conclusions

The conversations revealed how, as different occupations apply their knowledge to their work, they all echo many of the features of clinical mindlines. Obviously, there were exceptions, demonstrating that context can affect not only how knowledge is applied but also how it is acquired. Social aspects of mindlines, such as collective learning, were curtailed in some occupations, for example, by cultural, financial, or organisational considerations. Nevertheless, what emerges is a constellation of features that, while they vary across the different occupations, all share some "family resemblance" (Wittgenstein 1953) – a cluster of overlapping similarities with the key features of mindlines.

In other words, what the mindlines model uncovered about how clinical practitioners use knowledge is part of a wider picture across a very wide range of occupations. We are back where we started on page 1 – describing something that is obvious and yet enigmatic. It is surely unsurprising that people need to meld many different types of knowledge when doing complex tasks, that they often have to bend the rules and take shortcuts to get things done, to supplement what they are taught by learning from experience and by interacting with others, to blend tacit and explicit knowledge, and so on. Yet the social and psychological processes that enable these phenomena to happen remain mysterious. There are many unanswered questions: For example, how does the melding occur, not only individually but collectively? What is the philosophical status of knowledge-in-practice-in-context? How can we ensure that 'System-1½' thinking (See Chapter 14) is as error-free as possible? What are the implications for how we organise work, how we educate and train practitioners, how we produce and promote practical guidance for complex, contextually-bound tasks, how we monitor performance? There remain many challenges, and not just within the clinical sphere where the mindlines story started.

One last question: why did the mindlines model strike such a chord in the world of health and social care? Perhaps the answer is that the model is itself a contextually-rooted social construct; it came about because it helped explain a situation in which healthcare found itself at the end of the 20th century, torn between the cherished but often flawed art and craft of professional judgement and the understandable attempts to push practitioners towards the scientific rationalism of evidence-based practice. Maybe in our enthusiasm to improve healthcare, we all needed to be reminded to take account of something so obvious (and probably universal) as mindlines.

Summary

- Through informal but focused conversations, we have explored how knowledge is learned and put into practice by an architect, a barrister, two butchers, a cabinet maker, a classical musician, a hospital discharge coordinator, a district judge, a fishmonger, a head teacher and schools' inspector, a helpline volunteer, an investment banker, an international-project evaluator, a jazz musician, a motor mechanic, a pharmacist, two roofers, a solicitor, and a tank driver.
- We found that across all the occupations there were strong echoes — 'family resemblances' — of all the main features of the mindlines model that we have described in health and social care. The phenomenon of mindlines is widespread across all types of occupational practice, albeit with contextual adjustments in how mindlines are acquired and used.

- The model is both obvious – in that it is immediately recognisable – and enigmatic – in that we still need to understand much more about the social and psychological underpinnings of mindlines.
- The mindlines model may have resonated in health and social care because it highlights and confirms how misguided it may be to drive a wedge between scientific rationalism and professional judgement and always privilege the former. In practice, mindlines meld the two.

References

Bârsan VA, Bondreia I. 2015. 'Study about the theories and models in collaborative engineering'. *Revista Academiei Forțelor Terestre* Nr., 1(77): 102–112. https://www.armyacademy.ro/reviste/rev1_2015/BARSAN.pdf

Bruce T. 2017. 'Introduction from the editors', in T Bruce, P Hakkarainen, M Bredikyte (Eds.) *The Routledge international handbook of early childhood play*. Abingdon and New York: Routledge.

Cain T, Brindley S, Brown C, Jones G, Riga F. 2019. 'Bounded decision-making, teachers' reflection and organisational learning: How research can inform teachers and teaching'. *The British Educational Research Journal*, 45: 1072–1087. https://doi.org/10.1002/berj.3551

Fennell DA. 2022. 'The tourism knowledge translation framework: bridging the canyon between theory and practice'. *Current Issues in Tourism*, 25(5), 674–691. https://doi.org/10.1080/13683500.2021.1887099

Kantola A, Harju AA. 2021. 'Tackling the emotional toll together: How journalists address harassment with connective practices'. *Journalism*, 1–19.

Wittgenstein L. 1953. *Philosophical investigations* (Trans. GEM Anscome, R Rhees, 1976 edition). Oxford: Basil Blackwell.

INDEX

NB: This index excludes the names of authors. It also excludes some general topics that suffuse most of the chapters, such as 'implementation', 'interaction', 'knowledge', 'learning', 'practice', 'qualitative research' and of course 'mindlines', as well as generic terms for key actors, such as doctors, nurses, and patients.